D.H. Patterson
(MJ-NJ 76

1500

A Course in Renal Diseases

A Course in Renal Diseases

GEOFFREY M. BERLYNE
MD, FRCP
Director, Department of Nephrology,
Soroka Medical Center, Beersheba
Professor of Medicine,
Ben-Gurion University of
the Negev, Beersheba.

FOURTH EDITION

BLACKWELL SCIENTIFIC PUBLICATIONS
OXFORD LONDON EDINBURGH MELBOURNE

© 1966, 1968, 1971, 1974 Blackwell Scientific Publications
Osney Mead, Oxford,
8 Nottingham Street, London WI,
9 Forrest Road, Edinburgh,
P.O. Box 9, North Balwyn, Victoria, Australia.

All rights reserved. No part of this publication may be reproduced, stored in a retrieval system, or transmitted, in any form or by any means, electronic, mechanical, photocopying, recording or otherwise without the prior permission of the copyright owner.

ISBN 0 632 09600 4

First published 1966
Second edition 1968
Third edition 1971
Fourth edition 1974

German edition 1969
Portuguese edition 1973
Spanish edition 1974
Japanese and Polish
editions in preparation

Distributed in the U.S.A. by
F. A. Davis Company, 1915 Arch Street,
Philadelphia, Pennsylvania

Photoset in Malta by
St Paul's Press Ltd.
Printed in Great Britain by
Compton Printing Ltd.
Aylesbury,
and bound by
Kemp Hall Bindery, Oxford

In Memory of my father-in-law,
Hugh Selbourne

Contents

	Foreword to First Edition	ix
	Introduction to First, Second Third and Fourth Editions	x
	Use of this book	xiii
1	Anatomy of the Kidney	1
2	Renal Physiology	15
3	Renal investigations – Biochemical	45
4	Renal investigations – Morphological	74
5	Glomerulonephritis	108
6	Nephrotic Syndrome	135
7	Pyelonephritis	169
8	Acute Renal Failure	185
9	Chronic Renal Failure	205
10	Collagen Diseases and the Kidney	228
11	Diabetes Mellitus and the Kidney	248
12	Polyuria	257
13	The Kidney and Pregnancy	268
14	The Kidney and Hypertension	279
15	Renal Tubular Disorders	295

16	Congenital and Inherited Diseases of the Kidney	321
17	Focal Nephritis and Miscellaneous Nephritides	335
18	Surgical Diseases of the Kidney	346
19	The Bones and the Kidney	355
20	Drugs and the Kidney	371
21	Renal Transplantation	385
	Appendix	394
	Index	399

Foreword to first edition

This book offers to anyone who wants to learn more about renal diseases a relatively new method of instruction which recognises the lamentable truth that the simple desire to learn is not at all times sufficient; so that it must be fortified by attention-compelling devices, of which the challenging question is the most effective. This has long been known, in its oral form, to teachers; but even the best teachers cannot be there all the time, and this method of 'programmed learning' allows the student to work when he likes, and to hold his interest while he is doing so. Nephrology is losing neither intricacy nor importance with the passing of the years; and it may be that some who start to study it as an examination subject may remain to practise it in all its fascinating depth.

The author has already published a number of papers, but this is his first essay in book form. It is always embarrassing to speak well of a colleague (though not quite so embarrassing as to speak ill) and I may perhaps content myself with saying that Dr Berlyne's memory, like the heart of Byron's hero, is 'wax to receive and marble to retain'. When he was an undergraduate in this school, it was a touchstone of intellectual integrity in members of the staff that they would accept his filling-in of their information. This book will make his didactic skill available to a wider audience, and – hubris or not – I predict for it a considerable success.

Douglas Black

Introductions

To first edition

This book has been written in a scrambled format with questions and answers at the end of each paragraph so as to give the reader the best possible chance of assimilating the information. It is written as if the reader were having a tutorial course on renal disease. Because of the scrambling of the paragraphs it is difficult to read without answering the questions, so the chance of day-dreaming through a chapter is reduced.

This book is intended for post-graduates studying for the MRCP to give a background knowledge of renal disease, and for the advanced undergraduate who wishes to acquire further knowledge of renal diseases. It is not meant to replace any of the standard monographs on renal disease, but it could be read with profit before going on to the monographs for more detailed information.

In writing this book I had to choose between writing a fully programmed book with one question per fact and writing a compromise semi-programmed book with one question for several facts. I chose the latter for two reasons:

1 'One fact – one question' would require about 300,000 words on glomerulonephritis alone.

2 Because much about renal disease is unknown it is impossible to give a logical step-by-step programme: one is obliged to jump from one known fact to another. This is not therefore a suitable subject for full programming.

The questions at the end of each paragraph have been chosen not necessarily to include the most important fact but to include facts which, in my experience, students usually find difficult to remember.

The format of the book has been chosen so as to make it, in effect, a type of pocket teaching machine. All possible steps have been taken to reduce the cost to the minimum while at the same time presenting the information in a legible and pleasant form.

Before submitting this book to the publishers, I have had individual chapters read by the following colleagues to whom I am indebted:

Professor Sir Robert Platt, Professor D. A. K. Black, Dr A. J. Ralston, Dr A. B. Shaw, Dr Anne Holmes, Dr Jacqueline Woolcock, the house physicians on the professorial medical unit at Manchester Royal Infirmary, and several medical students. Dr C. J. Dickinson has been subjected to the entire manuscript and for his valuable criticisms I am deeply indebted. It is due to his advice that I have included a small section on surgical renal diseases of interest to physicians. I wish to thank Dr Ian Isherwood of the Department of Radiology, Manchester Royal Infirmary for the radiographs used throughout this book and the Department of Medical Illustration for preparing the photographs. Dr E. J. Watson-Williams was kind enough to provide me with facilities for micro-photography.

Mr Per Saugman of Blackwell Scientific Publications has been particularly encouraging and helpful throughout the eighteen months cyesis of this book, and to him and his colleague, Mr John Robson, my thanks are due.

To second edition

Nephrology is an expanding subject. Advances are being made at remarkable speed. I have attempted to make this second edition as up-to-date as possible, having made changes in virtually every chapter. A new chapter has been added on drugs and the kidney, and an addition has been made to the appendix in which details are given of the behaviour of commonly used drugs in advanced renal failure, and the recommended dosage of antibiotics. Several photomicrographs have been added so that the reader should find some of the facts easier to remember. My thanks are due to Dr J. Ransom of Lange Publications, for his valuable suggestions. I would like to thank my colleagues from this country and abroad for their encouragement, and useful comments in private letters and published reviews. I would like to thank Mr Per Saugman and Mr John Robson for publishing the manuscript in the shortest possible time.

To third edition

In this edition much new material has been added to bring the work up to date, some of it being so new as to be unpublished. In any work of this type the aim has to be to give the reader a working knowledge of basic nephrology, and sometimes detail has had to be pruned to permit the reader to see the principles. The bulk has been reduced so that the book is still small enough to carry in a raincoat pocket. Throughout the preparation of this edition I have been mindful of the views of the reviewers of the previous edition, and have made changes which appear reasonable to me. I hope that the reader will enjoy using the book as I have in writing it. The improvement in format and paper quality is necessary to permit the reader to see the details of the microphotographs. The book remains an inexpensive teaching machine.

To fourth edition

In this edition I have removed much out of date material and replaced it with the latest material available at the time of writing (December 73). There have been great advances in our understanding of the different types of nephrotic syndrome, with a new classification which has a clear cut histological basis. The understanding of the action of vitamin D and the pathogenesis of renal osteodystrophy have made considerable progress. I have avoided the temptation to insert much material dealing with some of the newer artificial kidneys which are as yet not in widespread use. There is always the tendency to enlarge a book by increasing its size until it is too large to hold or to put in the pocket. This I have with difficulty resisted, because I believe that the usefulness of this book would be diminished if it gets much larger. I have accepted many suggestions for improvements in the text by my colleagues. I am particularly indebted to my colleague Professor D. N. S. Kerr for his constructive criticism. Where other advances have clarified knowledge I have corrected the text to fit in with our present day theories. Textbooks of kidney disease become out of date within 2 or 3 years at most. For this reason I have produced a new edition every 2 to 3 years. I hope that advances in our knowledge will continue to make this necessary and that this book's format will contribute to the spread of knowledge of renal disease in an efficient and at the same time as pleasant a manner as possible.

G. M. Berlyne

Beersheba, December 1973

How to Use This Book

1 Read chapters 1, 2, 3, 4, in that order. Then you can pick chapters as you feel like it: it is better to work straight through a chapter than to stop work halfway through. So as to give you a rough idea of the length of time an MRCP candidate takes to read a chapter, I have put at the head of each chapter the average time taken by 3 or more MRCP students. This is only a rough guide, depending on your prior knowledge and speed of learning.

2 Start at the first paragraph in each chapter, answering the questions at the end of each paragraph to the best of your ability, and **follow the instructions there. Do not read straight on from the first paragraph to paragraph 2, etc.**

Time for this chapter: 20 minutes

Chapter 1
Anatomy of the kidney

1.1 The kidneys lie most frequently opposite the bodies of the 1st and 2nd lumbar vertebrae, in relation to the twelfth rib as shown in Fig. 1.1a. They move caudally with inspiration. They weigh about 150 g each. The kidney is buried in perirenal fat which is itself enclosed by perirenal fascia. The renal capsule is a thin, though fibrous layer which covers the surface of the kidney cortex; in health the capsule can be smoothly separated with ease from the underlying cortex. The kidney proper (see Fig. 1.1b) consists of an outer layer, the cortex, wrapped round an inner layer, the medulla. The cortex and the medulla both about on to the renal pelvis; the cortex sends down columns of cortical tissue known as columns of Bertin separating the medullary renal pyramids. There are about 12 to 14 medullary pyramids in each kidney; some are single, others are fused to their neighbours. They terminate in the papillary tips which project into the calyces, which are infoldings of the renal pelvis wrapped around the papillae.

You have now read the first paragraph. Now choose what you think is the correct answer to the following question from the three answers given. Go on to the paragraph indicated by your answer.

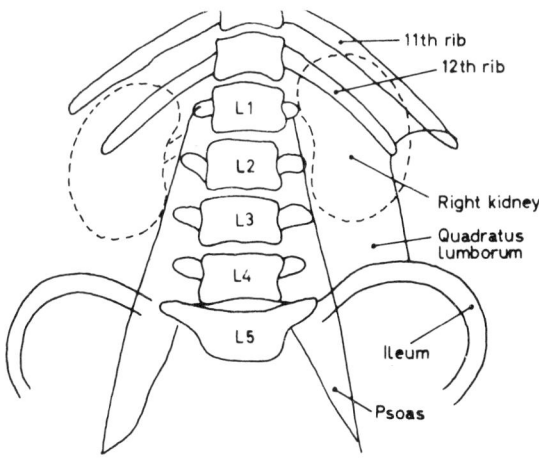

Fig. 1.1a

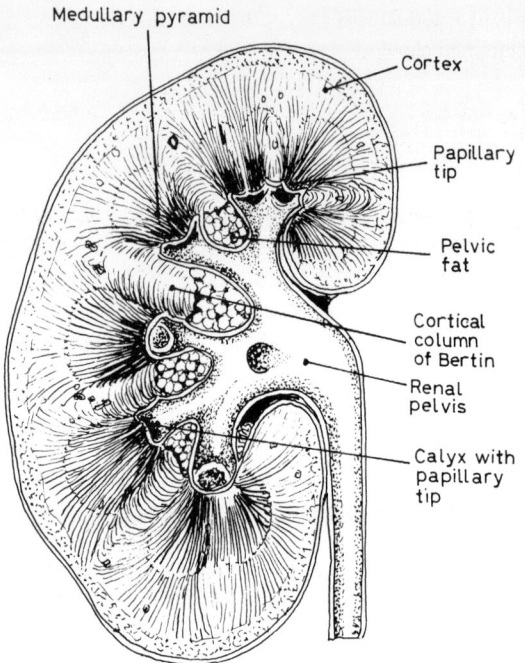

Fig. 1.1b

Question Do any parts of the renal cortex come into contact with the renal pelvis?

Answer 1. No. Go on to **1.3**
2. Yes. Go on to **1.7**
3. Don't know. Read **1.8**

1.2 You should not be going on to read this paragraph. Go back to **1.1** and re-read the instructions at the end of it.

1.3 Your answer – no part of the cortex comes into contact with the pelvis. You are wrong.

You have not read **1.1** properly. The columns of Bertin are cortical columns which pass down through the medulla proper. Go back to **1.1** and make the correct choice.

1.4 Your answer – the efferent arterioles provide the arterial supply to the glomeruli.

No. Efferent arterioles take blood from the capillary plexus of the glomeruli. Read **1.7** again and choose the correct answer.

1.5 Your answer – the afferent arterioles bring arterial blood to the glomeruli. This is correct. Go on to read **1.10**.

1.6 Your answer – the vasa recta bring arterial blood to the glomeruli.
    This is wrong. The vasa recta bring blood from the efferent juxtaglomerular arterioles into the renal pyramids. Read **1.7** again and answer the question again.

1.7 Your answer – part of the cortex comes into contact with the renal pelvis. You are correct.
    You are now ready to deal with the structures at the hilum of the kidney. They are the renal artery, renal vein and ureter. The vein is anterior to the artery and the ureter is the most posterior of the 3 structures. The renal arteries are frequently multiple, up to 1 person in 4 having more than 1 renal artery on each side. They usually come as small multiple branches from the aorta, and frequently supply the poles of the kidneys. These small arteries are of great importance in hypertension due to stenosis of the renal arteries which will be discussed in a later chapter. The renal arteries in the kidney break up into arching branches known as the arcuate arteries which run in the region of the cortico-medullary junction: they are end arteries, anastomosing solely through capillary channels. The intralobular arteries branch off the arcuate arteries and run at right angles towards the renal capsule, traversing the cortex and branching again at right angles into the afferent arterioles supplying the glomeruli; some branches go down into the medulla, first passing through the juxta-medullary glomeruli and then becoming large straight vascular channels known as vasa recta which pass down into the depths of the renal pyramids, and then bend back up to reach the arcuate veins at the cortico-medullary junction. The tips of the papillae have a special arterial supply of their own from spiral arteries, branches of the interlobular arteries in the pelvis of the kidney.
    In the cortex the afferent arteriole breaks up into a 20–40 capillary loops in each glomerulus, which rejoin to form the efferent arteriole. This then splits up again to form a second capillary network which surrounds the tubules, both proximal and distal; this network itself empties into interlobar veins.

Question What blood vessels bring arterial blood into the glomeruli?

Answer 1. The efferent arterioles. Go on to **1.4**
2. The afferent arterioles. Go on to **1.6**
3. The vasa recta. Go on to **1.6**
4. Don't know. Go on to **1.9**

1.8 Your answer – I don't know if any part of the cortex comes into contact with the pelvis.

If you don't know either you have not read the text of **1.1** or you have not looked at Fig. 1.1b. Let us have a look at it. You can see the cortical columns of Bertin coming down between the renal pyramids in the figure. Therefore the answer to the question is Yes. Now go on to **1.7**.

1.9 Your answer – I don't know which vessels bring arterial blood to the glomeruli.

Well, bear in mind that the arteriole going *to* the glomerulus, bringing arterial blood to it, is called afferent; the efferent one takes blood *from* the glomerulus to either the peritubular venous plexus in the cortex or the vasa recta of the medulla. Re-read **1.7** with more attention and try the answers again.

1.10 We can now begin a more detailed study of the structure of the kidney. The unit of which the kidney is constructed is the nephron. This consists of a glomerulus with proximal convoluted tubule, loop of Henle, distal convoluted tubule and collecting duct (see Fig. 1.10). Individual intact nephrons can be dis-

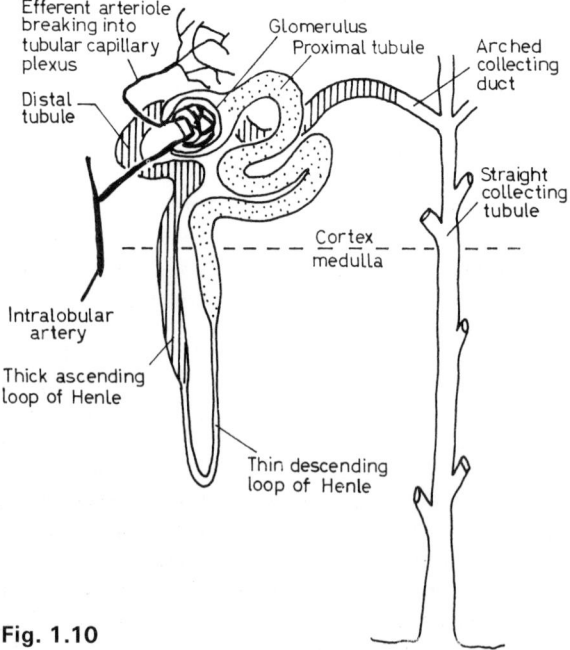

Fig. 1.10

sected out by the method pioneered by Jean Oliver, using kidneys previously macerated in strong mineral acid. The length of the nephron is about 5 cm but is variable. There are approximately 1 million nephrons in each kidney. The majority of the glomeruli are in the cortex; some are in the juxta-medullary region. The proximal and distal convoluted tubules and blood vessels constitute the bulk of the non-glomerular cortical tissues. The medulla is composed of some loops of Henle, vasa recta and a mass of collecting tubules. In man, only 1 loop of Henle in 7 is long and descends far into the renal pyramids. In desert animals such as the kangaroo rat a far higher proportion of long loops of Henle go down into a very long papilla; this is an important structural factor responsible for the water conservation required of desert animals. Now answer the question below.

Question In man what proportion of long loops of Henle dip far down into the renal pyramids?

Answer 1. One in seven loops dip down. Go on to **1.12**.
2. All dip down. Go on to **1.14**.
3. None dip down. Go on to **1.15**.

1.11 Your answer is – the foot processes are extensions of the parietal epithelial cells.

You are not clear about the difference between parietal and visceral epithelial cells. Let us take the pleura as analagous to the epithelial cells lining Bowman's capsule. The parietal pleura lines the pleural cavity in much the same way that the parietal epithelial cells line Bowman's capsule. Similarly, the glomerular tuft can be compared to the lung: the lung is covered with visceral pleura; the glomerular tuft is covered with visceral epithelial cells. It is these visceral epithelial cells which send down foot processes to the basement membrane. Now read **1.12** again and give the correct answer to the question after looking carefully at figures **1.10** and **1.12**.

1.12 Your answer – one loop in 7 dips down into the medulla.

You are correct. The glomeruli are specialised invaginations of the proximal convoluted tubules. There is a 'urine'-containing space between the glomerular capillary tuft and Bowman's capsule. Both sides of Bowman's capsule are lined with epithelial cells, the parietal epithelial cells being flatter and less noticeable than the larger, pale staining visceral epithelial cells which line the outer side of the capillary tuft. The epithelial cells lie on a basement membrane which is continuous with that of the proximal tubule. Electron microscopy (see Fig. 1.12) of the glomerulus reveals that the epithelial cells do not lie in close apposition to the basement membrane; extensions of the cytoplasm of the cell, called 'foot processes' or podocytes, come into contact with the basement membranes at inter-

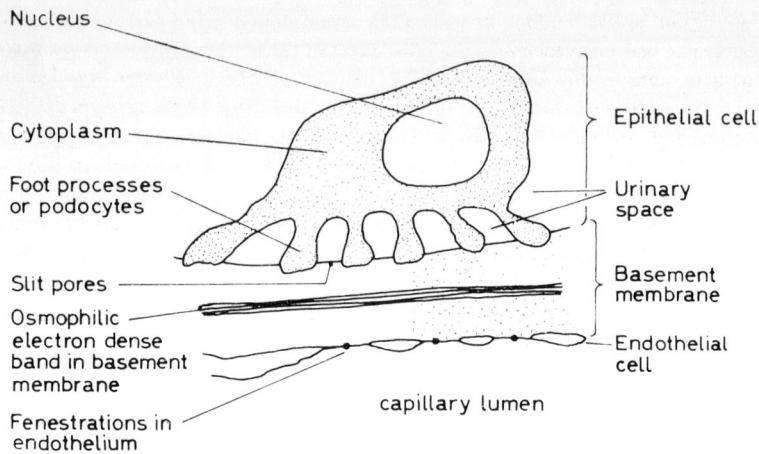

Fig. 1.12

vals, leaving many areas of basement membrane surfaces free of epithelial cell contact. These areas have a mean width of 400 Å and are known as slit pores. Look at Fig. 1.12 then answer the question.

Question What are the foot processes?

Answer 1. Extensions of the parietal epithelial cells. Proceed to **1.11**.
2. Extensions of the visceral epithelial cells. Proceed to **1.16**.
3. Don't know. Go on to **1.17**.

1.13 Your answer – pores are visible in the basement membrane in man.

No. Although it behaves as if it contains pores none are visible. This error means that you have not read **1.16** with enough care. Go back to it, re-read it and then answer the question in detail.

1.14 Your answer is – all loops of Henle go down into the renal pyramids in man.

This is wrong. Very few do. Re-read **1.9** and answer the question correctly.

1.15 Your answer was that no loops of Henle dip down into the medulla in man.

This is wrong. The medulla is composed of loops of Henle, collecting ducts and blood vessels. In man one loop of Henle in seven sends down a long loop into the renal pyramids. In desert animals a far higher proportion of loops go down into the medulla. This is important in the setting up of a counter-current multiplier system which we shall discuss later. Now answer the question in **1.9** correctly.

1.16 Your answer – foot processes are extensions of visceral epithelial cells. Good. The basement membrane can be seen by special stains on light microscopy but it is more readily visible with the higher magnifications obtained by electron microscopy. It runs through all the capillary walls, sandwiched between the foot processes of the epithelial cells on the one side and the endothelial cells on the other. It is continuous with the basement membrane of the tubules. Its thickness is 3000 Å in man and 800 Å in the mouse. There is a central electron dense band in the basement membrane of the tubules. No pores are visible in the basement membrane, but it behaves as if it had pores of 75–100 Å in diameter. Now answer the question.

Question Are pores visible in the basement membrane in man?

Answer 1. Yes. Go on to **1.13**.
2. No. Go on to **1.18**.

1.17 Your answer was 'don't know'. In that case you must have failed to read **1.12** properly. Look at Figs. 1.10 and 1.12; read the legends of each carefully, and then go on to answer the question. If you still are unable to answer the question you are not concentrating. Try again **1.12**.

1.18 Your answer – No pores are visible in the basement membrane.
This is quite right. Let us now consider next the structure of the endothelial cells; go on to **1.19**.

1.19 Look at Fig. 1.19. The capillary walls are lined by endothelial cells which

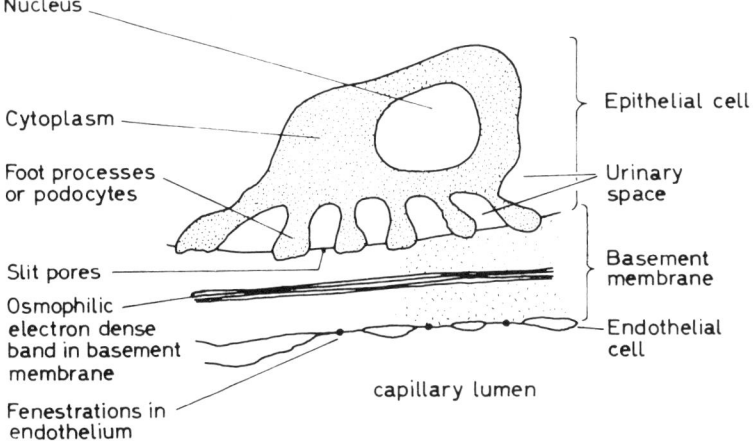

Fig. 1.19

lie on the basement membrane. These cells are flat and completely cover the basement membrane, unlike the epithelial cells which come into contact with the basement membrane only at the foot processes. There are fenestrations in the endothelial cells with an average diameter of 600 Å. They are closed by a diaphragm. The endothelial cells of the glomeruli are continuous with the endothelial lining of the efferent and afferent arterioles. The axial or mesangial cells are intercapillary endothelial cells which form a syncytium in the capillary wall between adjacent loops. The mesangial cells are embedded in a mesangial matrix resembling basement membrane.

Question What cells line the lumen of the capillary loops of the glomerulus?

Answer 1. Epithelial cells. Go on to **1.20**.
2. Endothelial cells. Go on to **1.22**.
3. Axial or mesangial. Go on to **1.24**.

1.20 Your answer – the epithelial cells line the capillary lumen. All capillaries, indeed all blood vessels, are lined by flat cells known as endothelial cells. The endothelial cells in the capillaries of the glomeruli are specialised. The epithelial cells lie on the opposite side of the basement membrane to the capillary lumen, lining both visceral and parietal layers of Bowman's capsule. Now re-read **1.19** and go on to answer the question again.

1.21 Your answer – the juxta-glomerular apparatus is in the wall of the efferent arteriole.

You have confused efferent and afferent. The juxta-glomerular apparatus is in the wall of the afferent arteriole which takes blood *to* the glomerulus; it is possible that the juxta-glomerular apparatus is sensitive to the height of the blood pressure in the afferent arterioles. This will be discussed later. Now go on to answer the question in **1.22** correctly.

1.22 Your answer – the capillaries of the glomeruli are lined by endothelial cells. Good. Now let us examine the arterioles of the glomeruli in greater detail. There are two arterioles to each glomerulus (1) afferent and (2) efferent.

The afferent arteriole takes blood *to* the glomerulus; the efferent takes blood *from* it. In the juxta-medullary region some arterioles appear to have no glomeruli, each plunging straight into the medulla as an arteria recta vera; but careful microdissection demonstrates that there are atrophic glomeruli on many of these arterioles.

The afferent arteriolar wall is composed of an inner layer of endothelium in contact with a smooth muscle layer; at the point where the distal convoluted tubule is in contact with the afferent arteriole, the latter contains the juxtaglomerular apparatus (see Fig. 1.22), a series of granular cells believed to be the source of the enzyme renin which will be described later in Chapter 14 on

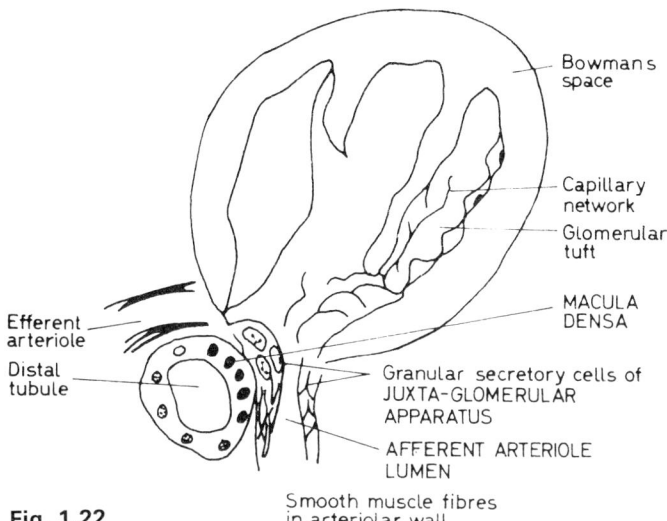

Fig. 1.22

'Hypertension and the Kidney.' The efferent arteriolar wall is composed of smooth muscle with an endothelial lining: it has no juxta-glomerular cells. The efferent arteriole breaks up into a capillary network surrounding the tubules. These finally join up to form the interlobar veins. These capillaries are completely surrounded by a basement membrane which lies close to the tubular basement membrane. The endothelium lining the capillaries has fenestrations 600 Å in size. The structure of the peritubular capillaries is such as to promote ready exchange of materials between the tubular cells and the capillaries.

Question Where is the granular, renin producing juxta-glomerular apparatus?

Answer 1. In the wall of the afferent arteriole. Go on to **1.25**.
2. In the wall of the efferent arteriole. Go on to **1.21**.
3. In the peritubular capillaries. Go on to **1.23**.

1.23 Your answer – the juxta-glomerular apparatus is in the peritubular capillaries. You are wrong. Re-read **1.22**.

1.24 Your answer – axial or mesangial cells line the capillary loops – is not completely true. The endothelial cells line the capillary loops but they are closely related to the mesangial or axial cells which may actually differentiate into the endothelial cells in certain circumstances. Proceed now to **1.22**.

1.25 Your answer – the juxta-glomerular apparatus is in the wall of the afferent arteriole.

Correct. The proximal tubules are confined to the cortex of the kidney: they connect the glomerulus proximally with the descending limb of the loop of Henle distally. The cells of the proximal tubule are cuboidal or columnar, having a distinctive brush border in contact with the lumen of the tubule.

The brush border consists of numerous villi, about 150 per square micron, which increase the absorbing surface area enormously. There are a large number of mitochondria and ribosomes in the cytoplasm of the cells, indicative of the metabolic activity of these cells. There is also a characteristic infolding of the plasma membrane of the base of the cell which interdigitates with those of neighbouring cells. The basement membrane of the proximal tubular cells is in close contact with that of the peritubular capillaries, facilitating exchange of substances from tubule to capillary and vice versa. Now answer the question below.

Question Where is the brush border of the proximal tubular cell?

Answer 1. In contact with the tubular lumen. Go on to **1.27**.
2. In contact with the basement membrane. Go on to **1.30**.

1.26 Your answer – the cells at the U bend of the loop of Henle are flat squamous epithelial cells.

You are correct. You are now ready to study the distal convoluted tubule.

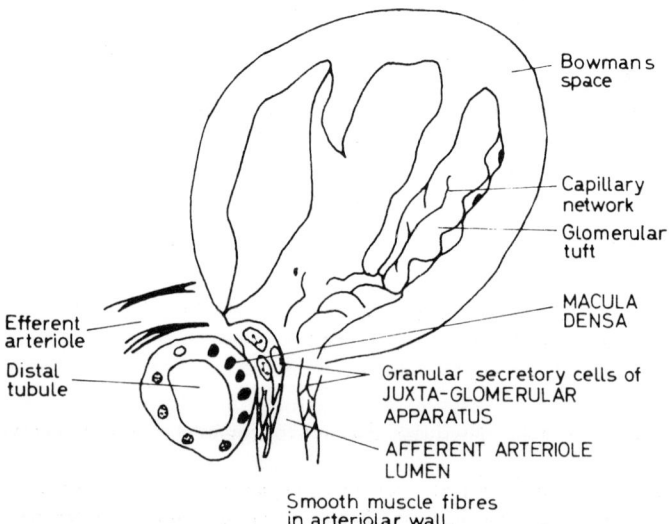

Fig. 1.26

There is no clear-cut place at which the thick ascending limb of the loop of Henle becomes the distal convoluted tubule. The epithelium of the distal convoluted tubule is columnar, the surface being covered with numerous microvilli; as the collecting duct is approached the cell height becomes smaller, giving way to the cuboidal cells of the collecting ducts. At the point at which the distal convoluted tubule approaches the vascular pole of the glomerulus the nuclei of the epithelial cells become crowded closer together and appear darker staining than in other parts of the distal tubule; this hypernuclear area is known as the macula densa. Look at Fig. 1.26.

Question What part of the nephron is known as the macula densa?

Answer 1. The juxta-glomerular apparatus. Go on to **1.28**.
2. Part of the distal convoluted tubule close to the vascular pole of the glomerulus. Go on to **1.29**.
3. The loop of Henle. Go on to **1.33**.

1.27 Your answer — the brush border of the proximal tubular cell is in contact with the tubular lumen.

You are correct. Let us now consider the loop of Henle which is shaped like a U tube connecting proximal and distal convoluted tubules, dipping down a variable distance into the medulla. There is a thick-walled straight descending segment which terminates in a thin-walled segment; the thin segment running down into the medulla bends in a U shape then turns back to run up to the cortex, joining the distal convoluted tubule. The cells of the thick descending limb have a clear cytoplasm and a few coarse brush border extensions, much fewer than the proximal tubular cells. The thin segment is composed of flat squamous cells with starfish-like cytoplasmic extensions resting on a basement membrane. The cells of the thin limb change to a thicker and wider cell as the distal convoluted tubule is approached, the cytoplasm containing numerous mitochondria with multiple infoldings of the basal plasma membranes.

Question What type of cell structure is present at the 'U bend' in the loop of Henle?

Answer 1. Flat cells. Go on to **1.26**.
2. Cuboidal cells. Go on to **1.32**.
3. Don't know. Go on to **1.34**.

1.28 Your answer — the juxta-glomerular apparatus is known as the macula densa.

This is wrong. The juxta-glomerular apparatus is in the afferent arteriolar wall, whereas the macula densa is the distal convoluted tubular cells closely applied to the afferent and efferent arterioles where they enter and leave the glomerulus. Now read **1.26** again and answer the question.

1.29 Your answer — the macula densa is part of the distal convoluted tubule close to the vascular pole of the glomerulus.

You are correct. The cortical collecting ducts are a continuation of the distal convoluted tubules. They run into the collecting ducts of the medulla. The cells of the cortical collecting ducts are cuboidal in shape, and the majority are 'dark' intercalated cells, the remainder being 'light' cells. The *'dark'* cells have large numbers of perinuclear mitochondria, a luminal surface covered with microvilli and a very large nucleus. The *'light'* cells have few mitochondria, a large nucleus and some granules. The cortical collecting tubules join the collecting ducts in the medulla. These cells of the latter have a cuboidal shape, with light cytoplasm relatively free of mitochondria: they resemble the 'light' cells of the cortical collecting tubules. The collecting ducts run into the papillary ducts of Bellini; in the papillary ducts the cells are columnar in shape, having a basal nucleus and few mitochondria. The ducts of Bellini join the renal pelvis, which is covered with transitional epithelium.

Question Where are the intercalated or dark cells?

Answer 1. In the cortical collecting tubules. Go on to **1.35**.
2. In the collecting tubules of the medulla. Go on to **1.37**.

1.30 Your answer — the brush border of the proximal tubule is in contact with the basement membrane of the cell.

You have not read **1.25** with enough care. Go over it again and you should be able to answer correctly the question in **1.25**.

1.31 This paragraph is meant to test your knowledge of renal anatomy which you have just reviewed in this chapter. Answer the questions after due thought or you may find yourself starting again at the beginning.

Question Look at the following statements, some of which are true and some of which are false, and pick out the appropriate answer from the answers listed below.

Statement 1 There are 1 million nephrons in the normal adult's kidney.
Statement 2 The juxta-glomerular apparatus consists mainly of granular cells.
Statement 3 The collecting tubule has a large brush border.

Answers 1. All the statements are true. Go on to read **1.41**.
2. Statements 1 and 2 are true. Go on to read **1.36**.
3. All the statements are false. Go on to read **1.38**.
4. Statements 1 and 3 are true, statement 2 is false. Go on to read **1.39**.

5. Statement 2 and 3 are true. Go on to read **1.40**.
6. Statement 1 is true, 2 and 3 are false. Go on to read **1.42**.
7. Statement 2 is true, 1 and 3 are false. Go on to read **1.43**.
8. Statement 3 is true, 1 and 2 are false. Go on to read **1.44**.

1.32 Your answer – the loop of Henle at the 'U bend' is formed of cuboidal cells.
This is not correct. There are cuboidal cells in the thick descending portion of the loop of Henle which become thin squamous flat cells long before the U turn. The thin segment is of variable length depending on whether the loop of Henle is one of the 16 per cent that dip down deep into the medulla. The cells remain flat until, approaching the cortex, they become cuboidal or columnar before merging into the distal convoluted tubule. Now answer the question at the end of **1.27** again, this time correctly.

1.33 Your answer – the macula densa is the loop of Henle.
This is wrong. Read **1.26** and try again.

1.34 Your answer – I don't know what is the histology of the cells at the bend of the loop of Henle.
You are not learning adequately. Go back over **1.27** again and see if you get the correct answer this time.

1.35 Your answer – the 'intercalated' or 'dark cells' are in the cortical collecting tubules.
This is correct. Now go on to read **1.31** with great care. Think about the answers before deciding which of them is correct because this paragraph tests the knowledge you have gained in reading this chapter.

1.36 Your answer – Statements 1 and 2 are true. This is correct. You can go on to **1.45**.

1.37 Your answer – the intercalated or dark cells are in the collecting tubules of the medulla.
Most of the intercalated cells have disappeared by the time the collecting tubule of the medulla is reached, almost all the cells being 'light' in type. The intercalated cells are dark cells similar to those found in the distal convoluted tubule; read **1.29** again and answer the question.

1.38 Your answer – all the statements are false. No. Only Statement 3 is false. There are 1,000,000 glomeruli in each kidney and the juxta-glomerular apparatus is a granular structure with, in all probability, endocrine functions. Re-read **1.22** and go on from there.

1.39 Your answer — 1 and 3 are true, 2 is false.
Statement 1 is true, but 3 is false and 2 is true. Re-read **1.22**.

1.40 Your answer — 2 and 3 are true.
The answer is partly correct in that 2 is true, but Statement No. 3 is false. Similarly 1 is also true, not false. This means you need to read **1.1** again; it is better to realise you don't know something and remedy the defect in your knowledge than to deceive yourself that you have a good knowledge of the subject.

1.41 Your answer — all the statements are true.
The collecting tubule has not got a large brush border, so you are wrong about Statement 3 being true. You are confusing the collecting tubule with proximal tubule. Read **1.29** again.

1.42 Your answer — only Statement 1 is true.
You are right about Statement 1 but Statement 2 is also true. Read **1.26** again and then go on to **1.45**.

1.43 Your answer — only Statement 2 is true. You are wrong about Statement 1. Go back to **1.1** and read through to **1.26** then go on to **1.45**.

1.44 Your answer — only Statement 3 is true. You are wrong on all points. Better go back to **1.1** and read through the chapter again.

1.45 Before leaving the chapter you may wish to refer to more advanced work on the subject of renal anatomy:
Rhodin's articles in Renal Disease, (edited by D. A. K. Black, 2nd edition, Blackwell 1967) and in Diseases of the Kidneys, (edited by M. B. Strauss & L. G. Welt, Little, Brown 1963) are models of clarity with fine illustrations.
Now read Chapter 2.

Time for this chapter: 55 minutes

Chapter 2
Renal physiology

2.1 The kidneys are remarkable organs, maintaining the composition of the internal environment within narrow limits in spite of great variations in intake and metabolic activity. How the kidneys are able to do this is not completely understood, although there is a host of information available about the simpler functions of the kidneys. First of all let us consider the functions of the kidney as being divided into glomerular and tubular parts. The glomeruli filter about 180 litres of fluid each day although only $1\frac{1}{2}$ litres are passed as urine. The fluid in Bowman's space is the result of ultrafiltration of plasma from the capillary lumina through the capillary wall of endothelium and basement membrane and through the visceral epithelial cells. This theory of ultra-filtration was propounded first by Carl Ludwig, the great German physiologist, in 1844, but remained an hypothesis until the fluid in Bowman's space of the frog was actually sampled and analysed by means of micropuncture by Richards in 1923. Since then Bowman's space fluid has been obtained in necturus, the rat and ultimately in the dog by Berliner and colleagues in 1964, and latterly, in the monkey. These workers showed that there was only a slight trace of protein in the glomerular filtrate, as would be expected if the glomerular tuft ultra-filtered the plasma. Similarly, the fluid in Bowman's space had the composition of a filtrate when the osmolality, pH, electrical conductivity, sodium, potassium and chloride concentrations were measured, allowing appropriate corrections for changes due to the difference in protein concentration.

Question What type of filtration of plasma is carried out by the normal glomerulus?

Answer 1. Ultra-filtration. Go on to **2.5**.
2. Simple filtration. Go on to **2.7**.

2.2 Your answer – the renal clearance of inulin was 100 ml/min.
This is correct.

The usual method of determining inulin, radioactive sodium iothiomalate, radio-chromium E.D.T.A. and thiosulphate clearance is by intravenous infusion at a constant rate of the substance with accurate timed collections of urine and plasma samples. The use of urethral catheterisation for the purpose of obtaining accurately timed and complete urine collections is an unnecessary hazard, and should be avoided. Because of the difficulties inherent in accurate urine collections some workers prefer to measure the rate of disappearance from the plasma of an injected intravenous load of, say ^{51}Cr EDTA, and calculate from this GFR. This is an indirect method which is best avoided if accurately timed samples can be obtained. It is necessary if urinary incontinence or obstructive uropathy is present. The chemical analyses for inulin and thiosulphate, though tedious, are not difficult to perform; these are the most accurate methods of determining GFR. Endogenous creatinine clearance is less reliable, endogenous creatinine being reabsorbed by the renal tubules in congestive heart failure and in infancy; in some people it is secreted by the renal tubules. It is a convenient clinical index of progress in that it does not require an infusion, although its relationship to GFR is inconstant. The ideal substance for measuring GFR has not yet been discovered but should have the following properties:

(1) Filtered completely by the glomerulus.
(2) Not secreted and not reabsorbed by the tubules.
(3) Not protein bound.
(4) Does not require infusion intravenously.
(5) Easily measured.

GFR varies according to the size of the subject, a 90lb. 4ft. 6 in. man having a smaller GFR than a 200lb. 6ft. man, but the relationship of GFR to body surface area is reasonably constant. It is usual to correct GFR for body surface area by means of nomograms, the result being expressed as ml/min/1.73 m². The nomogram for conversion of heights and weights to surface areas is in the appendix (p. 394).

Question A man 160 cm in height and 50 kg in weight has a GFR of 75 ml/min as measured by inulin clearance. Using the nomogram on p. 394 determine his GFR corrected to 1.73 m² of surface area.

Answer 1. About 87 ml/min. Go on to **2.8**.
2. About 75 ml/min. Go on to **2.4**.
3. About 65 ml/min. Go on to **2.11**.

2.3 Your answer – TmG means active transport.
This is not quite correct.
Active transport requires energy, and this is provided by enzyme systems which have a limit on the amount of energy which can be provided per unit time; thus active transport is rate limited and reaches a maximum: now read **2.8** again.

2.4 Your answer – the GFR corrected for body surface area is 75 ml/min.
You have not used the nomogram to determine this man's surface area which is about 1.5 m². Now repeat the calculation at the end of **2.2**.

2.5 Your answer – the plasma is ultrafiltered by the glomerulus.
This is correct. The next subject to be discussed is the glomerular filtration rate usually referred to by the abbreviation of GFR. This is defined as the amount of plasma being filtered by the glomeruli per minute. In man the normal GFR is 127 ml/min/1.73 m² of body surface, or 180 litres/day. In women the figure is slightly lower. To understand how GFR is measured, it is necessary to be familiar with the concept of renal clearance rates. The clearance rate of a substance is the amount of plasma cleared per minute of the substance. This is expressed mathematically as

$$C_x = UV/P$$

Where C_x = renal clearance of substance x
 U = urine concentration of x in mg/100 ml.
 V = volume of urine passed per minute
 P = plasma concentration of x in mg/100 ml.

Some substances are secreted *into* the tubular urine by the cells of the renal tubules; others are reabsorbed *from* the tubular urine by the renal tubular cells; many undergo reabsorption at one site and secretion at another. If we want to measure GFR we need to use one of the few substances which are neither secreted nor reabsorbed by the renal tubular cells. Usually GFR is measured by inulin clearance, the clearance of endogenous creatinine, radioactive iodine-labelled sodium iothiomalate, radioactive chromium labelled E.D.T.A., or thiosulphate. Now answer the question, using paper and pencil.

Question What is the renal clearance of inulin in a patient passing urine at 4.2 ml/min; the plasma inulin concentration is constant at 25 mg/100 ml and the inulin concentration in the urine specimen is 600 mg//100 ml?

Answer 1. About 100 ml/min. Go on to **2.2**.
 2. About 6 ml/min. Go on to **2.6**.
 3. About 100 mg/ml. Go on to **2.9**.

2.6 Your answer – the renal clearance of inulin is about 6 ml/min.
You have used the formula incorrectly. The clearance of a substance x is obtained by taking the amount of x excreted in the urine per unit time and dividing this by the mean plasma concentration; this gives the amount of plasma cleared of x by the kidneys per unit time. You have not done this in your calculation. Repeat it, using the formula, $C_x = \dfrac{UV}{P}$ and choose the correct answer to the question at the end of **2.5**.

2.7 Your answer – plasma undergoes simple filtration by the glomerulus.

This is wrong. If simple filtration occurred, the fluid in Bowman's space should be loaded with protein; micropuncture studies in the frog and dog have shown just a trace of protein. Ultrafiltration is filtration without protein passing through into the filtrate. Now re-read **2.1** again and answer the question again.

2.8 Your answer – the corrected GFR is 87 ml/min/1.73 m².

This is correct. Now we are going to consider functions of the tubules; first of all, *tubular reabsorption*. Many substances are found in the glomerular filtrate during micropuncture experiments which are absent or very much reduced in concentration in the bladder urine; these substances must have been absorbed by the renal tubules. Reabsorption may be an active process, with passage of the material *against* an electrochemical gradient; or passive, with passage of substances *down* an electrochemical gradient. Active transport energy is provided by the action of the appropriate enzymes inside the tubular cells. Because there is a limit to the amount of energy which can be supplied for any process inside the cell, there is a limit to the maximum amount of a substance that can be actively transported; this maximum rate of transport of any substance from the tubular lumen is known as *tubular maximum rate of reabsorption*. Similarly, in active transport of substances into the tubular lumen *from* the blood plasma the term *tubular maximum rate of secretion* is used. In practice both these terms are rarely used, being replaced by the symbol T_m or tubular maximum transport rate, the question of secretion or reabsorption being ignored. Thus T_mG refers to tubular maximal rate of *reabsorption* of glucose and T_mPAH to tubular maximal rate of secretion of para-amino hippurate.

Question What does T_mG mean?

Answer 1. Tubular maximum rate of glucose *reabsorption*. Go on to **2.10**.
      2. Active transport. Go on to **2.3**.
      3. Tubular maximum rate of glucose *secretion*. Go on to **2.15**.

2.9 Your answer – the renal clearance of inulin is 100 mg/min.

Your answer is partly correct in that you employed the clearance formula correctly, but the units in which the answer is expressed are wrong. The clearance of a substance is defined as the *volume* of plasma cleared of that substance per minute. Your answer should therefore be 100 ml/min. Now go on to **2.2**.

2.10 Your answer – T_mG means tubular rate of glucose reabsorption.

You are correct. T_mG is determined by measuring the rate of tubular reabsorption of glucose while increasing the plasma glucose concentration so a point is reached where the proximal tubular cells attain their maximum reabsorptive capacity for glucose; once the load of glucose filtered by the glomeruli exceeds the maximal tubular reabsorptive capacity of the tubules, glucose appears in the urine. This is shown in Fig. 2.10. Look at it carefully.

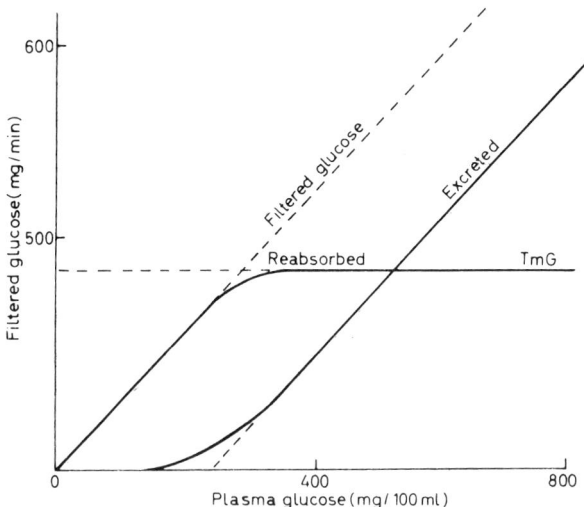

Fig. 2.10

The mean value of T_mG is 375 mg/min/1.73 m² for men and 303 mg/min/1.73 m² for woman.

In some people glucose is excreted at normal plasma levels. This condition is known as *renal glycosuria* and is due either to a low T_mG in all nephrons or a T_mG which varies from nephron to nephron. It will be discussed further in the chapter on proximal tubular disorders.

Question What is the name of the condition where glucose appears in the urine at normal blood sugar levels?

Answer 1. Diabetes mellitus. Go on to **2.14**.
2. Renal glycosuria. Go on to **2.12**.
3. Diabetes insipidus. Go on to **2.17**.

2.11 Your answer — GFR correct for surface area is 65 ml/min/1.73 m².

You are not correct. Having found from the nomogram that the surface area of the man is 1.5 m², you have multiplied the actual GFR by $\dfrac{1.5}{1.73}$ instead of $\dfrac{1.73}{1.5}$, which will give you the correct answer. Work out the problem again at the end of **2.2**.

2.12 Your answer — renal glycosuria is a condition where glycosuria is associated with a normal blood sugar concentration.

You are correct.

Micropuncture studies have shown that glucose is reabsorbed in the proximal tubule. Phlorizin is a glucoside which was shown to induce glycosuria by von Mering in 1899. The clearance rate of glucose rises to equal that of inulin when phlorizin is given to the dog; this shows that there is a complete block of tubular reabsorption of glucose induced by phlorizin. Xylose, fructose and galactose also compete with glucose in active transport out of the tubular lumen into the proximal tubular cells; phlorizin blocks the tubular reabsorption of these carbohydrates. Inulin is a fructose polymer obtained from the dahlia tuber and the Jerusalem artichoke. It is neither reabsorbed nor excreted by the tubular cells and is consequently used for measuring the GFR.

Question What is the effect of phlorizin on proximal tubule handling of glucose?

Answer 1. Depressed tubular reabsorption of glucose. Go on to **2.13**.
2. Increases tubular reabsorption. Go on to **2.18**.
3. Don't know. Go on to **2.20**.

2.13 Your answer — Phlorizin depresses tubular reabsorption of glucose.

You are correct.

Now let us consider the proximal tubular reabsorption of amino acids. Amino acids are found in the urine in small amounts normally and are identified readily by chromatography. Glycine, arginine and lysine have a tubular maximum reabsorption rate, but many others such as histidine, methionine, tryptophane, leucine and phenylalanine have very efficient reabsorptive mechanisms without a measurable maximum value. There are several mechanisms for the reabsorption of different groups of amino acid. (1) The basic amino acids (arginine, histidine and lysine): members of this group compete with each other for reabsorption. (2) The carboxylic acid group of leucine and isoleucine: they also compete with each other for reabsorption. (3) Glycine appears to be absorbed independently of the other two groups.

Question Where are amino acids reabsorbed?

Answer 1. Proximal tubule. Go on to **2.16**.
2. Distal tubule. Go on to **2.19**.

2.14 Your answer — glucose appears in the urine with normal blood sugar levels in diabetes mellitus.

You are wrong. In diabetes mellitus there is an elevated blood sugar level before glycosuria appears. In some families renal glycosuria is followed by diabetes mellitus, but this is very unusual Read **2.10** again and pay attention to the text.

2.15 Your answer — T_mG means tubular maximum rate of glucose *secretion*.

Glucose is reabsorbed in the renal tubule. There would be glucose in normal urine if glucose were predominantly secreted rather than reabsorbed. Read **2.8** again and answer the question.

2.16 Your answer – amino acids are reabsorbed in the proximal tubule.

This is correct. Now let us look at the reabsorption of phosphate in the proximal tubule. First of all let us examine what types of phosphate exist in the glomerular filtrate and tubular fluid. Inorganic phosphate can exist in solution as as $(H_2PO_4)^-$ and $(HPO_4)^{--}$; the ratio of $H_2PO_4^-$ to HPO_4^{--} is determined by the pH of the fluid. The glomerular filtrate is at pH 7.4 and the ratio $HPO_4^{--}/H_2PO_4^-$ is 4/1. As the urine in the tubule changes in pH this ratio alters. Compared to the phosphate concentration in the glomerular filtrate there is very little phosphate in the urine which is in the bladder, indicating that the bulk of filtered phosphate is reabsorbed in the tubules: stop flow experiments have shown that most of the phosphate reabsorption is in the proximal tubule. In man a tubular maximum rate of phosphate reabsorption has been demonstrated. Phosphate reabsorption is influenced by parathyroid hormone activity: injected parathormone causes a decreased tubular phosphate reabsorption and an increased phosphate excretion in the urine, leading to a depressed plasma phosphate. In the detection of patients with parathyroid tumours the decreased tubular reabsorption of phosphate is used as an important test, but it is difficult to interpret unless phosphate dietary intake has been rigidly controlled for several days.

Thyrocalcitonin injection causes in man an increase in P and Ca excretion in the urine and a fall in plasma calcium. It inhibits the release of calcium from the bone and inhibits the conversion of 25 (OH) vitamin D_3 to its biologically active form 1:25 dihydroxy Vit D_3 in the kidney. It appears at present that $1:25 (OH)_2 D_3$ formed in the kidney is active in mobilizing calcium from bone.

Urates are also reabsorbed in the proximal tubules, but reappear distally due to secretion at other sites in the nephron.

Question How is phosphate reabsorption affected by injection of parathyroid hormone?

Answer 1. Decreases phosphate reabsorption. Go on to **2.24**.
2. Increases phosphate absorption. Go on to **2.27**.
3. Don't know. Go on to **2.23**.

2.17 Your answer – diabetes insipidus is a condition where glycosuria occurs with a normal blood sugar.

This is quite wrong. Diabetes insipidus has nothing to do with glucose metabolism. You have not been concentrating. Read **2.10** again and answer the question.

2.18 Your answer – phlorizin increases tubular reabsorption of glucose.

Phlorizin is an enzyme poison which reduces the amount of energy available for active transport of glucose from the proximal tubular lumen into the tubular cell and then into the blood. It therefore cannot increase tubular reabsorption of glucose. Now read **2.12** again and answer the question.

2.19 Your answer – amino acids are reabsorbed in the distal tubule.
This is incorrect. Amino acids are reabsorbed in the proximal tubule. Read **2.13** again.

2.20 Your answer – I don't know what the effect of phlorizin is on tubular reabsorption of glucose.
If you do not know you have not read **2.12** carefully. Go back and read **2.12** now without day-dreaming and then answer the question at the end of it correctly.

2.21 Your answer – ERPF = 600 ml/min.
You are correct.
Now we can discuss the measurement of Tm of PAH – ie. tubular maximum rate of PAH secretion. If the plasma PAH concentration is increased to between 30 and 50 mg/100 ml, the tubules reach a maximum rate of secretion above which no further increase in secretion rate is possible: this is TmPAH and is comparable to the reabsorption Tm of glucose. At high plasma levels of PAH, protein binding of PAH must be taken into account because only the non-protein bound plasma PAH can take part in transfer from plasma to tubular fluid, and therefore the non-protein bound PAH concentration is used in all calculations of TmPAH. The average value of the non-protein bound fraction is 78 per cent of the total PAH concentration: in all calculations of TmPAH the plasma PAH concentration should therefore be multiplied by 0.78.

Now let us have a look at the calculation of TmPAH. It is more complicated than the calculation of Tm glucose; we measure TmPAH at high plasma concentrations of PAH, and at these concentrations, urinary PAH excretion is the sum of PAH filtered at the glomerulus and that secreted by the tubules. This is expressed by the formula

$$UV = GC_{PAH} + T_{PAH} \tag{1}$$

Where U = urinary concentration of PAH (mg/100 ml)
V = urinary vol./min
GC_{PAH} = glomerular filtration of PAH in mg/min
T_{PAH} = tubular secretion of PAH in mg/min

Now 78 per cent of PAH is not bound to plasma protein, so that
$$GC_{PAH} = C_{in} \times 0.78 \times P \tag{2}$$

Where C_{in} = GFR measured by inulin clearance (ml/min)
= plasma PAH concentration (mg/100 ml)

Where T_{PAH} has reached its maximum value,

$$UV = (0.78 \, P \times C_{in}) + TmPAH.$$
Therefore $TmPAH = UV - (0.78 \, P \times C_{in})$

The usual value of TmPAH in man is about 80 mg/min/1.73 m²; in woman 77 mg/min/1.73 m². Now let us apply this formula to a problem.

Question Calculate the tubular maximum rate of secretion of PAH from the following data:
Plasma level of PAH = 40 mg/100 ml
Inulin clearance = 120 ml/min
Urinary excretion of PAH = 117 mg/min
Non-protein bound fraction of PAH = 78 per cent of total plasma PAH concentration.

Answer 1. About 80 mg/min. Go on to **2.32**.
         2. About 155 mg/min. Go on to **2.22**.
         3. About 70 mg/min. Go on to **2.30**.

2.22 Your answer – TmPAH is about 155 mg/min.
This is incorrect due to your having added the filtered load of PAH *to* the urinary excretion of PAH; you should go over the formula (3) of **2.21**. Now repeat the calculation.

2.23 Your answer – I don't know the effect of parathyroid hormone on phosphate reabsorption.
In that case you are not learning properly. The point of reading this section is to become acquainted with the fundamentals of renal physiology and you have to remember what you read and not browse through this like a novel. Now go back and read **2.16** again.

2.24 Your answer – tubular reabsorption is reduced by parathyroid hormone injection.
This is correct. The next subject to be dealt with is *tubular secretion*. This involves a similar set of concepts to those discussed earlier when dealing with reabsorption: there are enzyme systems involved in tubular secretion which have a maximum rate of transfer or 'tubular maximum' – Tm. Let us take para-amino hippurate (PAH) as an example of secretion. If PAH is given intravenously so that it has a low plasma concentration (2 mg/100 ml) almost all the PAH entering the kidney through the renal artery has disappeared by the time the renal vein is reached. There is a little left, some of the blood not traversing glomeruli but going to pelvis, capsule etc. and some of the PAH being protein-bound. If the clearance of PAH is compared to that of inulin it will be found that the PAH clearance is about 600 ml of plasma per minute compared to 127 ml/min for inulin. This must indicate that tubular secretion of PAH occurs and other studies have shown

that this occurs in the proximal tubule. The renal plasma flow (RPF) is measured using PAH extraction by the kidneys at low plasma PAH concentrations: accurate RPF determinations depend on the Fick principle where renal arterial and renal venous blood samples are obtained and the extraction of PAH measured.

$$\text{RDF} = \frac{UV}{P_a\text{PAH} - P_v\text{PAH}} \quad (1)$$

Where U = urine concentration of PAH
V = volume of urine
P_aPAH = renal artery concentration of PAH
P_vPAH = renal vein concentration of PAH

In practice it is not convenient to obtain renal venous blood, and as P_aPAH is usually equal to systemic venous PAH concentrations we get the formula:

$$\text{ERPF} = \frac{UV}{P} \quad (2)$$

where ERPF = estimated RPF
P = PAH concentration in systematic venous plasma

If renal disease is present, or in infancy, formula 2 leads to errors because extraction of PAH by the kidneys is less efficient; formula 1 is more accurate, although it is difficult and usually unjustifiable to obtain renal vein blood for PAH determinations.

Question What is the ERPF in a man excreting 12 mg of PAH per minute in his urine, if his plasma PAH concentration is 2 mg/100 ml?

Answer 1. 2400 ml/min. Go on to **2.26**.
2. 600 ml/min. Go on to **2.21**.
3. 600 mg/ min. Go on to **2.28**.

2.25 Your answer – filtration fraction is 72,000 ml/min.

You are wrong. You have not used formula (1) in **2.32** correctly. Read **2.32** again and answer the question using the appropriate formula.

2.26 Your answer – 2400 ml/min.

You are incorrect.

You have multiplied the plasma concentration of PAH by the urinary minute excretion. If you look at formula (2) in **2.24** you will see that ERPF = UV/P UV = 12 mg/min. P = 0.02 mg/ml.

Now work out the result again and choose the correct answer at the end of **2.24**.

2.27 Your answer – parathyroid hormone injection increases tubular phosphate reabsorption.

You are incorrect. Remember that parathyroid tumours are associated with a hyperphosphaturia and hypophosphataemia. These changes are due to the decreased proximal tubular reabsorption of phosphate. Now read **2.16** again and answer the question correctly.

2.28 Your answer – ERPF = 600 mg/min.

You have done the calculation correctly but your result is expressed in the wrong units. Renal plasma flow is expressed as ml of plasma per minute. Now re-write the answer correctly and choose the appropriate answer at the end of **2.24**.

2.29 Your answer – the loop of Henle is a counter current multiplier system. You are correct. The next subject to be discussed is the concept of *free water*.

'Free water' is a convenient term referring to the water which is present in urine but which is in excess of the volume of water needed to produce urine at the osmolality of plasma: this 'free water' is known as non-osmotically obligated water. If the urine is more dilute than plasma, the free water clearance (C_{H_2O}) will be positive: if the urine is more concentrated than plasma, C_{H_2O} will be negative. 'Free water clearance' is a misnomer, because it is not a true clearance in that it does not express the volume of plasma cleared of water per minute. This can be more readily understood by looking at the formula expressing this:

$$V = C_{H_2O} + \frac{U \text{ osm } V}{P \text{ osm.}}$$

Where V = urine vol/min   U osm = urine osmolality
C_{H_2O} = free water clearance   P osm = plasma osmolality

The amount of free water clearance can be up to 15 ml/min in water diuresis. The entire concept of 'free water' excretion is bedevilled by a varying terminology: in the presence of urine hypertonic to plasma the negative free water clearance is frequently referred to as a positive figure known as $T^c_{H_2O}$, tubular reabsorption of free water. This is expressed in the formulae

$$V = \frac{U osm\ V}{Posm} - T^c_{H_2O}$$

$$T^c_{H_2O} = -C_{H_2O}$$

If an osmotic diuresis is taking place due to mannitol being given intravenously with antidiuretic hormone, then $T^c_{H_2O}$ reaches a maximum reabsorption rate, $T_m{}^c_{H_2O}$. This has a value of about 5 ml/min in the normal adult; it is one of the readily measurable indices of the functioning mass of the distal tubules and is analagous to $T_m PAH$ and TmG which give a rough indication of the functioning mass of the proximal renal tubules. If saline is used to produce an osmotic diuresis rather than mannitol, no T_m value is reached; $T^c_{H_2O}$ rises progressively.

Question When the urine which is being secreted is more concentrated than plasma, is C_{H_2O} positive or negative?

Answer 1. Positive. Go on to **2.41**.
2. Negative. Go on to **2.45**.
3. Don't know. Go on to **2.48**.

2.30 Your answer – TmPAH is about 70 mg/100 ml.

You have neglected the protein binding of PAH which makes the filtered load of PAH 0.78 of the figure you used. Repeat the calculation taking this into account.

2.31 Your answer – filtration fraction of 0.2.

You are correct. Let us consider next the absorption of water. This is a remarkably efficient mechanism, the daily urine volume varying according to the requirements of the body in health from 500 ml to 3 or 4 litres: usually the average urine volume is about 1500 ml. The volume of water filtered by the glomeruli each day is about 180 litres, so that about 99 per cent of the filtered water is reabsorbed. Most of this water (70–80 per cent) is reabsorbed passively in the proximal tubule pari-passu with sodium reabsorption, the tubular fluid remaining isosmotic, ie. same concentration as plasma. What happens in the loop of Henle and beyond depends on whether anti-diuretic hormone (ADH) is being secreted from the neurohypophsis into the blood stream and thus stimulating the renal medulla to produce a concentrated urine. First of all let us deal with the condition of water diuresis when ADH secretion is shut off and very dilute urine is being formed: under these circumstances water can pass out through the wall of the thin part of Henle's loop but not through the thick portion of the ascending loop. The urine in the distal convoluted tubule is hypotonic; in the absence of ADH the urine remains dilute as it passes down into the collecting ducts and so on into the renal pelvis, ureter and bladder. Before we go on to the more complicated mechanism of urine concentration, answer the question below.

Question How much water is reabsorbed in the proximal tubule irrespective of whether the final urine is concentrated or dilute?

Answer 1. 70–80 per cent. Go on to **2.36**.
2. Don't know. Go on to **2.39**.

2.32 Your answer – TmPAH is about 80 mg/min.

This is correct. The renal tubules secrete, in addition to PAH, diodrast (which is a radio-opaque iodine-containing contrast medium), phenol red and penicillin. Their excretion is reduced by caronamide or benemid. These two drugs also reduce tubular reabsorption of urate in man. It is probable that phenol red, PAH, diodrast and penicillin share a common mechanism of secretion.

Before leaving the subject of tubular secretion the term 'filtration fraction' should be explained. The filtration fraction (FF) is the fraction of renal plasma flow which is being filtered by the glomeruli, i.e., the ratio of the glomerular filtration rate to the renal plasma flow. This is expressed as:

$$FF = \frac{C_{in}}{C_{PAH}}$$

In man, changes in RPF are associated with changes in afferent and efferent arteriolar tone tending to maintain the glomerular filtration rate constant: this means that $FF = \frac{K}{C_{PAH}}$ where K is a constant.

Question Calculate FF in a man whose inulin clearance is 120 ml/min and renal plasma flow = 600 ml/min.

Answer 1. 72,000 ml/min. Go on to **2.25**.
2. 0.2. Go on to **2.31**.
3. 0.2 ml/min. Go on to **2.34**.

2.33 Your answer − the osmolalities are similar in water deprivation in both Henle's loop tip and the distal tubule.
You are wrong.
Read **2.40** properly and answer the question correctly.

2.34 Your answer − filtration fraction is 0.2 ml/min.
You are partly correct but you have used the wrong units. The filtration fraction is the ratio of two clearances, GFR and RPF, and therefore the filtration fraction is a ratio without any units being necessary. Now go on to read **2.31**.

2.35 Your answer − the distal convoluted tubule and the tip of Henle's loop have a different osmolality.
You are correct. Henle's loop urine has a high osmolality under conditions of ADH secretion but the urine in the distal convoluted tubule is always hypotonic to plasma whatever the state of ADH secretion.

The mechanism which accounts best for the phenomenon of urine concentration as far as data have been accumulated is that of the counter-current multiplier system. You are probably already familiar with the common engineering concept of a counter-current heat exchanger used so commonly in the chemical industry in which incoming cold gases are heated by the hot effluent exhaust gases, so reducing the energy lost to the system. The capillary loops of the medulla have a comparatively low blood flow, and the exchange of gases and solutes can occur between the arterial and venous limbs: they function as counter-current exchangers, conserving a high content of solute and CO_2 (and a low content of O_2) in the deeper zone of the medulla. The long loops of Henle themselves are thought to be counter-current multiplier systems. What is this? Now look at Fig. 2.35 where there is represented a loop of Henle with a membrane down the middle. The cells forming the efferent limb are capable of pushing sodium across the membrane until there is a maximum difference between the two sides of say 50 mEq/1 beyond which passive back diffusion reduces the concentration difference back to 50 mEq/1 again. This is shown in Fig. 2.35 parts (a) and (b). In (a) the multiplier is not working. The urine enters (a) at a concentration of 280 mOsm/kg; the multiplier is activated by ADH which causes the sodium ion to be pumped out of the lower segment (b) so that is has a concentration of 255 mOsm/kg, whereas the upper compartment has a concentration of 305 mOsm. In (c) more urine has entered as flow continues and some of the fluid from the upper compartment has gone down to the lower compartment; at the tip the osmolality is 305 mOsm on both sides. In (d) we see the new concentrations where the sodium pump has been at work again. The papillary tip is now 330 mOsm in the upper limb sodium having been pumped from the extreme right end of the lower limb reducing that to 280 mOsm and keeping the difference in concentrations across adjacent parts of the membrane at 50 mOsm/kg. In (e) fresh urine has entered pushing the 330 mOsm urine round the tip and by (f) another 50 mOsm/kg concentration difference between adjacent portions of upper and lower tubes has been set up. The osmolality is now 355 in the tip of the upper tube. This osmolality can go on increasing in this manner, being limited by the integrity of the sodium pump mechanism, the availability of sodium and the presence of a circulation in the medullary vessels tending to wash away the increased concentration of solutes in the medulla. Fortunately the medullary circulation is relatively sluggish and appears to be specially adapted to prevent such a washout of solute from the medulla. When the urine leaves the loop of Henle to reach the distal convoluted tubule it is dilute; however it becomes concentrated again as the urine passes in the collecting tubules through the hyperosmotic medulla since the walls of the collecting ducts are permeable to water under the influence of ADH. Thus urine is produced in a concentrated form by a counter-current multiplier system.

The sodium concentration falls progressively in the ascending limb of the loop of Henle from the hairpin bend to the distal tubule. This has been demonstrated by micropuncture in the rat by Berliner and his colleagues, so giving direct experimental confirmation to the counter-current multiplier hypothesis with a sodium pump in the thin segment of the ascending loop of Henle. Lever has suggested that the site of the multiplier mechanism is in the vasa recta, but this theory has been demolished by Berliner by both experimental proof and on theoretical grounds. It is likely that the vasa recta are the site of a counter-current exchanger mechanism responsible for the maintenance of the high medullary osmolality, preventing the washout of the high medullary osmolality by the blood flow in the vasa recta.

Question What is the type of system for concentrating the tubular fluid in the loop of Henle?

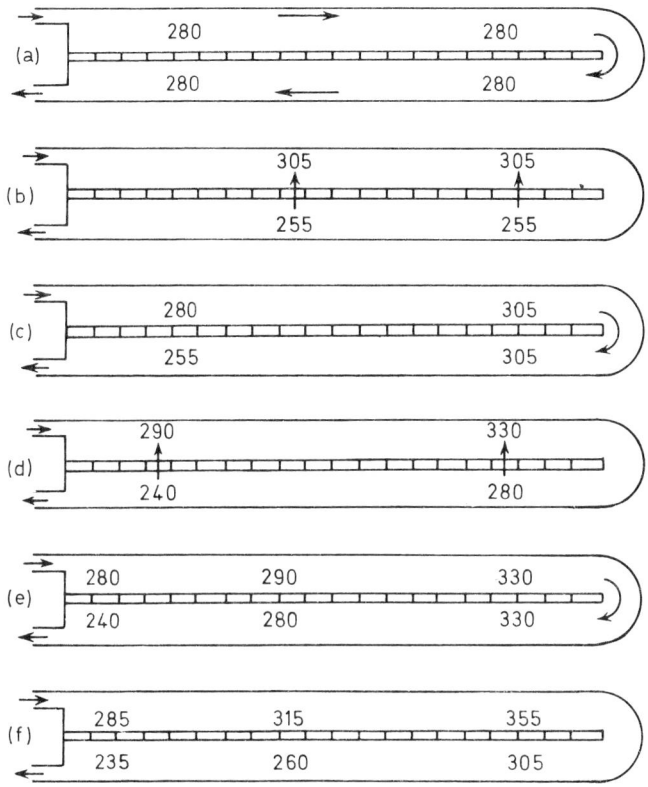

Fig. 2.25 After R. W. Berliner.

Answer 1. Counter-current exchanger system. Go on to **2.42**.
2. Counter-current multiplier system. Go on to **2.29**.

2.36 Your answer – 70–80 per cent of the water is reabsorbed in the proximal tubule.

You are correct.

Before we can go into a detailed discussion of how urine is concentrated, you must be acquainted with the terminology which is used. First of all, the degree of concentration of a solution is expressed in terms of osmolality of a solution rather than the specific gravity with which you are probably familiar. *Osmolality* of a solution is a term indicating the number of osmotically active particles per *kilogram of solvent*. *Osmolarity* is often used and it describes the number of osmotically active particles *per litre of solution*. The difference between osmolality and osmolarity is very small and much less than the minimum 1 per cent error inherent in determination of osmolality by freezing point depression (cryoscopy). Now a solution of sodium chloride containing 1 gram molecule per kilogram of solvent will contain 1 osm/kg of sodium ions and 1 osm/kg of chloride ions, giving a total osmolality of 2 osm/kg. Similarly calcium chloride gives three osmotically active particles per molecule. Molecular size does not affect osmolality; thus 1 gram molecule of a large molecule like albumin with a molecular weight of 70,000 has just the same osmotic activity as 1 gram molecule of a tiny proton (H^+) one seventy thousandth of its weight. Because biological solutions are often very dilute, the term milliosmol, i.e. one thousandth of an osmol, is used. Plasma osmolarity is about 285–290 milliosmols/litre. Human urine produced under conditions of water deprivation may have an osmolarity as high as 1400 milliosmols/litre. Under conditions of ingestion of large volumes of water a very dilute urine may be produced with an osmolarity of 37 milliosmols/litre. Specific gravity of 1010 corresponds to an osmolarity of 285 milliosmols/litre.

Question What is the osmolality of a solution containing 0.25 gram molecules of potassium chloride per kg of solvent?

Answer   1. 250 milliosmols/kg. Go on to **2.37**.
          2. 500 milliosmols/kg. Go on to **2.40**.
          3. Don't know. Go on to **2.38**.

2.37 Your answer – a 0.25 g-mol./kg solution of KC1 has an osmolality of 250 milliosmols/kg.

You are not quite right. Osmolality refers to the number of osmotically active particles and each molecule of KC1 dissociates into K^+ and Cl^- ions, that is 2 ions per molecule. Therefore there are 2 osmols per mol. of KC1 in solution. Now answer the question in **2.39** correctly.

2.38 Your answer – I don't know how many osmols there are in a 0.25 g-mol./kg solution of KC1.

In that case you have not followed **2.39** carefully. Read **2.37** then **2.39** again and choose the right answer.

2.39 Your answer — I don't know how much water is reabsorbed in the proximal tubule.

If you don't know you have not been reading **2.31** with enough care. This is a difficult subject to read for the first time so please pay more attention and read **2.31** again.

2.40 Your answer – A 0.25 mol./kg solution of KC1 has an osmolality of 500 milliosmols/kg.

You are correct.

We shall consider the known facts about the composition of tubular urine and the tissues of the kidney under conditions of water deprivation, i.e., ADH stimulation, before going on to understand the theory which has been developed to account for these data.

Under conditions of water deprivation the solute content of tissue slices of the medulla is much higher than that of the cortex. Solute concentration increases progressively as the tip of the renal pyramid is approached. The osmolarity of the tissue at the papillary tips is about the same as that of the concentrated urine passing out of the collecting ducts into the pelvis, while the cortex has the same osmolarity as plasma. In desert rodents with a long papillary tip, the tip of Henle's loop has been found by micropuncture to have a very high osmolarity like that of the surrounding papillary tissues; the blood in the vasa recta here at the papillary tip also has a high osmolarity. The tubules are next accessible to micropuncture techniques in the distal convoluted tubule where the tubular fluid is *hypotonic* to plasma both in water diuresis and in water deprivation. The urine in the collecting ducts has a high osmolarity, corresponding to the osmolarity in the papillary peak in water deprivation. In water diuresis, although the tissue osmolarity in the medulla is higher than in the cortex, the urine produced is hypotonic to plasma.

Question In conditions of water deprivation, is the osmolarity of tubular urine the same in the tip of Henle's loop and in the distal convoluted tubule?

Answer 1. Yes. Go on to **2.33**.
2. No. Go on to **2.35**.

2.41 Your answer — in urine which is concentrated C_{H_2O} is positive.
You are wrong. C_{H_2O} is defined by the formula

$$V = C_{H_2O} + \frac{U \text{ osm } V}{P \text{ osm}}$$

Now if U osm is greater than P osm the expression $\frac{U \text{ osm } V}{P \text{ osm}}$ is greater than V, say $V + k$.
So that $C_{H_2O} = V - (V + k)$
$= -k$

Therefore C_{H_2O} is negative.
Now read **2.29** again and answer correctly.

2.42 Your answer — the loop of Henle is a counter-current exchanger.
No. The counter-current exchanger system is a simple mechanism present in the medullary capillaries. The loop of Henle is thought to be the more complex counter-current *multiplier* system where the concentration difference between

efferent and adderent fluids is *multiplied* so that very high osmolarities are reached at the tip of the loop of Henle. Read **2.35** again and answer correctly.

2.43 Your answer – the greater part of the filtered sodium is reabsorbed in the proximal tubule, you are correct.

The mechanism of absorption of sodium in the ascending loop of Henle is by means of a sodium pump located in the tubular cells. There is some evidence that this is dependent on aerobic metabolism, in that there is a direct relationship between the amount of sodium reabsorbed by the kidney tubules, and the oxygen consumption of the kidney. The sodium pump is thought to receive energy by the conversion of ATP to ADP. This conversion is carried out by an enzyme known as sodium and potassium sensitive adenosine triphosphatase or Na-K ATPase which is found in large amounts in the renal medulla and which is inhibited by ouabain and reduced in amount by furosemide. The presence of both sodium and potassium ions are necessary for its activity. The administration of both ouabain and furosemide is followed by a sodium diuresis i.e. sodium reabsorption is inhibited by them. Microdissection studies indicate that the ascending limb of the loop of Henle is particularly rich in Na-K ATPase; this is the probable site of the sodium pump so essential in the counter current multiplier theory of urine concentration that you have read earlier in this chapter. Now reread this paragraph because the subject matter is difficult; then answer the following question.

Question What enzyme is present in the sodium pump in the kidney?

Answers 1. ATP. Go on to **2.50**.
          2. Na-K ATPase. Go on to **2.44**.
          3. ADP. Go on to **2.55**.

2.44 Your answer: Na-K ATPase is an enzyme present in the sodium pump in the kidney. You are correct. Potassium is the next cation to be considered. There is good evidence from micropuncture and stop flow experiments that potassium is both reabsorbed and secreted by the renal tubule. 'Stop flow' is a type of experiment carried out frequently in dogs in which a ureter is exposed and cannulated under anaesthesia and then, commonly when an osmotic diuresis with mannitol is occurring, the ureter is clamped. It is released after a few minutes during which time the fluid in the various parts of the nephron is almost stationary and is acted upon by the adjacent tubular cells so that on release the fluid when taken in consecutive fractions has the exaggerated biochemical changes characteristic of the part of the nephron it has been in contact with. The site of the glomerulus is determined by injecting inulin a few seconds before release of the occlusion, the glomerular samples being the first samples containing inulin after removal of the ureteric occlusion. PAH is injected to give information about the site of the proximal tubule, the distal end of which is represented by the earliest samples containing PAH. Stop flow is somewhat crude because flow continues inside the nephron in spite of ureteric obstruction, but it has yielded a great deal of information about tubular function.

Question How does one know which stop flow specimens are from the proximal tubule?

Answer 1. Inulin is present in them. See **2.46**.
2. PAH is present in them. See **2.52**.

2.45 Your answer − in urine which is concentrated C_{H_2O} is negative.

You are correct. The next subject to be discussed is the absorption of small ions − first of all, sodium.

The consumption of oxygen by the kidney is closely related to the amount of sodium which is being reabsorbed. Micropuncture studies have shown that sodium reabsorption initially is *against* an electro-chemical gradient and therefore is an *active* process, sodium bicarbonate being actively reabsorbed in the initial part of the proximal tubule. This is an isosmotic reabsorption, i.e., water is reabsorbed along with sodium in a Na/H_2O ratio equal to that found in a protein free filtrate of plasma. As a result the concentration of chloride rises in the remaining fluid in the proximal tubule, and so sodium may be reabsorbed accompanying chloride down a chemical concentration gradient. 75−80 per cent of the sodium reabsorption occurs in the proximal tubule, the sodium concentration of the tubular fluid being maintained close to that of plasma throughout the proximal tubule owing to the simultaneous reabsorption of water. About 10 per cent of sodium reabsorption is thought to occur in the loop of Henle, where under the stimulus of ADH, the sodium ejected into the medullary interstitium is an important factor contributing to medullary hypertonicity and hence to the formation of a concentrated urine by the counter-current multiplier system.

Distal tubular reabsorption of sodium occurs both in the distal convoluted tubule and in the collecting ducts; it is an efficient process which can render the urine almost free of sodium. Part of the distal sodium reabsorption is an active transport process but some is reabsorbed by an ion-exchange system, in which sodium is exchanged for hydrogen ions and/or potassium ions. Sodium reabsorption is dependent on several factors such as the GFR, aldosterone, and corticosteroids such as cortisone and hydrocortisone which cause an increase in sodium reabsorption. It is now very likely that another powerful mineralocorticoid exists, with 18 OH DOC as a precursor in the adrenal cortex. Its identity is at the moment unknown. Mercurial diuretics, chlorothiazide, and the carbonic anhydrase inhibitors cause a reduction in sodium reabsorption. Recently a new naturally occurring sodium excreting factor has been described. It is known as 'Third factor,' but its very existence is in some dispute. It is responsible, if it exists, for the sodium diuresis caused by expansion of the extra cellular fluid (ECF) by infusion of isotonic saline.

Question Where is the greater part of the filtered sodium reabsorbed?

Answer 1. Proximal tubule. Go on to **2.43**.
2. Distal convoluted tubule. Go on to **2.49**.
3. Collecting system. Go on to **2.47**.

2.46 Your answer – the proximal tubule samples in stop flow experiments are indicated by the presence in them of inulin.

You are not correct in thinking that inulin in the specimens indicates that they are proximal samples; inulin indicates which is the first glomerular sample although there is some movement of fluid from the glomerulus down into the proximal tubule during the stopped part of the stop-flow experiment. The specimens immediately before the inulin containing sample are usually acceptable as proximal tubular samples. Now read **2.43** again and answer the question.

2.47 Your answer – the greater part of the filtered sodium is reabsorbed in the collecting system duct.

You are incorrect. Only a small amount of the filtered sodium is absorbed in the collecting system. Read **2.45** again and answer the question correctly.

2.48 Your answer – I don't know if C_{H_2O} is positive or negative if concentrated urine is being formed. If C_{H_2O} is defined by the formula

$$V = C_{H_2O} + \frac{U \text{ osm } V}{P \text{ osm}}$$

then $C_{H_2O} = V - \frac{U \text{ osm } V}{P \text{ osm}}$

and $\frac{U \text{ osm}}{P \text{ osm}}$ is greater than one if the urine is concentrated.

Therefore C_{H_2O} will be negative. Go back and re-read **2.29**.

2.49 Your answer – the greater part of the filtered sodium is reabsorbed in the distal convoluted tubule.

You are wrong. 75 per cent of the filtered sodium is reabsorbed in the proximal tubule, only a small amount being left for reabsorption in the distal tubule, although this fraction is often very important in determining the final sodium concentration of the urine.

Read **2.45** again and answer the question.

2.50 Your answer – ATP is the enzyme present in the sodium pump. No, you have not appreciated that ATP is not an enzyme but actually is the high energy phosphate containing substance known as adenosine triphosphate. The enzyme is a sodium and potassium sensitive adenosine triphosphatase. The ase indicates that this is an enzyme. Read **2.43**.

2.51 Your answer – sodium ion is exchanged for potassium ion.
You are partly correct but hydrogen ion is also involved. Read **2.52** again.

2.52 Your answer – the earliest specimens with PAH in them are from the proximal tubular region.
Quite right. Now we can return to potassium. There is some evidence that potassium is absorbed proximally, the urine reaching the distal tubular site of secretion being almost free of potassium. Secretion of potassium is thought to occur in the distal tubule by a mechanism of ion exchange, sodium ions being absorbed in exchange for potassium ions. Potassium conservation in the kidney is less efficient than sodium conservation, the urine still containing appreciable concentrations of potassium in the absence of potassium in the diet. Hydrogen ion secretion appears to compete with potassium ion in exchange for sodium reabsorbed in the distal tubule. During the administration of chlorothiazide and under the influence of aldosterone, distal potassium secretion is enhanced.

Question In the distal tubular ion exchange for sodium ion, what other ions are involved?

Answer 1. Potassium ion. Go on to **2.51**.
2. Hydrogen ion. Go on to **2.53**.
3. Potassium and hydrogen ion. Go on to **2.54**.

2.53 Your answer – hydrogen ion is exchanged for sodium ion.
You are partly correct but potassium ion competes with hydrogen ion as well. Read **2.52** more carefully.

2.54 Your answer – potassium and hydrogen ions are exchanged for sodium ions in the distal tubule.
You are correct. The next subject to be considered is acidification of the urine and the closely related bicarbonate reabsorption. It was once thought that acidification of urine took place at a distal tubular site only, but micropuncture studies have shown that the tubular fluid becomes more acid than plasma in the *proximal* tubule. Large amounts of hydrogen ion are being secreted into the proximal tubule: it is probable that the secretion of hydrogen ion into the proximal tubule is one of the mechanisms by which much bicarbonate is removed from the proximal tubular fluid; thus

$$HCO_3^- + H^+ \rightleftharpoons H_2CO_3 \rightleftharpoons CO_2 + H_2O$$

The CO_2 can be readily reabsorbed and reconverted rapidly in the cells to carbonic acid and bicarbonate.

Question Is proximal bicarbonate reabsorption connected in any way with hydrogen ion secretion?

Answer 1. Yes. Go on to **2.56**.
2. No. Go on to **2.59**.

2.55 Your answer – ADP is the enzyme present in the sodium pump. No. You have not read **2.43** carefully enough. ADP is the substance adenosine diphosphate. It is not an enzyme. Read **2.43** again carefully. Do not hurry over it.

2.56 Your answer – proximal bicarbonate reabsorption is connected with hydrogen ion secretion.

You are correct.

The hydrogen ion coming from the tubular cells is exchanged for sodium ions which are actively transported into the cell. The source of the hydrogen ion, according to Pitts and Alexander, is carbonic acid: in the presence of carbonic anhydrase the following reactions occur

$$H_2O + CO_2 \xrightleftharpoons[\text{anhydrase}]{\text{carbonic}} H_2CO_3 \rightleftharpoons H^+ + HCO_3^-$$

The bicarbonate ions inside the cell, together with sodium ions, enter the interstitial fluid and then the peritubular capillaries. Look at Fig. 2.56.

The diagram shows how bicarbonate coming down into the proximal tubule combines with hydrogen ion produced in the tubular cell by hydration of carbon dioxide and ionization of the resulting carbonic acid. The CO_2 produced in the lumen of the tubule can diffuse rapidly into the cells to provide hydrogen ion. One bicarbonate ion is produced intracellularly for each bicarbonate ion which is destroyed by combination with hydrogen ion in the tubular lumen. The bicarbonate ion passes from the tubular cell into the interstitial fluid with sodium ion. In fact this is a simplification of the process which goes on, for an ion exchange of intracellular H^+ for tubular Na^+ would not require the demonstrated active transport of sodium.

Look at the figure 2.56, carefully.

Question What is the source of hydrogen ion produced by the proximal tubular cell?

Answer 1. Water and carbon dioxide. Go on to **2.58**.
2. Bicarbonate. Go on to **2.60**.
3. Carbonic acid. Go on to **2.62**.

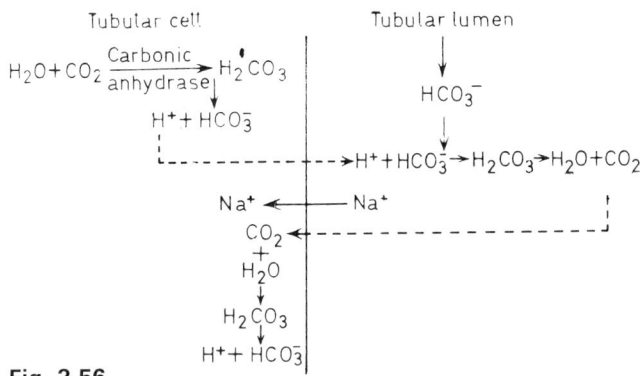

Fig. 2.56

2.57 In addition to reacting with bicarbonate, hydrogen ion will combine with buffers, and also with ammonia to form ammonium ion. A little hydrogen ion remains free in solution. The combination of hydrogen ion with buffer is measured as 'titratable acidity.' This is defined as the amount of alkali in mEq required to titrate the urine to a pH of 7.4. Titratable acidity is a measure of the hydrogen ion taken up by the two buffers, phosphate and creatinine. In the proximal tubule bicarbonate is the most important buffer, but it is reduced in concentration by the hydrogen ion secreted into the tubular fluid; by the time the distal tubule is reached there is little bicarbonate left: at urine pH below 6.0 the bicarbonate concentration is so small it can be ignored for all practical purposes. In the distal tubule, phosphate and creatinine are the two most important buffers. Ammonia is produced by mechanisms in the tubular cells which will be dealt with later, but when it diffuses into the tubular urine it reacts with free hydrogen ion to form ammonium ion (NH_4^+). This NH_4^+ cannot diffuse freely back through the tubular cell wall and so urinary ammonium ion is a measure of part of hydrogen ion secretion.

$$H^+ + NH_3 \longrightarrow NH_4^+$$

The total amount of hydrogen ion secreted in the distal tubule may be arrived at by adding ammonia and titratable acid and subtracting bicarbonate excretion thus:

$$\Sigma H^+ = NH_4^+ + T.A. - HCO_3^-$$

where ΣH^+ = total hydrogen ion
NH_4^+ = ammonium ion ⎫
T.A. = titratable acid ⎬
expressed as mEq/litre
HCO_3^- = bicarbonate ion m Mol/litre.

Total hydrogen ion excretion is usually expressed as a rate, i.e. the amount excreted per minute or per day. Because the amount of hydrogen ion excreted per minute is small it is usually expressed as micro-equivalents/min (μEq/min) rather than milli-equivalents/min (mEq/min). Total hydrogen ion excretion per day is expressed as mEq/day.

Question If a man excretes 30μ Eq of ammonia per minute in his urine and 16μ Eq of titrable acid at a urinary pH of 4.9, what is his hydrogen ion excretion per minute.

Answer 1. 46μ Eq/min. See **2.64**.
2. 14μ Eq/min. See **2.61**.
3. Can't say because you have not given HCO_3^- excretion. See **2.65**.

2.58 Your answer – hydrogen ion in the tubular cell is produced from water and carbon dioxide.

You are correct although you have presumed one step. Hydrogen ion is generated as follows:

$$H_2O + CO_2 \xrightarrow[\text{anhydrase}]{\text{carbonic}} H_2CO_3 \longrightarrow H^+ + HCO_3^-$$

The carbonic anhydrase inside the cells causes a very rapid combination of water and carbon dioxide to form carbonic acid. In the tubular lumen CO_2 produced by the action of H^+ on bicarbonate has no carbonic anhydrase to speed up the production of carbonic acid. CO_2 can diffuse rapidly into the cells from the tubular lumen. Now go on to **2.57**.

2.59 Your answer – there is no connection between hydrogen ion secretion and proximal bicarbonate reabsorption. Go back to **2.54** and read it again.

2.60 Your answer – hydrogen ion in the tubular cell is produced by bicarbonate.
You are wrong. Don't be discouraged. This type of material is difficult to digest. Go and read **2.56** again and see if you can answer the question.

2.61 Your answer – hydrogen ion excretion is 14 Eq/min. No. You have not used the formula in **2.57** correctly. Go back and do this again in **2.57**.

2.62 Your answer – hydrogen ion in the tubular cell is produced from carbonic acid. You are right. Now go on to read **2.57**.

2.63 Your answer – NH_4^+ can diffuse as quickly as NH_3 through the tubular cell plasma membrane.

You are wrong. The principle of non-ionic diffusion is that non-ionised substances can readily pass through the lipid cell walls whereas ionised substances are more insoluble in lipid and unable to pass through the cell wall with such speed, unless there are special transport mechanisms; re-read **2.64** again.

2.64 Your answer – hydrogen ion output is $46\mu\text{Eq/min}$.

You are correct. Micropuncture studies have revealed that ammonia is added to the tubular fluid not only in the distal tubule and collecting system, but also in the proximal tubule. The amount of ammonia leaving the kidney in the renal vein blood is larger than that in the blood entering the kidney through the renal artery: this proves that ammonia is *formed* in the kidneys. It is formed mainly from the amide nitrogen of glutamine in the presence of the enzyme 'glutaminase,' and to a lesser extent by deamination of glycine, alanine, aspartic acid, and leucine. In the rat after prolonged acidosis caused by administration of ammonium chloride, there is an increase in the amount of glutaminase in the kidney, although in the dog such a rise does not take place. The amount of ammonia excreted in the urine is related to the pH of the urine. When free NH_3 diffuses into acid urine from the tubular cells it combines with free hydrogen ion to form ammonium ion, thus

$$NH_3 + H^+ \longrightarrow NH_4^+$$

The tubular cell membranes are thought to have a lipid outer layer which will permit non-ionised substances to pass through them: this is known as *non-ionic diffusion*. Ionised substances cannot pass as readily through the lipid layer as non-ionic substances, so NH_4^+ cannot diffuse back into the tubular cells although non-ionised NH_3 diffuses out. In acid urines a concentration difference is established between NH_3^+ in the cells and in the tubular fluid. This leads to a rapid loss of NH_3 into the urine as NH_4^+. If less hydrogen ion is available eg. in alkaline urine, the free ammonia will not become NH_4^+ in the tubular lumen and to a large extent will be free to diffuse back into the tubular cell through the lipid cell membrane.

Question Can ammonium ion (NH_4^+) diffuse as quickly as NH_3 through the tubular cell plasma membrane?

Answer 1. Yes. See **2.63**.
2. No. See **2.66**.
3. Don't know. See **2.68**.

2.65 Your answer – can't do it because you have not given (HCO_3^-) concentration.

You are strictly correct but at pH of 4.9 urine contains virtually no bicarbonate, so taking this as (HCO_3^-) = 0, go on to calculate the answer to the question in **2.57**.

2.66 Your answer – NH_4^+ cannot diffuse as quickly as NH_3 through the tubular cell plasma membrane.

You are quite correct.

Before leaving the physiology of urinary acidification there are a few more facts you must know. First of all the urine pH in man can vary from about pH 8.4 after an alkaline load or potassium feeding, to a pH of 4.6 after an acid load. With intravenous infusion of sodium sulphate to give a large amount of non-reabsorbable anion, it is possible to get a urine pH of 4.1. In the presence of carbonic anhydrase inhibitors, there is a reduction in hydrogen ion secretion and the plasma bicarbonate falls. The urinary leak (i.e. loss) of bicarbonate varies with the plasma bicarbonate level; in the normal person the urine is acid and free of bicarbonate when the plasma bicarbonate is low: as the plasma bicarbonate rises to 27 or 28 mEq/1, bicarbonate appears in the urine. Further intravenous infusions of bicarbonate do not raise the plasma level very much, mainly increasing the urinary bicarbonate excretion. If the P_{CO_2} is elevated, tubular bicarbonate reabsorption is enhanced. This is the cause of the high plasma bicarbonate in patients with CO_2 retention and a high P_{CO_2} due to pulmonary disease. Respiratory alkalosis caused by overbreathing, say, causes a fall in tubular bicarbonate reabsorption, with an increase in bicarbonate excretion in the urine.

Question What effect will an intravenous infusion of bicarbonate raising the plasma bicarbonate to 35 mmols/1 have on the urine bicarbonate in a normal man.

Answer 1. Augment it. See **2.70**.
2. Reduce it. See **2.72**.

2.67 You have now finished the chapter on renal physiology: if you would like to read more about the subject of renal physiology here are some references:

Articles

Robinson J. R. (1962) Principles of renal physiology, in Black D. A. K. (ed.) Renal Disease, p. 30. Blackwell, Oxford.

Berliner R. W. (1971) Renal physiology in Strauss M. B. & Welt L. G. (eds.) Diseases of the Kidney. Churchill, London. 2nd Edition.

De Wardener H. E. (1958) The Kidney, chapters on renal function. Churchill, London.

Various chapters in Renal Symposium, Am. J. Med. June 1964.

Chapter by Berliner R. W. in Symposium on ADH, Am. J. Med. May 1967.

Monographs

Hamburgers et al. Structure & function of the kidney 1971 Saunders London.

Pitts R. F. (1968) Physiology of the Kidney and Body Fluids. Year Book Publishers, Chicago. (2nd Edition, 1968).

Smith, Homer (1956) Principles of Renal Physiology. Oxford University Press, New York.

Valtin H. (1973). Renal Function. Little, Brown, Boston.

Smith, Homer (1951) The Kidney. Oxford University Press, New York.

Now go on to the next chapter.

2.68 Your answer — I don't know if NH_4^+ can diffuse as quickly as NH_3 through the tubular cell plasma membrane.

You have not read **2.64** properly. Read it again and answer the question correctly.

2.69 Your answer — a low protein diet decreases maximal attainable urine concentration.

You are quite right. Now answer the next question:

Question What is the effect of vasopressin on the permeability of the collecting ducts to urea?

Answer 1. Decreases it. See **2.78**.
2. Increases it. See **2.76**.
3. No effect. See **2.74**.
4. Don't know. See **2.73**.

2.70 Your answer — augmenting the plasma bicarbonate will increase the urine bicarbonate loss in normal man.

You are correct.

Urea is a remarkable substance. It can diffuse very rapidly into most tissues, with the exception of the central nervous system and also certain parts of the nephron. Urea is an important substance in the medullary interstitium, contributing to the high osmolality during the formation of a concentrated urine, as well as being the major urinary solute. In man or animals on a low protein diet the maximum concentrating ability and $T_m{}^cH_2O$ are diminished; addition of urea or protein to the diet has been shown to increase the concentrating power; the change in urine concentration is not solely due to the amount of urea present because the non-urea constituents are reduced in concentration as well.

About 40–50 per cent of the filtered urea diffuses out of the proximal tubule by a passive process. In the descending loop of Henle urea enters the tubular fluid from the medullary interstitium and collecting ducts, so that by the time the distal convoluted tubule is entered the tubular fluid once again contains an amount of urea equal to that present in the glomerular filtrate. As the tubular fluid passes down the collecting ducts a large amount of urea is lost into the medullary interstitium. In the presence of vasopressin the distal tubules and collecting ducts have an *increased permeability to urea* so that when a concentrated urine is being formed an increased amount of urea diffuses into the medullary interstitium so increasing its osmolality, and thus abstracts water from the loop of Henle. This results in increasing the concentration of non-urea solutes in the loop of Henle.

Question What is the effect on the maximal attainable urine concentration of giving a low protein diet?

Answer 1. Decreases maximum attainable urine concentration. Go on to **2.69**.
2. Increases urine concentration. Go on to **2.71**.

2.71 Your answer – a low protein diet increases maximal attainable urine concentration.

You are wrong. Go back and read **2.70** again, bearing in mind that this is a difficult paragraph requiring all your attention.

2.72 Your answer – augmenting the plasma bicarbonate concentration will reduce the urine bicarbonate in a normal man.

In normal people the urine remains free of bicarbonate when the plasma bicarbonate concentration is below 27–28 mMol/1. As soon as this threshold level is exceeded bicarbonate appears in the urine in increasing amounts. Now answer the question in **2.66** correctly.

2.73 Your answer – I don't know what is the effect of vasopressin on the permeability of the collecting ducts to urea.

You should read **2.70** again and concentrate, then answer the question in **2.69**.

2.74 Your answer – vasopressin has no effect on the permeability of the collecting ducts to urea.

You have not absorbed the information about this topic properly. Go back and read **2.70** again and answer the question in **2.69**.

2.75 Your answer – all the statements are true. You are wrong.

Urine is *not* concentrated solely by a counter current exchanger although there is one at work in the vasa recta keeping the sodium and urea in high concentration in the medulla. The main concentrating mechanism is a counter-current multiplier system. Go back to **2.35** and work back through the paragraphs. You will then realise why statement 3 is also wrong.

2.76 Your answer – vasopressin increases the permeability of the collecting ducts to urea.

You are correct. You are now ready to answer a group of questions to test the knowledge of renal physiology you have acquired in reading this chapter. The questions should be carefully thought about before you choose the answer. If an important defect in your knowledge is disclosed you may find yourself back in the early paragraphs in this chapter, having to work your way through again. Now go on to **2.80**.

2.77 Your answer — all the statements are false.

You are right about statements (1) and (3) being false but statement (2) is true — go back to **2.45** and work through from there.

2.78 Your answer — the effect of vasopressin is to decrease the permeability of the collecting ducts to urea.

No, vasopressin increases the permeability of the collecting ducts to urea; this is one of the mechanisms of building up a high medullary osmolality. Read **2.70** again and answer the question in **2.69** correctly.

2.79 Your answer — 1 and 3 are true only.

You are wrong. Both 1 and 3 are false. Go back to **2.35** and work through from there.

2.80 This question contains several statements. Read them carefully, then choose the appropriate answer.

> **Statement 1** The urine is concentrated by a counter current exchanger system.
>
> **Statement 2** Most of the filtered sodium is reabsorbed in the proximal tubule.
>
> **Statement 3** Bicarbonate is present in large amounts in acid urine.

Answer 1. All the statements are true. Go on to **2.75**.
2. All the statements are false. Go on to **2.77**.
3. 1 and 3 are true only. Go on to **2.79**.
4. 1 is true only. Go on to **2.83**.
5. 1 and 2 are true. Go on to **2.82**.
6. 2 and 3 are true. Go on to **2.84**.
7. 3 is true only. Go on to **2.85**.
8. 2 is true only. Go on to **2.81**.

2.81 Your answer — only 2 is true.

You are quite right. Go on to **2.67**.

2.82 Your answer — 1 and 2 are true. You are correct about 2 but 1 is not quite true; urine is concentrated by a counter current *multiplier* system. Read **2.35** again and then go on to **2.67**.

2.83 Your answer — 1 is true.

You are wrong. 1 and 3 are false. Go back to **2.35** and read the paragraph carefully.

2.84 Your answer — 2 and 3 are true.

You are correct about 2 being true, but statement 3 is not true. Go back to **2.56**.

2.85 Your answer – only statement 3 is true. You are wrong. Only statement 2 is true. Go back to **2.45**.

Time for this chapter: 50 minutes

Chapter 3
Renal investigations: 1. Biochemical

3.1 The biochemical investigation of renal function in clinical medicine will be discussed in this chapter. First of all let us consider examination of the urine. The most obvious abnormality is proteinuria, the significance of which has been known since Richard Bright's monograph published in 1827, a book remarkable for its prescience. Protein is normally found in urine in amounts up to a total of 150 mg a day: if this normal protein is concentrated by dialysis or evaporation and then examined by immunoelectrophoresis it is found to be predominantly albumin and IgG with the addition of globulins of fairly small molecular weight identical with those found in the serum. In addition there are proteins produced in the tubules (notably the mucoprotein known as Tamm-Horsfall protein of which hyaline casts are composed) and β microglobulin and post γ microglobulin and also additions from the lower urinary pathways such as prostatic and urethral secretions. The normal proteinuria is so small in amount that it can be detected only if the urine is concentrated, appearing as a faint opacity on the addition of salicylsulphonic acid (sulfosalicylic acid).

Now answer this question.

Question Does normal urine ever contain any protein?

Answer 1. Yes. Go on to **3.6**.
   2. No. Go on to **3.8**.
   3. Don't know. Go on to **3.4**.

3.2 If you are reading this paragraph you are not following the instructions. The only purpose of a programmed course is that the programming is designed to help you learn, as if a teacher were there to help you. Go back to **3.1** and answer the question at the end of the paragraph. Always follow the instructions or you will get no benefit from using this book.

3.3 Your answer – considerable quantities of IgM in the urine indicate the presence of 'large size' pores.
You are correct. Now answer the following question.

Question At what temperature does the Bence Jones protein of myelomatosis precipitate out of the urine on heating?

Answer 1. 45–55°C. Go on to **3.5**.
2. 100°C. Go on to **3.9**.
3. Don't know. Go on to **3.13**.

3.4 Your answer – I don't know whether protein is ever found in normal urine.
The contents of **3.1** were meant to be read carefully, not glanced at. You have not been concentrating properly and are not learning. Read **3.1** again and answer the question correctly.

3.5 Your answer – Bence Jones proteins are precipitated by heat at 45–55°C.
You are correct.
There is a type of proteinuria associated with renal tubular diseases, such as the Fanconi syndrome. Tubular proteinuria consists of predominantly α_2 globulin, β microglobulin and post γ microglobulin with little albumin on electrophoresis of the urine.
The commonest type of proteinuria is orthostatic or postural proteinuria which occurs in about 3 per cent of adolescents and is usually not associated with disease: proteinuria is present in the urine produced in the upright posture but is absent from that produced when the patient is recumbent. Bull showed that postural proteinuria is associated with a lordotic erect position; this produces venous congestion and vasoconstriction in the kidneys. Occasionally postural proteinuria is not innocent, being found in such disorders as renal tubular disease, chronic glomerulonephritis and polycystic kidneys. At present an adequate study of the renal pathology of a large series of patients with postural proteinuria has not been carried out to elucidate the frequency of innocent and pathological varieties of postural proteinuria.
Functional proteinuria can be caused by fever, severe exercise, heat stroke, or severe cold; the pathogenesis of the proteinuria is obscure, although vasoconstriction is thought to be important.
Asymptomatic persistent proteinuria has been investigated by Kark and his colleagues in Chicago. They found that renal biopsy disclosed chronic proliferative glomerulonephritis, incipient nephrotic syndrome due to membranous glomerulonephritis, lupus glomerulitis, pyelonephritis, and occasionally nothing abnormal on light microscopy in this group of patients.

Question Postural proteinuria is a condition in which urine is protein-free when it is produced by the kidney in what position?

Answer 1. Recumbency. Go on to **3.7**.
2. Standing up. Go on to **3.11**.
3. Don't know. Go on to **3.22**.

3.6 Your answer – protein is found in normal urine.
You are correct. If more than 150 mg of protein/day are found in the urine

the proteinuria is pathological. The maximum amount of proteinuria which we have seen was 51 g/day; many patients with nephrotic syndrome have 10–20 g/day; usually this level of proteinuria exceeds the capacity of the body to synthesize albumin, so that hypoalbuminaemia results. The composition of the proteinuria depends on the disease producing it. Diseases of the glomeruli produce a proteinuria in which albumin predominates with smaller amounts of the serum globulins which are filtered at the diseased glomeruli. If the glomerular filters are very abnormal with large 'pores,' larger molecules such as Gamma-1-macroglobulin (β_2M or IgM, mol. wt. 900,000), β lipoprotein (molecular weight 1,250,000 to 2,500,000) are found in the urine, as well as the smaller molecules such as 7s γ globulin, (IgG) (molecular weight 150,000) which can get through smaller pores. In myelomatosis, abnormal globulins are found in the urine which can be detected regularly by electrophoresis of urine proteins: they usually give a sharp peak which migrates electrophoretically as a γ globulin or somewhere between β and γ globulins. The protein can be demonstrated on heating the urine in about half the patients suffering from myelomatosis; it is known as Bence Jones protein; on heating urine the Bence Jones proteins are precipitated at 45–55°C, and re-dissolve at 95–100°C.

To understand what Bence Jones proteins are, we must first know a little about the constitution of γ globulin. The 7s γ globulins are composed of linked long and short polypeptide chains referred to as L and S or B and A chains. In myelomatosis abnormal globulins are produced and there is either over-production of some of the B chain polypeptides or failure of their incorporation into the γ globulins. These B chain polypeptides spill over from the blood stream into the urine and they are known as Bence Jones proteins. In some very rare diseases the Bence Jones proteins are A chain polypeptides.

Question If IgM is found in considerable amounts in the urine, are large size 'pores' likely to be present in the diseased glomeruli?

Answer 1. Yes. Go on to **3.3**.
2. No. Go on to **3.10**.
3. Don't know. Go on to **3.42**.

3.7 Your answer – the urine in postural proteinuria is protein free when formed in the kidneys of the recumbent patient.

You are correct.

Before leaving the question of proteinuria it is necessary to describe the tests commonly used for qualitative detection of proteinuria.
These are:

(1) **Heat in an acidified specimen**. A few drops of acetic acid are added to the urine which is boiled; a cloudy opalescence forms if protein is present. Some prefer to boil the urine first, then add acetic acid to any cloud which forms, so differentiating protein from phosphate which comes down on boiling and redissolves on addition of the acid.

The disadvantage of this test is that heating is required so making it inconvenient in domiciliary visiting.

(2) **Salicylsulphonic acid (25 per cent)**, which produces turbidity in a protein containing solution: to 5 ml of urine in a test tube a few drops of 25 per cent salicylsulphonic acid (sulfosalicylic acid in the USA) are added, the amount of turbidity produced being related to the protein concentration. This test will detect 10 mg of protein/100 ml of urine. Its advantage is simplicity – there is no need to heat the urine.

(3) **Stick tests employing tetrabromphenol blue**. In these tests (eg. Albustix) the cardboard stick is dipped into the urine: in the presence of protein the colour of the stick becomes green, varying according to the amount of protein present. The colour change depends on the displacement of the transformation range of indicators by protein solutions. This is known as 'protein error of indicators' and was described first by Sorensen in 1909. The advantage of Albustix is its great sensitivity but it often gives false positives which are not confirmed on testing with salicylsulphonic acid.

Question What substance is present in a specimen of urine which becomes cloudy when a few drops of 25 per cent salicylsulphonic acid are added?

Answer 1. Glucose. Go on to **3.17**.
2. Protein. Go on to **3.20**.
3. Don't know. Go on to **3.15**.

3.8 Your answer – protein is *never* found in normal urine.

The point made in **3.1** is that protein is found in normal urine up to a total of about 150 mg a day. You have not absorbed this so you cannot be paying adequate attention to your learning. Go back and read **3.1**.

3.9 Your answer – Bence Jones protein is precipitated at 100°C on heating urine.

Bence Jones protein comes down at 45–55°C and then redissolves as heating goes on above 95°C. Read **3.6** again.

3.10 Your answer – If IgM protein is found in urine, then large pores are not likely to be present in the diseased glomeruli.

You are wrong. IgM is a large molecule, a macroglobulin with a molecular weight of 900,000. To allow a considerable amount of a big protein like this to pass there must be a substantial number of larger pores in the diseased glomeruli. Now go back and read **3.6**.

3.11 Your answer – in postural proteinuria the urine secreted standing up is protein free.

No. Bull demonstrated that the lordotic position so common in the erect posture was associated with proteinuria. Go back and read **3.5**.

3.12 Your answer – the blood urea level begins to rise when GFR falls below 25–30 ml/min.
You are correct.

Now let us consider urea clearance, a test which is used clinically very frequently. If there is a large urine flow (more than 2 ml/min) urea clearance is expressed by the formula:

$$C_{urea} = \frac{UV}{P}$$

Where C_{urea} = ml. of plasma cleared of urea per minute.
U = urine concentration of urea (mg/100 ml.)
V = volume of urine (ml./min.)
P = plasma urea (mg/100 ml.)

This formula gives a figure which is about 60 per cent of the GFR in health; as the GFR falls to very low levels, (say < 3 ml/min), the $\frac{urea\ clearance}{GFR}$ ratio rises to 1. If urine flow is low, the relationship to GFR is unpredictable due to the increased reabsorption of urea in the collecting ducts. Van Slyke invented a curious empirical formula to express urea clearance at flow rates below 2 ml/min; he called it 'standard clearance', this being defined as

$$SC = \frac{U\sqrt{V}}{P}$$

where SC = standard urea clearance in ml/min.
U = urine urea concentration in mg/100 ml.
V = urine minute vol in ml/min.
P = plasma urea concentration in mg/100 ml.

This formula is dubious because standard clearance is a mathematical device rather than a term corresponding to a physiological concept.

Van Slyke suggested that both urea clearance and standard clearance should be expressed as per cent of average normal. The 'normal value' for urea clearance is 75 ml/min and the 'normal value' for standard clearance is 54 ml/min. These figures are not usually corrected for body surface area. With all their drawbacks, the two urea clearances of Van Slyke (normal and standard) give some indication of renal function and are therefore useful in clinical practice.

Question Calculate the urea clearance, expressed as per cent of average normal, in a man passing urine at a rate of 4 ml/min, in whom the plasma urea level is 36 mg/100 ml, urine urea concentration is 675 mg/100 ml.

Answer 1. About 100 per cent. Go on to **3.14**.
2. About 75 per cent. Go on to **3.25**.
3. About 75 ml/min. Go on to **3.21**.
4. Don't know. Go on to **3.24**.

3.13 Your answer – I don't know at what temperature Bence Jones protein is precipitated on heating the urine. This temperature – precipitation relationship of the Bence Jones proteins is important in identification of this protein in the diagnosis of myelomatosis. You are not paying attention to reading the paragraphs properly. If you are being distracted by some external influence you cannot alter, stop reading rather than deceive yourself you are learning. If there are external distractions that you can correct, do so and then go back and read **3.6** carefully.

3.14 Your answer – urea clearance is 100 per cent average normal.

You are correct. Let us now turn to creatinine as a measure of glomerular function. The plasma creatinine bears a relationship to the glomerular filtration rate; the normal plasma creatinine is below 2.0 mg/100 ml, but when renal failure supervenes the plasma creatinine concentration rises, as shown in Fig. 3.14.

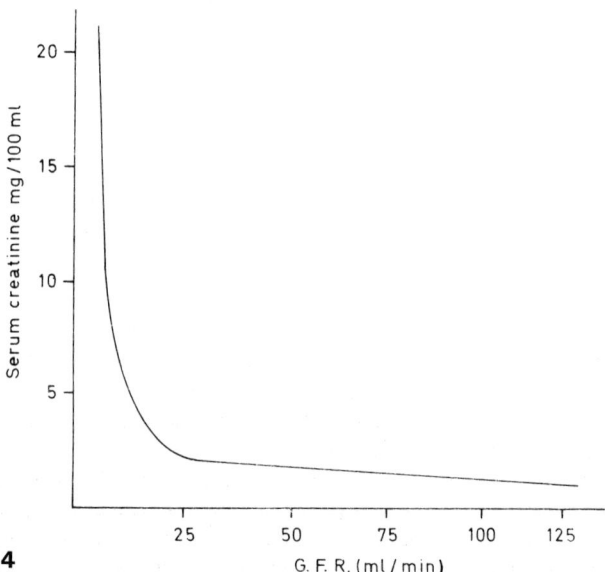

Fig. 3.14

Plasma creatinine is usually measured by a non-specific colorimetric reaction with alkaline picrate; unfortunately in the plasma of normal persons a proportion of the normal creatinine value is due to 'non-creatinine' chromogen of uncertain identity. As the plasma creatinine concentration increases, the amount of non-creatinine chromogen becomes of less and less significance and so fairly accurate measurements can be made of high plasma creatinine values. Total creatinine chromogen can be measured in the usual way; appropriate micro-organisms can then be added to destroy creatinine, and the non-creatinine chromogen can then be measured. The true creatinine concentration is the difference between the total creatinine chromogen and the non-creatinine chromogen. By this microbiological method very accurate measurements of true creatinine concentration can be made at all plasma concentrations. It should be noted that this microbiological method is not suitable for use as a routine renal function test. There are alternative methods of removing true creatinine from plasma based on absorbing true creatinine with fuller's earth while leaving the non-creatinine chromogen. These methods are useful at low plasma concentrations, but at high concentrations it is doubtful if anything is to be gained by using them in view of the smaller relative error introduced by non-creatinine chromogen as the true creatinine level rises.

Question If a patient has a serum creatinine concentration of 20 mg/100 ml, assuming he has a normal intake of protein, is his blood urea likely to be very high or normal?

Answer 1. Very high. Go on to **3.27**.
         2. Normal. Go on to **3.30**.
         3. Don't know. Go on to **3.32**.

3.15 Your answer – I don't know what substance is present in urine which goes cloudy on addition of 25 per cent salicylsulphonic acid.

You have not read **3.7** properly. Salicylsulphonic acid precipitates proteins from urine. Go back and read **3.7** again and answer the question properly.

3.16 The biuret test gives an accurate measurement of protein concentration.

You are correct. Let us now consider other indices of glomerular function, first of all the blood urea level. The normal blood urea level is 15–45 mg/100 ml. On a diet of normal protein content the blood urea level remains normal until the glomerular filtration rate has fallen to about 25 ml/min, after which it begins to rise, climbing steeply (see Fig. 3.16).

At a blood urea concentration of about 200 mg/100 ml of GFR is about 5 ml/min. A word of caution is necessary here, however. If the patient is on a very low protein diet the blood urea may be normal in the presence of a GFR of 5 ml/min. This will be discussed in a later chapter dealing with the dietary therapy of

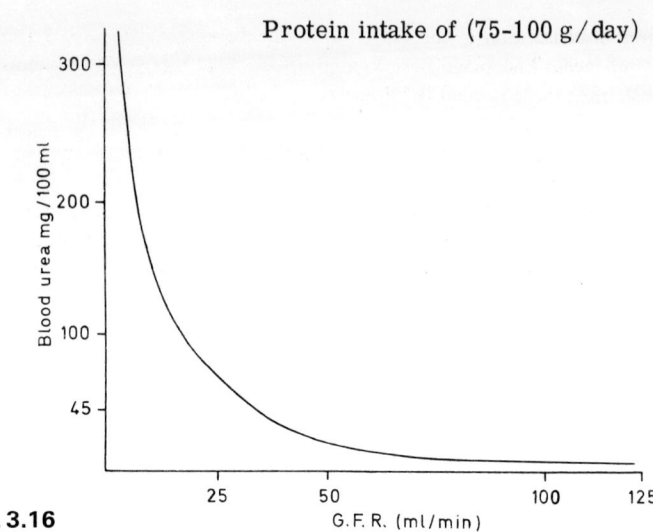

Fig. 3.16

chronic renal failure. If a patient with normal kidneys has a gastrointestinal haemorrhage, the blood proteins in the bowel are absorbed and this leads to an elevated blood urea level. In patients with minimal impairment of renal function in nephrotic syndrome the blood urea level is often elevated if corticosteroids are being given simultaneously. Another cause for a disproportionately high blood urea is the combination of dehydration plus cellular breakdown seen in acute infections. Apart from these exceptions, the blood urea level is a reasonable clinical index of the glomerular filtration rate.

Question What is the level of GFR below which the blood urea is likely to begin to be elevated in a man with a normal protein intake?

Answer 1. Below 25 or 30 ml/min GFR. Go on to **3.12**.
2. Below 5 ml/min GFR. Go on to **3.18**.
3. Don't know. Go on to **3.23**.

3.17 Your answer – salicylsulphonic acid produces turbidity in urine because of the presence of glucose.

You are wrong. Protein is precipitated by salicylsulphonic acid. Read **3.7** again.

3.18 Your answer – the blood urea will begin to be elevated with a GFR of 5 ml/min.

You are only partly correct. A GFR of 5 ml/min indicates a considerable degree of renal failure; the blood urea should be somewhere around the 200 mg/100 ml level. The blood urea begins to rise when the GFR has dropped below 25–30 ml/min. Now read **3.16** again.

3.19 Esbach's test gives more accurate information about urine protein concentration than the Biuret method.

You are wrong. Esbach's test is a crude method of estimating protein content by the bulk of the precipitate from the urine. It is semiquantitative but has become hallowed by usage. Much nursing time would be saved if the daily Esbach test were abandoned and replaced by an accurate once weekly measurement of a day's protein excretion by means of the biuret test. Now go on to **3.16**.

3.20 Your answer – addition of salicylsulphonic acid to urine causes turbidity in the presence of protein.

You are correct. *Quantitative* methods of estimating protein are:

(1) Esbach's picric acid – citric acid reagent. This produces a precipitate, the volume of which is read off directly in grams per litre. This test is particularly inaccurate although it offers a very rough guide to urine protein content for use by nursing staff.

(2) Salicylsulphonic acid. This test can be used in a similar way to the quantitative test, although 3 per cent salicylsulphonic acid is used, and the turbidity produced read in a nephelometer, a standard protein solution being employed at the same time. It is not as accurate as the two tests which follow but is quick and convenient.

(3) Biuret test. This gives accurate values for protein concentrations but is more difficult to carry out than salicylsulphonic acid estimations.

(4) Kjeldahl estimations of nitrogen can be very accurate but are time-consuming and tedious to perform.

Question If you want to estimate the protein concentration of urine, will the biuret test or the Esbach test give you more accurate information?

Answer 1. Esbach's. Go on to **3.19**.
2. Biuret. Go on to **3.16**.

3.21 Your answer – urea clearance is 75 ml/min.

You are perfectly correct but the Van Slyke urea clearance is usually expressed as per cent of average normal, for reasons of long continued usage. As 75 ml/min is regarded as 100 per cent 'average normal,' the answer is 100 per cent average normal. Go on to read **3.14**.

3.22 Your answer – I don't know what is the relationship between proteinuria and standing upright in postural proteinuria.

If you don't know you have not read **3.5** carefully. Read it again and answer the question correctly.

3.23   Your answer – I don't know below what level of GFR the blood urea begins to rise.

Ced begins to rise when the GFR drops below 25–30 ml/min, unless the patient is on a low protein diet. Go back and read **3.16** carefully.

3.24   Your answer – I don't know the urea clearance.

You have not read **3.12** properly. It is not particularly easy to understand, so read it again. Remember that urea clearance is a real clearance concept, but that in the standard urea clearance one gets a value of $\sqrt{V}$ close to 1 and so obtains figures which are to all intents and purposes a ratio of urine/plasma urea concentrations. Now go over **3.12** again and concentrate carefully.

3.25   Your answer – Urea clearance is 75 per cent of average normal.

You are not quite right, although you have done the calculation correctly. Clearance figures are expressed as ml/min and your answer derived by applying the formula $C_{urea} = \dfrac{UV}{P}$ is 75 ml/min. Now this has to be turned into the per cent of 'average normal' taking 100 per cent as 75 ml/min. Thus your answer should be $\frac{75}{75} \times 100$ per cent average normal = 100 per cent average normal. Go on to **3.14**.

3.26   Your answer – in vitamin D resistant rickets tubular phosphate reabsorption is unchanged.

You are wrong. Tubular reabsorption of phosphate is depressed so that the serum phosphate level falls due to the loss of phosphate in the urine. Now read **3.36** more carefully.

3.27   Your answer – the blood urea will be very high if the plasma creatinine concentration is 20 mg/100 ml.

You are correct. Creatinine clearance is often used as a renal function test. In man, *endogenous* creatinine clearance is used, which should be differentiated from that used in animal investigations such as the dog, where *exogenous* creatinine loading is employed. Now from **3.14** you will remember that is well nigh impossible to measure plasma creatinine exactly, unless the difficult microbiological methods are used. Hence it is difficult to get accurate results for creatinine clearance

$$C_{cr} = \dfrac{UV}{p}$$

Where C_{cr} = endogenous creatinine clearance
      U = urine concentration of creatinine

$$V = \text{volume of urine/minute}$$
$$p = \text{plasma creatinine concentration}$$

because p is imprecisely measured.

Several series of imprecise endogenous creatinine clearance results have been found to give values similar to inulin clearance figures (Cin) in man, although more careful work has shown that in the presence of proteinuria in relatively mild renal diseases causing the nephrotic syndrome, C_{cr} may be up to 2 or 3 times greater than inulin clearance, indicating that creatinine is being secreted by the renal tubules. In infants and patients with congestive cardiac failure the $\frac{C_{cr}}{C_{in}}$ ratio is less than 1, indicating that tubular reabsorption of endogenous creatinine is taking place. There has been a tendency in the past decade to equate the creatinine clearance with the GFR in man, this being mainly due to the convenience of any method of GFR measurement which does not require an intravenous drip at constant rates such as Inulin, thiosulphate, or ^{51}Cr EDTA clearances. However convenience cannot hide the imperfections of endogenous creatinine clearance, which, because of its variable relationship to GFR is useful as an index of clinical progress but not as equivalent to the GFR.

Question In man is endogenous creatinine clearance identical with the glomerular filtration rate?

Answer 1. Yes. Go on to **3.28**.
2. No. Go on to **3.33**.
3. Don't know. Go on to **3.35**.

3.28 Your answer – in man creatinine clearance is identical with the glomerular filtration rate.

You are wrong. In infancy and congestive heart failure Miller and his colleagues in 1951 showed that C_{cr} was less than C_{in}, using a microbiological method of determining creatinine concentrations. They also found C_{cr} to be greater than C_{in} in several patients with heavy proteinuria. Now read **3.27** again and answer the question correctly.

3.29 Your answer – tubular reabsorption of phosphate in vitamin D resistant rickets is increased.

No. In vitamin D resistant rickets tubular reabsorption of phosphate is *decreased*. Read **3.36** again.

3.30 Your answer – if the serum creatinine concentration is 20 mg/100 ml, then he will have a normal blood urea.

The normal plasma creatinine level is below 2.0 mg/100 ml, so this patient is in advanced renal failure. If his protein intake is normal his blood urea level will be very high indeed. Go back and read **3.14** again and answer the question correctly.

3.31 Your answer – a simple method of measurement of GFR is by means of inulin-^{14}C.

You are correct that Inulin ^{14}C carboxylic acid is a very accurate measure of GFR. It is expensive and is most commonly used in micro work involving micropuncture. On the other hand radioactive vitamin B_{12}, although less well documented, measures GFR accurately and is simple, safe and cheap to use, but is variably protein bound. ^{51}Cr EDTA is very useful for it is not protein bound. Now go on to read 3.36.

3.32 Your answer – I don't know what the blood urea level is likely to be.

A plasma creatinine concentration of 20 mg/100 ml is about twenty times the normal value. The blood urea level in a person on a normal protein intake is a good index of renal function, therefore you should now be in a position to give the correct answer to the question at the end of **3.14**. Read **3.14** again and don't day dream or skip the lines.

3.33 Your answer – in man creatinine clearance is not identical with the glomerular filtration rate.

You are correct. The easiest and most reliable methods for measuring GFR are Tritiated Inulin, I^{131} sodium iothiomalate, radioactive chromium EDTA, and radioactive ^{57}Co labelled cyanocobalamin. The first three are not protein bound, whereas vitamin B_{12} is variably bound to the plasma proteins and this introduces difficulties and inaccuracies. Radioactive substances are easy to count accurately, and are cheap and reliable. They have to be given intravenously, and if the direct method involving urine and plasma sampling is used rather than relying solely on rate of disappearance from the plasma, then a constant rate infusion has to be given. Inulin-C^{14} carboxyl can be used but is usually reserved for micropuncture and stop flow studies. It is less stable than Tritiated Inulin, and is best avoided for human studies. Polyfructosan S or Inutest is a synthetic fructose polymer which is, unlike inulin, quite stable. It is easy to measure by automated apparatus and is very accurate but requires intravenous infusion. There is rarely any need in routine clinical care of a patient for an exact measurement of the GFR and for all practical purposes blood urea (with a normal protein intake) and urea clearance in water diuresis (i.e. with urine flows above 2 ml/min) are quite adequate. Creatinine clearance is a convenient method of assessing progress but it is little better than urea clearance, and in renal failure is quite certainly inferior to urea clearance.

Question What is a simple method of measuring GFR using radioactivity?

Answer 1. ^{51}Cr EDTA. Go on to **3.36**.

2. Inulin – ^{14}C. Go on to **3.31**.
3. Endogenous creatinine. Go on to **3.34**.

3.34 Your answer – the simple method of measuring GFR using radioactivity is endogenous creatinine.

You are wrong on several counts. First of all endogenous creatinine is not radioactive. Secondly creatinine is not an accurate measure of GFR, but it is cheap and simple. Read **3.33** again.

3.35 Your answer – I don't know what is the relationship of creatinine clearance to GFR.

Miller and his colleagues in 1951 showed that creatinine clearance is lower than inulin clearance in infancy and congestive heart failure; in nephrotic syndrome they found several patients who had creatinine clearances higher than inulin clearances. Thus the relationship of creatinine clearance to inulin clearance is variable. Now read **3.27** again and answer the question.

3.36 Your answer ^{51}Cr EDTA is used as a simple radioactive method of measuring GFR.

You are correct as far as experience with this method goes. Now let us look at proximal tubular function tests: these comprise phosphate reabsorption, phenolsulphonphthalein excretion, PAH excretion, glucose reabsorption and amino acid loss in the urine. Tubular phosphate reabsorption (TRP) is most commonly determined in the differential diagnosis of parathyroid disease. In hyperparathyroidism there is a decrease in tubular phosphate reabsorption, but the conditions of the determination in respect of phosphate content of diet are critical and make interpretation of the results difficult. Phosphate tubular reabsorption is reduced in vitamin D-resistant rickets as well as in rickets due to vitamin D deficiency; it is also reduced in the proximal tubular syndromes such as Fanconi syndrome, heavy metal poisonings, and Wilson's disease. In vitamin D resistant rickets the tubular phosphate reabsorption is so low that the patient develops hypophosphataemia; these features result in the disease being often referred to as hypophosphataemic rickets. Tm phosphate is rarely determined as a clinical test of renal function.

Question What happens to tubular phosphate reabsorption (TRP) in vitamin D-resistant rickets?

Answer 1. Unchanged. Go on to **3.26**
2. Increased. Go on to **3.29**.
3. Decreased. Go on to **3.38**.

3.37 Your answer – all the statements are true.

No. Statement 1 is true but you have missed the point of **3.56** and **3.61**.

In renal tubular acidosis the patient cannot acidify his urine, and the Stamey test is no use in the diagnosis of anuria. Start at **3.56** and work on.

3.38 Your answer — in vitamin D-resistant rickets TRP is decreased.

You are correct. Phenolsulphonphthalein (PSP) is used as a test of renal function which is frequently performed in the general hospital ward. It requires the minimum of technical skill and gives a rough assessment of renal function. PSP is secreted by the proximal renal tubules, and some by glomerular filtration; the binding of PSP to protein is so high that only a small percentage of the PSP passing through the glomeruli can be filtered. The PSP test is carried out by giving 6 mg of PSP intravenously and collecting urine after 15 minutes, 30 minutes, 60 minutes, and 2 hours. The most important collection time from the point of view of assessment of renal function is the first 15 minute collection, which should contain about 35 per cent of the injected dose (range 28–51 per cent). Within 2 hours 70 per cent of the PSP is excreted (range 63–84 per cent). Unfortunately, in renal disease although the 15 minute excretion may be below normal, the two hour excretion may be within normal limits, giving a false impression of good renal function.

Question A man is given 6 mg of PSP intravenously and the urine 15 minutes later contains 1 mg of PSP. Is his renal function normal or is it impaired?

Answer 1. Normal. Go on to **3.39**.
2. Impaired. Go on to **3.44**.
3. Don't know. Go on to **3.41**.

3.39 Your answer — renal function is normal if he excretes 1 mg of PSP in 15 minutes.

You are wrong. The lower limit of normal for PSP excretion 15 minutes after the dose has been given is 28 per cent of the injected dose. In the question 1 mg was excreted i.e., $\frac{1}{6} \times 100$ per cent = 16.7 per cent. This is less than the lower limit of normal. Read **3.38** again.

3.40 Your answer — there is proximal tubular damage in cadmium poisoning.

You are correct. Now let us turn to the distal tubular clinical function tests. The test which is most commonly used clinically is that of concentration and dilution of urine. First of all let us look at the concentration tests. As you will remember from Chapter 2, the concentration of urine may be expressed as either specific gravity (which is influenced both by the *number* and *nature* of the particles in solution) or as osmolarity (which is influenced solely by the *number* of particles in solution). The urine is concentrated by a counter-current multiplier mechanism, the final concentrating process being carried out in the collecting system. If the glomerular filtration rate is reduced grossly, or the solute load in the urine is reduced e.g. by a low salt diet, or if the patient is on a low protein diet, the ability to concentrate the urine may be impaired without any anatomical damage to the kidneys. In advanced renal disease of any type, with a reduced GFR, and in early pyelonephritis and hydronephrosis *without gross reduction of GFR* but with damage to the medullary tubules and vasculature, the ability to concentrate the urine may be grossly impaired. The concentrating ability may also be defective due to absence of vasopressin in true diabetes insipidus; in renal diabetes insipidus there is a renal inability to respond to ADH in the presence of adequate amounts of ADH in the serum. Renal diabetes insipidus may be a congenital abnormality (often sex-linked recessive in its mode of inheritance), or it may be acquired due to hypercalcaemia, hypokalaemia, pyelonephritis, or hydronephrosis.

Question In renal diabetes insipidus, is there any plasma ADH?

Answer 1. Yes. Go on to **3.49**.
2. No. Go on to **3.52**.
3. Don't know. Go on to **3.55**.

3.41 Your answer – I don't know if renal function is impaired or not.

If you don't know you can't have read **3.38** properly. If you had paid attention, you would have remembered that a normal person excretes at least 28 per cent of the administered dose within 15 minutes. Go back and read **3.38** carefully. Then answer the question correctly. Don't think about something else when you read the paragraph.

3.42 Your answer – I don't know if there are large numbers of large pores in the diseased glomeruli if IgM is found in the urine in considerable amounts.

You have not understood **3.6** or are not paying attention, although the subject matter is a little difficult if you are not familiar with protein biochemistry. IgM is a large molecule as the name implies, with a molecular weight of 900,000. Plasma proteins are generally globular in shape (with the exception of fibrinogen), and the larger the molecular weight the bigger the molecular size. Thus a large molecule, if found in the urine, must have come through a large 'pore' in the glomeruli, assuming the 'sieve' theory to be correct. Now go back to **3.6** and read it again, answering the question correctly.

3.43 Your answer – in cadmium poisoning there is not likely to be any proximal tubular damage.

You are not correct. Proximal tubular damage is common in poisoning with the heavy metals, particularly with lead and mercury (although a reaction to the latter may be acute tubular necrosis). In cadmium poisoning there may be renal amino-aciduria and renal glycosuria, due primarily to a defect in amino acid and glucose reabsorption caused by proximal tubular damage. Now answer the question at the end of **3.45** correctly.

3.44 Your answer – renal function is impaired if 1 mg of PSP is excreted within 15 minutes of the injection.

You are correct. The dose excreted is $\frac{1}{6} \times 100$ per cent = 16.7 per cent. This is less than 28 per cent of the injected dose which is the lower limit of normal, so one can deduce that the patient has impaired renal function. The remaining renal function tests involving proximal tubular function primarily or exclusively, are divisible into research investigations, such as TmPAH, TmGlucose, and more widely used clinical tests used in investigating glycosuria and aminoaciduria. Glycosuria can be determined by three main methods.

(1) Copper reducing agents such as Benedict's reagent and Clinitest tablets. Details of these tests are found in the appendix. These tests are not specific for glucose but give positive results with any reducing substance such as lactose.

(2) Glucose oxidase sticks, e.g. Clinistix. These are quite specific for glucose, but give false positives with glycosides quite frequently and all positives with this method require confirmation; false negatives are very rare if adequate time is allowed for the blue colour to develop, which may take up to one minute.

(3) Chromatography. The method of choice in investigating sugars which reduce Benedict's reagent but are not glucose as shown by Clinistix test is chromatography. The significance of glycosuria from the point of view of diabetes mellitus will not be considered here. Renal glycosuria is a common condition, due to an abnormality of the proximal tubule; it is important to differentiate it from diabetes mellitus. In renal glycosuria there is a failure to reabsorb glucose normally in the proximal renal tubule in spite of a normal blood sugar i.e., there is either a low T_mG or the T_mG varies from nephron to nephron. The best evidence at present is that the T_mG of some of the nephrons is lower than normal, so that even the filtered load of glucose at normal blood sugar levels exceeds the low T_mG and glucose appears in the urine. Renal glycosuria can be readily differentiated from diabetes mellitus by a glucose tolerance test in most patients; the glucose tolerance test (GTT) is usually normal in renal glycosuria. However, patients with renal glycosuria occasionally develop diabetes mellitus (which is itself a common disease affecting 1–2 per cent of the population) so that sometimes the GTT is diabetic in type. In these patients treatment with hypoglycaemic agents will still be associated with a continuing glycosuria in spite of the now normal blood sugar. Renal glycosuria may occur as an abnormality per se, frequently inherited as an autosomal dominant trait, or it may occur in the proximal tubular syndromes, such as Fanconi syndrome, heavy metal poisoning, Wilson's disease, Lowe's syndrome, myelomatosis and frequently in patients with heavy proteinuria in whom the proximal tubules are being presumably damaged by the protein available for absorption. The total loss of glucose in the urine per day in renal glycosuria is less than 30 g.

Question In a patient with uncomplicated renal glycosuria, what type of glucose tolerance test is found?

Answer 1. Normal. Go on to **3.45**.
2. Diabetic. Go on to **3.47**.

3.45 Your answer – in uncomplicated renal gylcosuria the glucose tolerance test is normal.

You are correct. Amino acids are found in the urine in varying proportions, over 99 per cent of the filtered load being reabsorbed in the proximal tubules with the exception of glycine (95–98 per cent reabsorbed) and histidine (90–95 per cent reabsorbed). They are usually tested for clinically by determination of urinary amino nitrogen excretion and by chromatography of the urine. The normal patterns of amino acids in the urine are of three main types:

(1) Glycine is the most prominent of the amino acids.

(2) Taurine is the most prominent or at least equal to glycine.

(3) β Amino isobutyrate is excreted in equal amounts to glycine; and histidine, serine, glutamine and alanine may all be identified by paper chromatography.

The main diseases in which amino acids appear in abnormal amounts in the urine are (a) cystinuria, in which cystine and lysine appear in the urine; (b) Lignac-Fanconi syndrome or cystinosis, a disease of infants in which the excretion of most amino acids is raised; (c) and adult Fanconi syndrome in which there is generalised amino-aciduria. In Lowe's syndrome (cerebro-ocular renal dystrophy) there is a generalised amino-aciduria. Renal aminoaciduria occurs due to damage to the proximal tubule by endogenous poisons in galactosaemia, Wilson's disease, myelomatosis and heavy proteinuria; exogenous poisons include the heavy metals (such as lead, mercury, cadmium, and uranium) and organic chemicals of the phenol group.

Question In a patient with cadmium poisoning is there likely to be any proximal tubular damage?

Answer 1. Yes. Go on to **3.40**.
2. No. Go on to **3.43**.
3. Don't know. Go on to **3.48**.

3.46 Your answer – a low protein diet without disease of the kidneys can reduce the concentrating ability of the kidneys.

You are correct. The usual methods of measuring concentrating ability are (1) deprivation of water, (2) injection of vasopressin. Let us examine these in more detail.

(1) Deprivation of water

If a normal person on a diet of normal protein content is deprived of water after 4 p.m. until 8 a.m. the next day, the urine osmolality will be at least

800 mOsm/kg. This corresponds to specific gravity of about 1024. If water deprivation is continued for 30 hours, the urine concentration in the normal reaches a maximum of 800–1400 mOsm/kg; at 22 hours at least 90 per cent of this figure will be reached. In the azotaemic patient a prolonged period of water deprivation can be dangerous; it should also be avoided in patients with diabetes insipidus, renal or otherwise, in view of the danger of serious dehydration occurring. Patients with advanced renal disease are unable to concentrate their urine much above 300 mOsm/kg and patients in acute renal failure due to acute tubular necrosis often have urines which are slightly hypotonic to (i.e., of lower osmolality than) plasma. In diabetes insipidus dehydration should be carried out in a hospital with the patient being weighed every hour. The test should be stopped when weight loss has reached 5 per cent of the initial weight (about 7 lb. in an average person) or after 24 hours, whichever is the sooner. In persons with normal kidneys who have been drinking vast amounts of fluid, say 10–11 litres a day, because of hysterical polydipsia or for experimental purposes, the ability to concentrate the urine will be impaired for some days after the drinking is stopped.

Question If you have a 70 kg patient with suspected diabetes insipidus and are asked to carry out an adequate concentration test by water deprivation, for how long would you continue to deprive him of water, collecting hourly urine specimens?

Answer 1. Until he had lost 10 kg in weight. Go on to **3.58**.
2. Until he had lost 3.5 kg in weight. Go on to **3.62**.
3. For 48 hours. Go on to **3.63**.

3.47 Your answer – in a patient with uncomplicated renal glycosuria a diabetic glucose tolerance curve is found.

You are wrong. In renal glycosuria, glucose appears in the urine at normal levels of blood sugar because the TmG is low in all or some of the nephrons; in diabetes mellitus glycosuria occurs due to the increased filtered load being greater than the TmG which itself is not low. Now read **3.44** again and answer the question correctly.

3.48 Your answer – I don't know if there is likely to be proximal tubular damage in cadmium poisoning. The paragraph you have just read (**3.45**) contains a lot of facts and you have missed the statement about exogenous proximal tubular poisons such as heavy metals causing renal amino-aciduria. Read **3.45** again, paying attention to every sentence.

3.49 Your answer – in renal diabetes insipidus there is plasma ADH.
You are correct. Now go on to answer the next question.

Question Can a low protein diet without disease of the kidneys reduce the ability to concentrate the urine?

Answer 1. Yes. Go on to **3.46**.
2. No. Go on to **3.53**.

3.50 Your answer — a pH of 6.2 in the urine in an acidification test is a normal result.
You are incorrect. The maximum normal pH in an acidification test is 5.3. If a pH of 6.2 is found and it is known that the ammonium chloride has been absorbed having produced a systemic acidosis then the patient has a defect in acidification. Now answer the question at the end of **3.56**.

3.51 Your answer — In isothenuria the urine SG is 1000.
You are wrong. Go back and read **3.60** again carefully.

3.52 Your answer — in renal diabetes insipidus there is *no* plasma ADH.
You are wrong. In renal diabetes insipidus the renal tubules are refractory to the action of circulating ADH which is being liberated from the posterior pituitary gland. You must read **3.40** again with more care, and then answer the question correctly.

3.53 Your answer — a low protein diet cannot reduce the ability to concentrate the urine.
You are not correct. A low protein diet can certainly reduce the ability to concentrate. It seems to be able to do this by two mechanisms (1) by reducing the concentration of urea in the urine; (2) the non-urea solutes are also reduced in concentration. The mechanism of the non-urea solute concentration being reduced appears to be that less urea is present in the interstitium of the medulla to attract water out of the distal tubules and collecting ducts in the final concentrating process. Now answer the question at the end of **3.49** again.

3.54 Your answer — in Pitressin Tannate in oil the Pitressin is in solution.
You are wrong. Pitressin tannate is insoluble in mineral oil but forms a crude suspension on shaking vigorously. Read **3.62** again.

3.55 Your answer — I don't know whether there is any plasma ADH in renal diabetes insipidus.
You have not understood **3.40** properly. In renal diabetes insipidus ADH is present in the plasma, being liberated from the posterior pituitary gland into the blood stream, but the end organ i.e. the kidney — is refractory to its action. Now go back and read **3.40** again.

3.56 Your answer – in isothenuria the urine SG is 1010.
You are correct.

Acidification of the urine is a distal tubular and collecting system function which can be tested for most simply by means of a pH determination on a freshly passed specimen of urine; if the pH is 5.1 or less there is usually little need to go on to more elaborate tests to investigate acidification.

The acidification test of Wrong and Davies employs a metabolic acidosis, induced by oral ammonium chloride (0.1 g/kg body weight) over a short period of time (6–8 hours). Normal persons respond with a minimal pH of 5.3 or less, an ammonium output of 33–75 μEq/min, a titrable acidity of 24–51 μEq/min, and a total excretion of hydrogen ion of 60–124 μEq/min.

The most important use of the test is in determining if a patient has a defect in urine acidification which occurs in distal renal tubular acidosis, (this will be discussed in detail in the chapter on tubular syndromes) in which urine pH is always higher than 5.3 even in early and mild cases. Details of how to carry out the Wrong and Davies acidification test are found in the appendix (p. 396). The alternative acidification test which is still frequently used involves giving large doses of ammonium chloride for at least 3 days to ensure maximal response to an adequate acidosis; the disadvantage of this type of test is that the duration of the test requires the patient to be hospitalized for a few days, whereas the short term test of Wrong and Davies can be performed on an outpatient basis.

Question If a patient is given ammonium chloride, 0.1 g/kg body weight in the Wrong and Davies acidification test, what would you conclude from the fact that the minimal urine pH was 6.2.

Answer 1. The patient is normal and acidifies well. Go on to **3.50**.
2. The patient cannot acidify his urine. Go on to **3.57**.

3.57 Your answer – a urine pH of 6.2 in an acidification test is *not* normal; the patient cannot acidify his urine normally.

You are correct. You should always check that the total plasma CO_2 has fallen during the test, indicating that absorption of ammonium chloride has occurred, before concluding that the distal tubules are refractory to the stimulus of acidosis. There are many causes of inability to acidify which can be grouped under the heading of renal tubular acidosis syndromes: these include the rare familial renal tubular acidosis, pyelonephritis, hydronephrosis, hypokalaemia, and hypercalcaemia.

The ability of the distal tubules to conserve sodium is tested by giving the patient a diet containing 10–20 mEq of sodium per day and collecting the urine daily for at least 5 days.

Persons capable of normal sodium conservation come into sodium balance within 5 days, i.e., sodium loss in the urine decreases until the urinary sodium excretion in equal to the sodium intake. In salt-losing nephritis (commonly) in renal failure of any cause or in pyelonephritis) the patient continues to lose large quantities of sodium in the urine in spite of the restricted sodium intake of the diet. The patient goes into negative sodium balance and may become seriously and dangerously depleted if the test is continued. This is manifested by an orthostatic hypotension, then by a generalized fall in recumbent blood pressure, tachycardia, faintness, loss of tissue turgor and fall in eye ball pressure. The latter is often very difficult to judge clinically and should not be relied upon by the novice. In patients with Addison's disease this test should not be carried out because of the risk of serious sodium depletion. Now answer the following question.

Question A patient is given 10 mEq of sodium a day for 5 days; on the fifth day the urine contains 50 mEq of sodium. What conclusion would you draw about the patient's sodium conserving ability?

Answer 1. Sodium conservation is normal. Go on to **3.69**.
2. Sodium conservation is impaired. Go on to **3.61**.

3.58 Your answer — deprive him of water until he has lost 10 kg of weight.

You are wrong. To go on as far as this is dangerous and could be fatal. You should only deprive a patient of water up to 24 hours in time or until he has lost 5 per cent of his body weight. Now 5 per cent of the body weight is 3.5 kg in a 70 kg man. Now answer the question again after reading **3.46** again.

3.59 Your answer — in Pitressin Tannate in oil, the Pitressin is in suspension.

You are partly correct. If you have a well trained nurse she will have warmed and shaken the ampoule before giving it to you. Remember that the Pitressin Tannate is a brown smudge on the side of the ampoule. The pitressin has to be agitated into a crude suspension in the oil. Now go on to **3.60**.

3.60 Your answer — Pitressin Tannate in oil forms a brown smudge on the glass of the ampoule.

You are correct. Dilution tests are of little value in the diagnosis of renal disease. The diluting ability is retained until the renal disease is extremely far advanced, long after the ability to concentrate urine above plasma tonicity has been lost. When the urine concentration is fixed at the osmolarity of plasma (about 280 to 295 mOsm/litre) the condition is known as isosthenuria corresponding to a specific gravity of 1010. Urines which are hypotonic to plasma are termed hyposthenuric. These terms are probably better replaced nowadays by the terms hypotonic to plasma, isotonic with plasma and hypertonic to plasma, or better still the actual osmolarities should be stated.

A common method of performing dilution tests is to drink up to 1 litre of water over about 45 minutes and collect the urine every 20 minutes in the next four hours.

The dilution tests are of value not in the diagnosis of renal disease but in the diagnosis of Addison's disease, hypopituitarism and cirrhosis of the liver, where there is a delay in the excretion of an oral water load. In normal health the urine osmolarity can fall as low as 35 mOsm/litre (SG 1000) during water diuresis.

When carrying out a dilution test care should be taken not to assume that the apparent absence of detectable albuminuria is very dilute specimens of urine means that the patient has no albumin in his urine under normal circumstances. The same caution applies to the interpretation of the urine sediment on microscopy.

Question What is the specific gravity of the urine in a patient with isosthenuria?

Answer 1. SG is 1010. Go on to **3.56**.
2. SG is 1000. Go on to **3.51**.

3.61 Your answer – if, on the fifth day, of a 10 mEq/day sodium diet, a patient excretes 50 mEq of sodium in his urine, his sodium conservation mechanism is impaired.

You are quite correct.

Potassium conservation is a good deal less efficient than sodium conservation and accordingly there is no comparable low potassium diet which will give readily interpretable results like those of the low sodium diets. The next subject to be discussed is:

Divided Renal Function Tests: by this is meant study of the renal function of each kidney separately, using ureteric catheters tightly fitting into both ureters. The ureteric catheters require cystoscopy for their insertion. Divided renal function studies are performed in the investigation of hypertension where it is suspected that unilateral renal arterial stenosis or pyelonephritis may be the cause of the hypertension. Stamey advocated an infusion of urea, PAH, and saline and at present puts a catheter into 1 ureter only, the cystoscope or bladder catheter collecting the urine from the other kidney. For hypertension to be caused by a reduced blood supply to one kidney the flow rates by the Stamey technique should be at least 3 times greater in the normal kidney than in the diseased kidney. PAH is included in order to give an index of renal blood flow: PAH concentration should be increased by at least 100 per cent in the urine from the ischaemic kidney compared with the normal side. Sometimes *branches* of the renal artery are stenosed; the renal arteries may be *multiple* and some of them may be stenosed. Segmental lesions of significance produce at most a urine flow of 50 per cent of that of the unaffected side and a 16 per cent increase in PAH concentration on the affected side.

Question If a patient having a Stamey test has urine of the following composition from both kidneys, what conclusions would you draw?

	From right kidney	From left kidney
Urine vol. ml/min.	3	0.7
Urine PAH concn. mg/100 ml.	60	329

Answer 1. Left kidney ischaemic. Go on to **3.64**.
2. Right kidney ischaemic. Go on to **3.65**.
3. Left segmental lesion. Go on to **3.66**.
4. Normal bilaterally. Go on to **3.67**.

3.62 Your answer – deprive him of fluid until he has lost 3.5 kg in weight.

You are correct. 3.5 kg is 5 per cent of 70 kg. If he loses weight slowly, terminate the water deprivation after 24 hours even if he has not yet lost 3.5 kg.

The more convenient test for urine concentrating ability is the vasopressin test. This is safer in advanced renal disease than water deprivation, and in working with out-patients it is very useful because one does not have to alter a patient's fluid intake overnight *before* he comes to the clinic. There are two forms of pitressin which can be used: the most commonly used is Pitressin Tannate in oil, the dose being 5 units. The drug lasts for up to 24 hours; it should be given i.m. and the doctor prescribing it should always warm the oil in the ampoule in his hands before vigorously shaking and tapping the ampoule: this is done to suspend the pitressin in the oil; otherwise it would be left in the ampoule as a brown smudge, and the patient would receive an injection of oil without pitressin and might be thought because of his lack of response to the injection, to be suffering from an impaired concentrating mechanism. The alternative Pitressin preparation is aqueous Pitressin 0.5 units in aqueous solution. This is given intramuscularly or subcutaneously and lasts for at least one hour, so that more than one specimen of urine can be obtained conveniently. The major drawbacks of Pitressin injections are, first, their possible danger in persons with coronary atheroma, in whom angina and even myocardial infarction may be induced due to coronary vasoconstriction; secondly, there is always a chance that the Pitressin may be no longer active; this applies particularly to aqueous Pitressin solutions. The maximum osmolality achieved after Pitressin injections is less than after water deprivation. An average figure is 700–800 mOsm/kg in the normal.

Question In pitressin tannate in oil, where is the Pitressin in the ampoule when it is brought from the drug cupboard?

Answer 1. In suspension. Go on to **3.59**.

2. In solution. Go on to **3.45**.
3. Brown smudge on the ampoule wall. Go on to **3.60**.

3.63 Your answer – deprive him of fluid for 48 hours.

No. It is dangerous to deprive this patient of water for 48 hours. You should deprive him of water for 24 hours or until he has lost 5 per cent of the body weight, whichever is the sooner. In a person passing 5–7 litres of urine a day, 48 hours' water deprivation might well prove fatal, and the adage to remember in medicine is 'primum non nocere' – 'FIRST DO NO HARM.' Now read **3.46** again.

3.64 Your answer – the left kidney is ischaemic.

You are correct. There are several drawbacks to the Stamey test. These are:

(1) The dangers of infection with any instrumentation of the urinary pathways.

(2) Oedema of the ureters after the instrumentation with large size ureteric catheters can cause temporary anuria. The ureteric catheters have to be large to prevent leakage around the catheters. Stamey has lately advocated that only one ureter should be catheterised, the other ureter draining into the bladder which is itself drained by a urethral catheter. This method avoids trauma to *both* ureters and the resultant anuria.

(3) The urea in the infusion has on occasion led to cerebral shrinkage and death from resultant intracranial bleeding.

The question of whether the information obtained from divided renal function tests is worth the hazard of the test is a moot point. In view of the low success rate of surgical intervention in proved cases of unilateral renal artery stenosis, and the convenience and safety of hypotensive agents, the place of divided renal function studies in the diagnosis of renal ischaemia is less certain then was thought some years ago.

Question What is the cause of anuria following a Stamey test?

Answer 1. Renal infection. Go on to **3.70**.
2. Oedema of ureters. Go on to **3.68**.
3. Reflex anuria. Go on to **3.72**.

3.65 Your answer – the right kidney is ischaemic.

You are wrong. An ischaemic kidney has a lower urine flow, less than one third of that of the normal kidney. Similarly, the PAH concentration in the urine from an ischaemic kidney is at least twice that of the normal side. You are therefore wrong. Go back and answer the question in **3.61** correctly.

3.66 Your answer – there is a left segmental lesion.

You are wrong. A segmental stenosis gives values of urine flow greater than those found in a main renal artery stenosis, but less than the flow from normal side. This patient has urine flows on the left less than one third of the flow rates on the right. Read **3.61** again carefully and answer the question correctly.

3.67 Your answer – the kidneys are normal bilaterally. You are wrong. It is most unusual for such discrepancies in urine flow and PAH concentration to be found with two normal kidneys. The difference between the urines from the two kidneys cannot be accounted for by leakage round the ureteric catheters during the collection of ureteric specimens because the PAH *concentrations* are also grossly discrepant and collection defects can be excluded. Read **3.61** again and choose the correct answer.

3.68 Your answer – anuria following a Stamey test is due to ureteric oedema.
You are correct. Probably more valuable and possibly less hazardous than a Stamey test is the measurement of renal vein renin from both renal veins. In renal arterial occlusion the ipsi-lateral renal venous blood has a high renin content, and this is readily compared to the renin concentration in the non-stenosed side.

If the renin concentrations in the renal vein blood on both sides are measured, and if the renin concentration on the side with the arterial stenosis is 1.5 or more times larger than on the normal side, then there is a good chance that a corrective operation on the stenosed artery will lead to a fall in blood pressure. Some authors do not find this test reliable i.e. Guedon 1972.

The last type of renal investigation to be considered is the radio-active renogram, i.e., the use of radio-active compounds injected intravenously whose passage into and through the kidneys can be measured by probes held over the kidneys; the resultant patterns of radio-activity can give valuable information as to the kidney function, blood supply of the kidneys and obstruction to the lower urinary pathways. The most commonly used compound is para-amino-hippurate labelled with ^{127}I (or ^{131}I) which has superceded diodrast ^{131}I because the former is less concentrated in the liver. γ ray sensitive counters held over the renal angles activate a rate meter which gives a tracing on a moving paper. The rate of initial uptake is related to the renal blood flow (a) on Fig. 3.68 (i); then comes a secretory phase where the PAH is taken up by the renal tubules (b) on Fig. 3.68 (i); the final slow descent (c) on this figure) is related to the unobstructed passage of the radio-active urine out of the

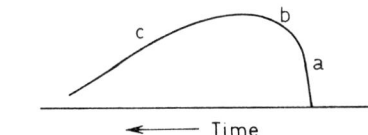

Fig. 3.68 (i) ⟵ Time

kidney. Obstruction to the ureter results in a renogram with a rising (c) instead of the normal fall-off (Fig. 3.68 (ii)).

In the presence of reduced blood supply unilaterally the climb a^1 is smaller on the affected side (Fig. 3.68 (iii)).

In Fig. 3.68 (iii) the (L) ischaemic blood supply is shown by a^1 being smaller than a, and the fall off is slower.

In bilateral parenchymatous renal disease such as glomerulone-phritis there is a rapid small rise due to the impaired blood supply phase, followed by a barely perceptible or absent secretory phase and a very slow fall-off. See Fig. 3.68 (iv). Now answer the question.

Question A man with a blood urea of 258 mg/100 ml has a bilateral radio-active renogram as in Fig. 3.68 (v).

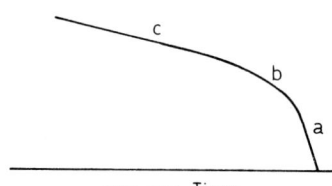

Fig. 3.68 (ii)

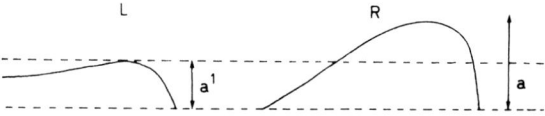

Fig. 3.68 (iii)

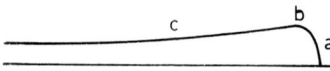

Fig. 3.68 (iv)

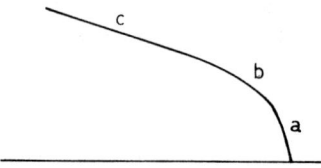

Fig. 3.68 (v)

What is the probable cause of this?

Answer 1. Renal artery stenosis. Go on to **3.74**.
2. Obstruction to urinary pathways. Go on to **3.75**.
3. Chronic glomerulonephritis. Go on to **3.76**.

3.69 Your answer – a patient on a 10 mEq sodium diet who excretes 50 mEq of sodium in the urine on the fifth day of the diet has normal sodium conservation.

You are wrong. The distal tubules and collecting system are quite remarkable in their ability to conserve sodium. The majority of normal people on a low salt diet reach an equilibrium state on or before the fifth day of the diet in which sodium loss in the urine is equal to the sodium in the diet (faecal sodium loss is negligible). Hence a normal person would be expected to lose 10 mEq of sodium each day in the urine on this diet, and certainly not 50 mEq of sodium on the fifth day. Now answer the question at the end of **3.57** again after re-reading **3.57**.

3.70 Your answer – anuria following a Stamey test is due to renal infection.

You are wrong. The large size of ureteric catheter causes trauma to the ureter whose lumen becomes occluded by the resultant oedema. Read **3.64** again.

3.71 Look at the following statements carefully, and then choose the appropriate answers. Remember that if you choose incorrectly and disclose a fundamental error of knowledge you may have to go back and start working through the chapter again.

Statement 1 On a normal diet the blood urea level remains normal until the GFR drops to below 25–30 ml/min.

Statement 2 A patient with renal tubular acidosis can reach a urine pH of 4.9 in the Wrong and Davies acidification test.

Statement 3 The Stamey test of divided renal function is useful in the diagnosis of anuria.

Answers 1. All the statements are true. Go on to **3.37**.
2. All the statements are false. Go on to **3.77**.
3. 1 is false, 2 and 3 are true. Go on to **3.78**.
4. 2 is false, 1 and 3 are true. Go on to **3.79**.
5. 3 is false, 1 and 2 are true. Go on to **3.80**.
6. 1 and 2 are false, 3 is true. Go on to **3.81**.
7. 1 and 3 are false, 2 is true. Go on to **3.82**.
8. 2 and 3 are false, 1 is true. Go on to **3.73**.

3.72 Your answer – reflex anuria is the cause of the anuria following the Stamey test.

You are wrong because passage of further ureteric catheters discloses urine secretion above the ureteric obstruction. Read **3.64** again.

3.73 Your answer – 2 and 3 are false, 1 is true.

You are correct. You can now proceed to Chapter 4, which deals with renal investigations of a morphological nature as opposed to the biochemical type discussed in the present chapter.

Books which can be consulted about individual tests are:
T. H. Stamey: Renal Artery Stenosis. Williams Wilkins, 1963. Reubi: Renal clearances. Thomas, 1962.
K. E. Britton and N. J. G. Brown: Clinical Renography. Lloyd-Luke, London 1971.

Articles:
  (1) Stamey, T. H. et al (1961) Medicine. Balt. **40** p. 347
  (2) Wrong, O. M. & Davies, H. E. F. (1959). Quart. J. Med. **28** p. 259
  (3) De Wardener and Barlow (1959). Ibid. **28** p. 235
  (4) Luke et al (1966). Ibid. **35** p. 237.
  (5) Marlow et al (1972) Clin Chim Act **28** 479
  (6) Earley, L.E. & Daughart, T.M. (1969). New England N. Med. **281**, 72
  (7) Stockigt et al (1972) Lancet *I*, 1194 (Renal vein renin)
  (8) Geudon, M. et al (1972) Rev Europ d'etudes clin. et biol. **17**, 757

3.74 Your answer – the renogram shows renal artery stenosis.

You are wrong. In renal artery stenosis the renogram is quite different. Look again at the figures in **3.68**.

3.75 Your answer – the renogram is due to obstruction to the urinary pathways.
You are correct. Now go on to **3.71**.

3.76 Your answer – the renogram shows chronic glomerulonephritis.
You are wrong. Go back and read **3.68** again.

3.77 Your answer – all the statements are false.

Statements 2 and 3 are false but statement 1 is true. The blood urea is below 45 mg/100 ml until the GFR has dropped to between 25 and 30 ml/min, assuming the patient is on a normal diet. Read **3.16** again, then go on to **3.82**.

3.78 Your answer – 1 is false, 2 and 3 are true.

You are wrong. How you can give such an answer is hard to understand if you have been working through the paragraphs. Look at the statements in **3.71** again. If you still give this same answer, start at **3.16** and go on from there.

3.79 Your answer – 2 is false, 1 and 3 are true.

You are correct about 1 and 2, but 3 is false. Read **3.61** and go on from there.

3.80 Your answer — 3 is false, 1 and 2 are true.

You are correct about 1 and 3, but wrong about 2. Go back to **3.56** and work on from there.

3.81 Your answer — 1 and 2 are false, 3 is true.

You are correct about 2 only, 1 and 3 are false. Go back to **3.16** and work through from there.

3.82 Your answer — 1 and 3 are false, 2 is true.

You are correct about 3, but incorrect about 1 and 2. Go back to **3.16** and work on from there.

Time for this chapter: 45 minutes

Chapter 4
Renal investigation: 2. morphological

4.1 In this chapter renal investigations will be discussed which are predominently morphological as opposed to the biochemical type of renal investigation described in Chapter 3. The morphological investigations include urine microscopy, renal radiology and renal biopsy.

Microscopical examination of the urine is the Cinderella of renal investigations. Whereas most self-respecting physicians will examine intravenous pyelograms themselves, only a minority routinely carry out microscopical examination of the urine. This omission is regrettable because much can be learned about renal lesions if one takes the trouble to examine the urine oneself. The necessary skill in using a microscope to recognise the cellular constituents of the unstained urinary deposit is readily acquired; use of a phase contrast microscope simplifies this task considerably. The technique of microscopical examination of the urine is as follows:

The urine specimen is looked at with the naked eye. If it is cloudy, smoky, or bloody, a drop of the *unspun* specimen is removed with a Pasteur pipette and placed on a clean slide and covered with a cover-slip. It is examined first with a $\frac{2}{3}$ inch objective then with a $\frac{1}{6}$ inch objective. In blood-stained urine the unspun specimen contains red blood cells in profusion. In acute pyelonephritis the unspun specimen contains large numbers of pus cells, and on phase contrast microscopy the organism responsible can often be seen. Phosphates appear as amorphous debris and may be so dense as to obscure the cellular deposits: such dense deposits of phosphate can be dissolved by the introduction of a drop of 3 per cent acetic acid to the urinary sediment in the test tube or directly on the slide under the cover-slip. The urine produced in severe oliguria due to acute tubular necrosis contains granular casts, pigment casts, tubular cells, a few red blood cells and pus cells, and a great deal of unidentifiable debris.

All the urine specimens, whether clear or otherwise, should be centrifuged and the urinary sediment examined. This is such an important part of the assessment of renal function that it is surprising how few clinicians are competent in the preparation of the sediment for microscopical examination or in the interpretation of what they are seeing under the microscope. The commonest mistake is to spin too fast for too long. Our standard technique is to place 10 ml of urine in a centrifuge tube and spin at 1000 revolutions per minute for 5 minutes. Faster and longer spinning may damage delicate casts and compress the sediment into a hard button which is then further damaged by the agitation necessary to resuspend it. After spinning, the sediment should be examined with the naked eye. Red cells show up as a reddish deposit: in contrast pus cells and amorphous phosphates look white or cream coloured: urates give a brick coloured deposit. The centrifuge tube should then be gently inverted, the supernatant urine being decanted off and saved for chemical testing. The drop of urine remaining in the centrifuge tube is agitated gently with a flick of the fingers and a drop removed and placed under a cover-slip and examined microscopically. Urine should be examined as quickly as possible after voiding, but there may still be identifiable casts, red cells and pus cells in urine 24 hours old; there is good evidence that, with time, casts and cellular constituents gradually disappear, particularly in alkaline specimens kept at room temperature. Before we go on to describe microscopical appearance of the urine sediment, answer the following question:

Question If the urine sediment in the centrifuge tube after spinning for 5 minutes is red, what is likely to be found when the sediment is examined microscopically?

Answer 1. White cells. Go on to **4.8**.
2. Red cells. Go on to **4.11**.
3. Amorphous phosphate. Go on to **4.5**.
4. Urates. Go on to **4.4**.

4.2 You should not be reading this paragraph. Please follow the instructions and go on to the paragraph indicated by the answer you have chosen in **4.1**.

4.3 Your answer — aspirin causes a 'telescoped' urine deposit.
You are wrong. A telescoped urine deposit is found in renal involvement in systematic lupus erythematosus. Read **4.19** again.

4.4 Your answer — a red deposit is due to urates. You are correct; the urate deposit is usually a uniform brick-red colour. Red cells give a red deposit which is a different colour but you will be able to recognise the difference if you centrifuge 0.1 ml of blood which has been added to 10 ml of urine and compare it to a urate deposit. Now go on to **4.11**.

4.5 Your answer — amorphous phosphates give a red urinary sediment.
You are wrong. Amorphous phosphates give the deposit a white or creamy colour. Read **4.1** again.

4.6 Your answer — Fig. 4.13 d shows a white cell.
You are correct. Urinary casts are an important feature of the urinary sediment. You will recall that hyaline casts are composed of Tamm-Horsfall protein, and are found in normal urine, particularly if it is a concentrated specimen. Some-

times these casts form long cylindroids. Hyaline casts are shown in Fig. 4.6 (i) which you should look at carefully.

The shape of the casts is thought to be governed by the shape of the tubular lumen in which they are formed.

Granular casts are almost always pathological with the exception of specimens taken immediately after heavy exertion. Granular casts are generally thought to be degenerated cellular casts (which will be described shortly), although this is unlikely. Look at Fig. 4.6 (ii).

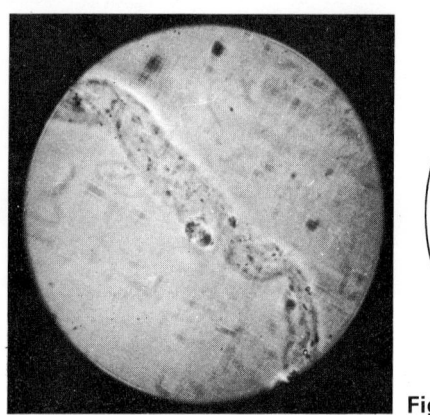
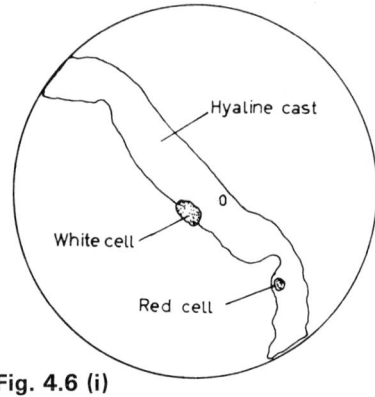

Fig. 4.6 (i)

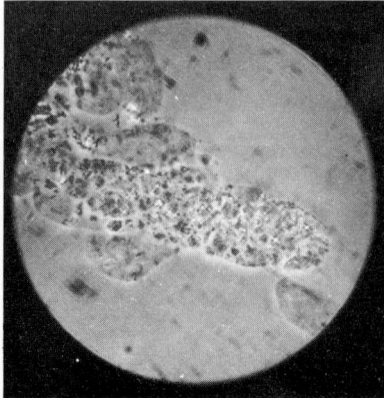
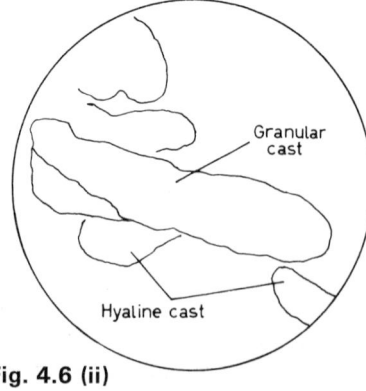

Fig. 4.6 (ii)

If the cast is formed in the wider tubules (such as the collecting system) due to low urine flow in renal failure, the casts tend to be very broad and are referred to as 'renal failure casts.' These are shown in Fig. 4.6 (iii). Look at it.

Now answer the following question.

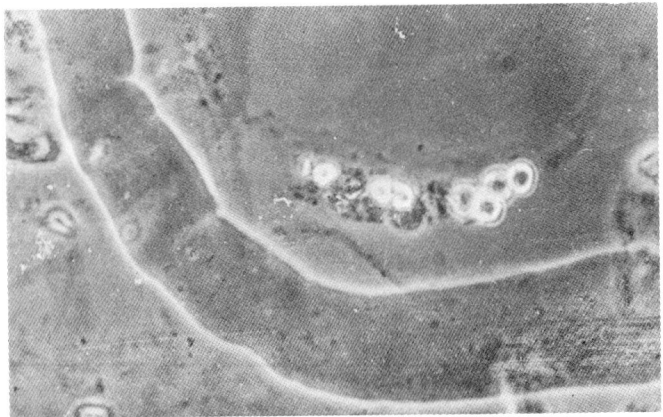

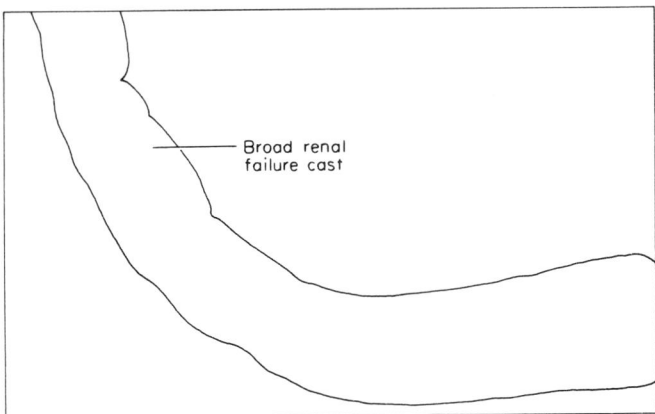

Fig. 4.6 (iii)

Question If you see a cast like that in Fig. 4.6 (iv), what would you conclude about the patient's kidneys?

Answer 1. Normal. See **4.24**.
2. Abnormal. See **4.19**.

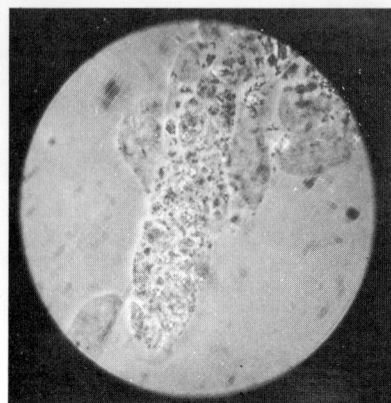

Fig. 4.6 (iv)

4.7 Your answer – the Addis count is compatible with normal health.

You are not correct. The Addis count is quite abnormal. Red cell excretion should be not more than 1,000,000/24 hours, white cells up to 2,000,000/24 hours; granular casts are rarely observed in health unless vigorous exertion has just taken place. Now read **4.11** again, look at the figure carefully as as to be able to recognise red cells when you see them.

4.8 Your answer – a red deposit in the centrifuge tube is associated with white cells in the urinary sediment.

You are wrong. Red cells give a red deposit, white cells do not. Read **4.1** again.

4.9 Your answer – aspirin causes an increased excretion of RBC's in the urine.

You are partly correct but only if such large amounts of aspirin are taken to lower the prothrombin concentration of blood sufficiently to lead to haematuria. Smaller doses of aspirin cause desquamation of tubular cells into the urine. Now go on to read **4.20**.

4.10 Your answer – Fig. 4.13d shows a squamous epithelial cell.

You are wrong. Go back to **4.13** and look at the figures carefully. Then answer the question correctly.

4.11 Your answer – a red deposit may be caused by red blood cells. You are correct. A deposit of brick-red colour may be caused by urates but there is rarely any reason to confuse the two deposits. Now let us turn to microscopical examination of the urine. The sediment should be examined with the $\frac{2}{3}$ inch and $\frac{1}{6}$ inch objectives by standard light microscopy and then with phase contrast microscopy if the apparatus is available. Red cells appear as circular objects without a nucleus. They are readily identified in Fig. 4.11 which is a photomicrograph of urine from a

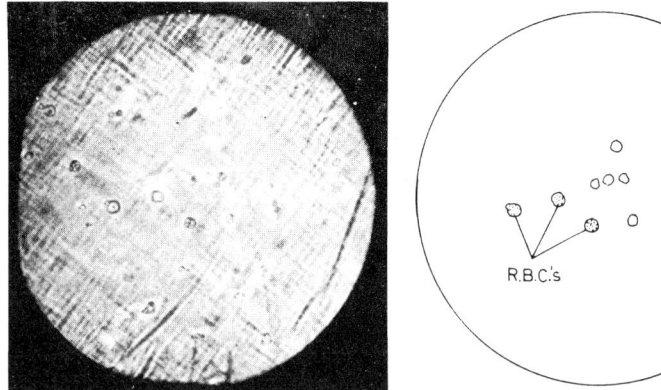

Fig. 4.11

patient who has focal nephritis. If the urine is very concentrated, the red blood cells crenate; if very dilute they will swell up and burst, leaving red cell 'ghosts' behind. The number of cells excreted per day may be estimated by several techniques:

(1) *The Addis count*, in which a 12 hour urine collection is made, the volume measured, and the number of red blood cells white blood cells, and casts measured using a haemacytometer counting chamber. The 12 hour excretion of cells can then be calculated. The normal values of the Addis count are:

    Red cells — up to 1 million per 24 hours.

    White cells — up to 2 million per 24 hours (including tubular epithelial cells).

    Casts — up to 10,000 per 24 hours — almost always hyaline (see below).

Cell counts greater than these values suggest the presence of renal disease.

(2) *2 hourly urine* collection for total cellular excretion. This is carried out in a similar way to the Addis count but over a 2 hour period: the normal red cell excretion may be up to 200,000 red blood cells per hour and white cells excretion is usually the same (up to 200,000 white cells per hour). A little arithmetic will make you realise that this gives a maximum normal red cell and white cell excretion of 24 × 200,000 cells/day = 4,800,000 cells/24 hours. This is far above the normal cellular excretion as established for the Addis count. There are two possible reasons for this discrepancy.

    (1) The cells may degenerate in the 12 hour collection of urine whereas they are fresh in a 1 or 2 hour collection.

    (2) Diurnal variation in cellular excretion may occur.

Now answer the following question

Question The results of an Addis count are as follows:
Excretion of red cells = 10,000,000 per 24 hours.
Excretion of white cells = 1,000,000 per 24 hours.
Granular casts = 1,000,000 per 24 hours.

What do these results indicate?

Answer 1. Normal health. Go on to **4.7**.
2. Renal disease. Go on to **4.13**.
3. Don't know. Go on to **4.14**.

4.12 Your answer – Fig. 4.13d shows a red cell.

You are wrong. Look at the figure in **4.11** which shows a red cell. Then look at **4.13** and study the figures before answering the question at the end of the paragraph.

4.13 Your answer – the Addis count indicates the patient has renal disease.

You are correct. Next let us turn to the appearance of white cells in the urine. White cells, like red cells, are found in normal urine in small numbers which were referred to in **4.11**. The white cells which originate in the *kidney* are said to be large pale staining cells with visible Brownian movement in the cytoplasm on supravital staining using a mixture of crystal violet and safranin (Sternheimer-Malbin stain); other white cells are smaller and darker staining. The large pale staining white cells are known as 'glitter' cells, but the very origin of these cells as distinct from other white cells is now in doubt because the appearance of 'glitter' cells depends on the urine osmolality. White cells in the urine can be readily differentiated from tubular epithelial cells, which are larger and have a compact nucleus. Look at Fig. 4.13, which shows (a) white cells and (b) tubular epithelial cells.

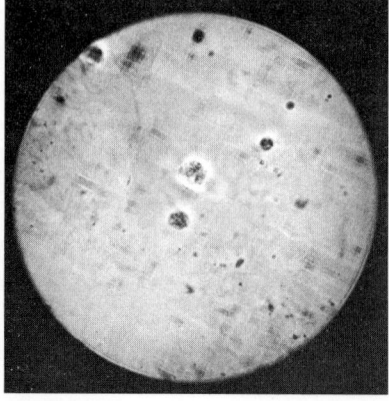
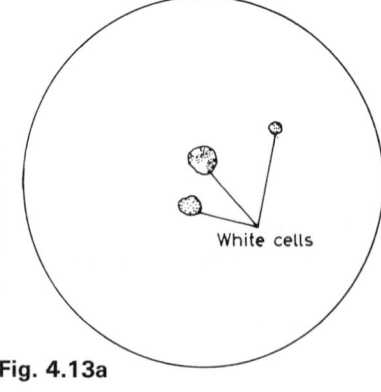

Fig. 4.13a

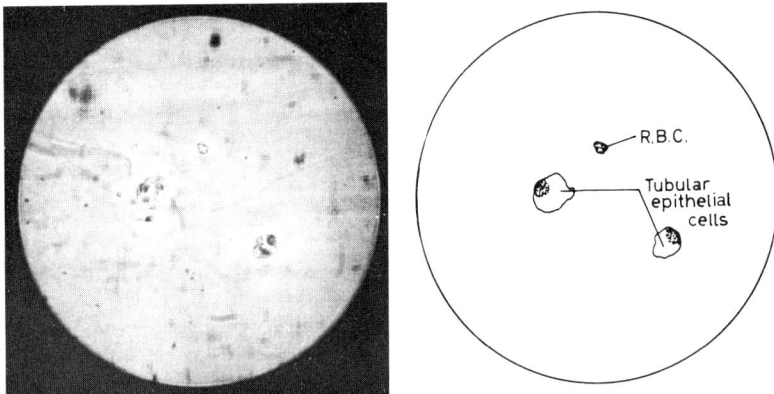

Fig. 4.13b

Squamous epithelial cells are quite different in appearance to tubular epithelial cells, originating in the squamous epithelium of the lower urinary pathways and, in women also in the vulva and vagina, as you can see in Fig. 4.13c.

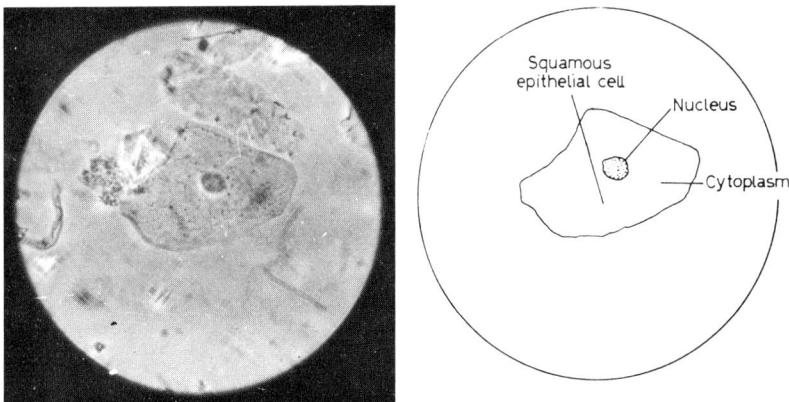

Fig. 4.13c

Question Look at Fig. 4.13d on page 82 and identify the cell.

Answer 1. White cell. Go on to **4.6**.
2. Tubular epithelial cell. Go on to **4.15**.
3. Red blood cell. Go on to **4.12**.
4. Squamous epithelial cell. Go on to **4.10**.

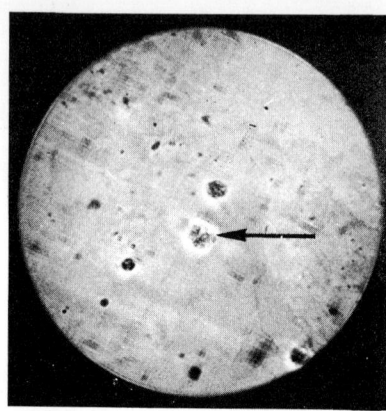

Fig. 4.13d

4.14 Your answer – I don't know what the Addis count indicates in this patient. You should read **4.11** again paying great attention to it. Avoid day-dreaming when you should be reading.

4.15 Your answer – a tubular epithelial cell is shown in Fig. 4.13d.
You are wrong. Go back and look at Figs. (a) and (b) in **4.13**. Then answer the question correctly.

4.16 Your answer – the blood urea is likely to be normal if IVP shows bilateral absence of function.
You are wrong. Read **4.20** again. Bear in mind that the presence of radio-opaque pelvic urine indicating renal function depends on the amount of contrast medium undergoing glomerular filtration and proximal tubular secretion: if the GFR is very low very little contrast medium will be excreted. Go back to **4.20** again.

4.17 Your answer – I don't know the blood urea level if the IVP shows no 'function'. If you don't know the answer you have not paid attention to **4.20**. Go back to it and read it properly; answer the question correctly.

4.18 Your answer – the normal length of the long axis of the kidneys is 12 to 13.5 cm. You are correct.

Having examined the plain film the intravenous injection of contrast medium is given and if the renal cortex is to be examined in detail films should be taken *every minute* for the first five minutes. The renal cortex can be seen clearly at this time before the urine in the calyces is opacified. The thickness of the cortex and its regularity can be assessed; the uniformly thinned cortex of chronic glomerulonephritis and the irregular moth eaten appearance of pyelonephritis and ischaemia can be detected at this stage. By 15 minutes there is adequate filling with the radiopaque medium of the calyces, pelvis, and ureters, making them clearly visible. The normal cupping of the calyces caused by the projection into them of the pyramids is shown in Fig. 4.18a; notice the shape of the calyces and renal pelvis. The next film is taken with compression of both ureters by external pressure over the abdomen. This compression improves contrast but makes the pelvis and calyces distorted.

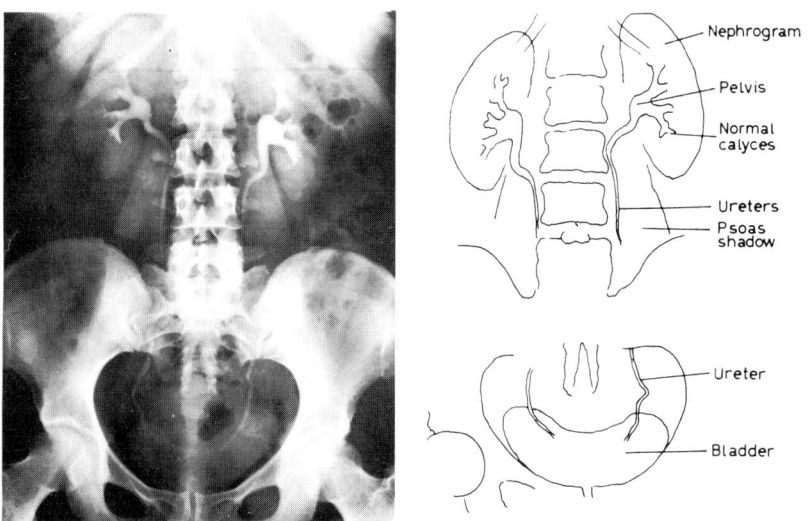

Fig. 4.18a

Space occupying lesions, such as cysts (either solitary or in polycystic-disease), hypernephromas, and abscesses, all produce a distortion of the calyceal pattern with 'silent' areas. In polycystic disease the distortion of the calyceal pattern is so widespread as to give a characteristic picture (see Fig. 4.18b).
Tuberculosis itself usually produces actual destruction of the calyces and pyramids often with calcification, the end stage being a destroyed and calcified kidney. If

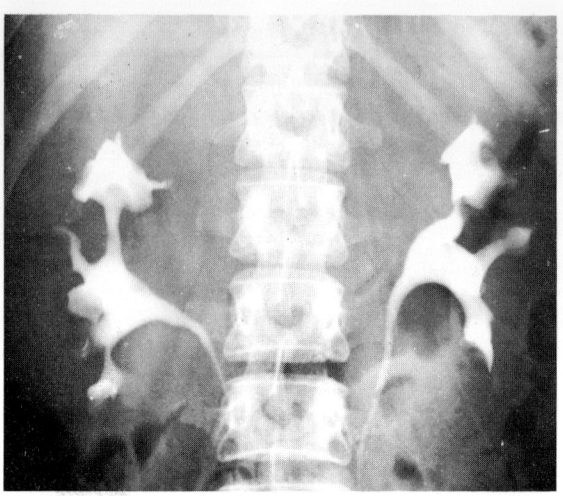

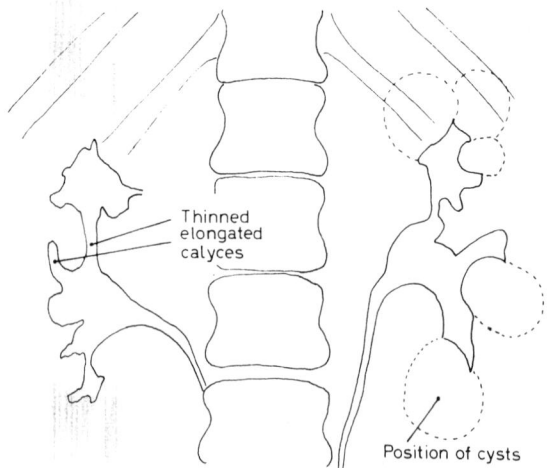

Fig. 4.18b

the external genitalia can be seen on the IVP the presence of calcification in the epididymis should be sought on cases of renal TB. Calcification of the ureter is commonly caused by tuberculosis. The size of the bladder should also be noted in view of the contracted bladder which results from advanced tuberculous disease. Look at Fig. 4.18c.

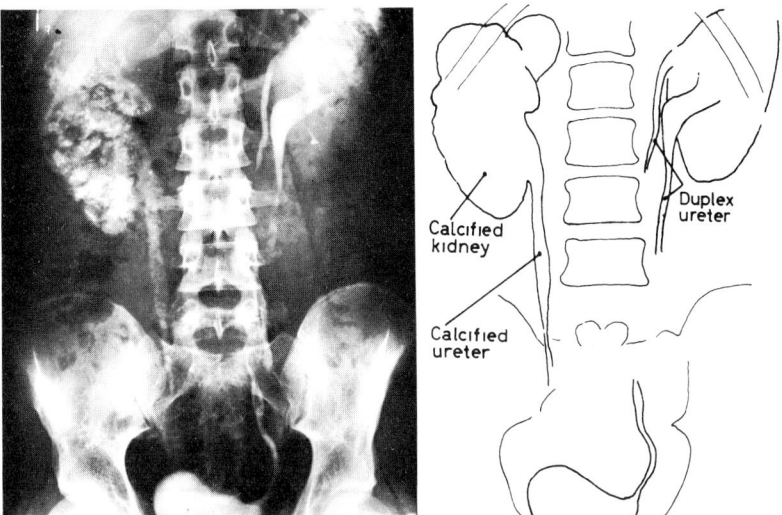

Fig. 4.18c

Hypernephromas give silent areas on IVP which are suggestive but not diagnostic. The X-ray (Fig. 4.18d) shows a typical IVP in a case of hypernephroma. A final film 35 to 45 minutes after the injection should be taken for details of bladder contour and extrinsic pressure defects. The volume of residual urine in the bladder can be assessed by a film taken after micturition.

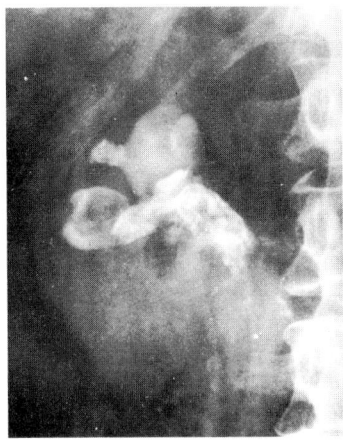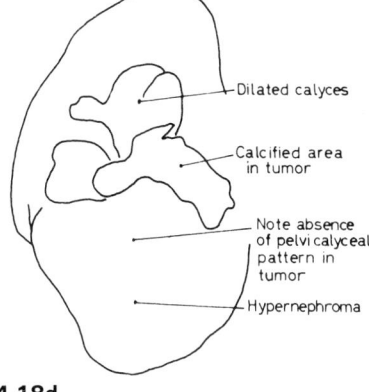

Fig. 4.18d

Question

What diagnosis would you make from this IVP?

Answer

1. Polycystic kidney.
   See **4.25**.
2. Normal.
   See **4.26**.
3. Hypernephroma.
   See **4.27**.

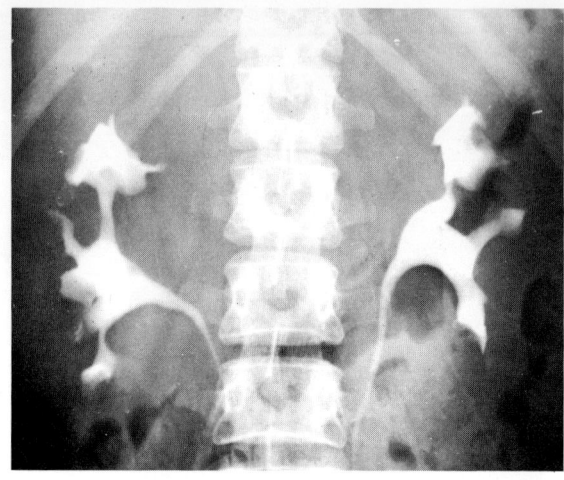

Fig. 4.18e

4.19 Your answer – the cast indicates an abnormal kidney.

You are right. The cast is a granular cast which is rarely found in normal urine.

Cellular casts are good evidence of abnormal tubules. The most striking cellular cast is the red cell cast, commonly found in acute nephritis and in any haematuria of glomerular origin. The red cells cling to the surface of the cast in large numbers. Look at Fig. 4.19a.

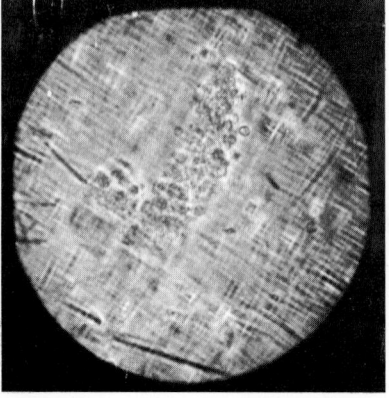 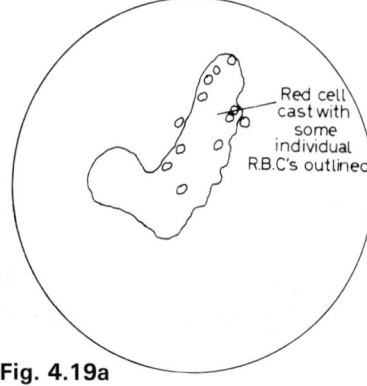

Fig. 4.19a

White cell casts are composed of leucocytes which are adherent to the cast surface (Fig. 4.19b).

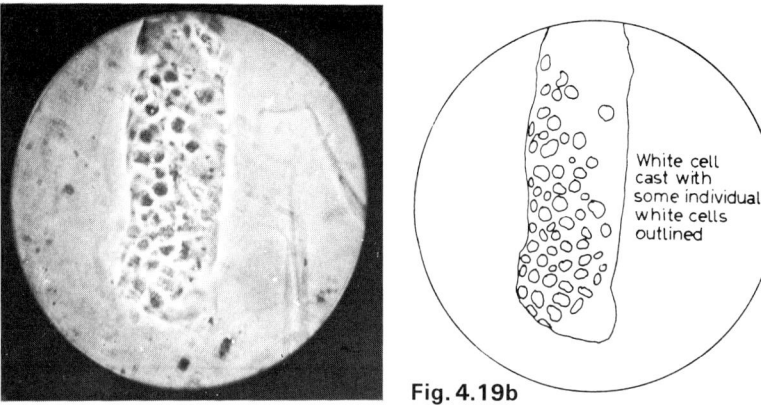

Fig. 4.19b

They are easy to identify if the leucocytes are not degenerated; if they are degenerated markedly, the cell type cannot be recognised with certainty. White cell casts are common in all diseases of the kidneys in which the glomeruli and tubules contain leucocytes eg. glomerulonephritis, systemic lupus erythematosus. Tubular cell casts are occasionally seen and are identified by the tubular cells on the surface of the cast. (Look at Fig. 4.19c).

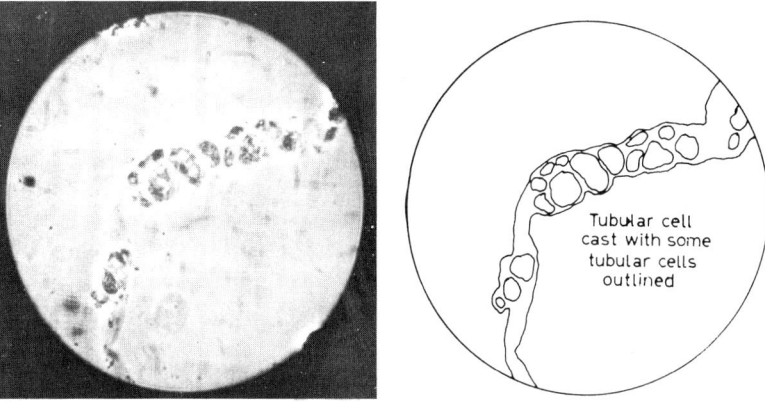

Fig. 4.19c

It is thought that degeneration of a cellular cast leads ultimately to the development of a granular cast. The origin of waxy casts (which look waxy as the name implies) is uncertain. Care should be taken to avoid confusing pus cells adhering together in clumps with white cell casts which are normally clearly delineated and roughly rectangular in shape. If all the cellular elements are present in one specimen of urine i.e. red cells, white cells, red cell casts, granular casts, white cell casts, broad renal failure casts and fatty casts, this is referred to as a 'telescoped urine deposit' which is associated with renal systemic lupus erythematosus but can also be found in other collagenoses. The excretion of tubular cells in the urine is increased as aspirin. Corticosteroids and bacterial pyrogens will cause a very large outpouring of leucocytes into the urine in chronic pyelonephritis and in some hypertensive patients. This fact is used in tests for chronic pyelonephritis; thus values of white cells excretion rates of 400,000/hour or more are considered as a positive result in the Pyrexal test in which Pyrexal (a bacterial pyrogen) is given intravenously. Unfortunately, false positives and negatives abound and, perhaps more important, the patients frequently experience such unpleasant chills and rigors from the injection of 'Pyrexal' that there is little justification for performing the 'Pyrexal' test. The use of prednisone in a dosage of 50 mg to stimulate urinary white cell excretion in the diagnosis of chronic pyelonephritis has been advocated, but its use has been occasionally associated with a flare-up of acute pyelonephritis and consequently it should not be employed as a test of renal infection.

Question What is the effect of aspirin administration on the urine cell excretion?

Answer 1. Increases tubular cell excretion in the urine. Go on to **4.20**.
2. Causes a 'telescoped' urinary deposit. Go on to **4.23**.
3. Increases red cell excretion in the urine. Go on to **4.9**.

4.20 Your answer – aspirin increases the excretion of tubular cells in the urine.
You are correct. The next subject to be considered is radiological examination of the kidney. This includes intravenous pyelography, retrograde pyelography, and renal arteriography. Intravenous pyelography (IVP) is one of the renal function tests which is all too frequently undertaken without adequate preparation and results in poor quality films which are difficult to interpret. Adequate preparation for an intravenous pyelogram requires (1) overnight dehydration in order to increase the concentration of the contrast medium in the urine. If the patient has dilute urine there will be a lower concentration of contrast medium in the pelvis, ureters, and bladder, which will thus be harder to define in detail on the X-ray film. (2) adequate purgation to remove as much bowel gas as possible: it is easy to obtain excellent abdominal films which are almost gas free in the ambulatory patient; in the ill patient, lying recumbent all day, it is very difficult to obtain gas-free films.

The contrast media are organic iodine compounds which enter the tubular fluid by glomerular filtration and proximal tubular secretion. In the presence of very diminished glomerular filtration so little of the contrast medium will enter the tubular fluid that the urine in the calcyes and pelvis will not be radio-opaque and so there will be no apparent 'renal function' on intravenous pyelography. It should be emphasised that absence of renal function on IVP does not mean that the kidneys are functionless: they may have a GFR on 10–15 ml/min and be able to sustain life for many years. Because it is rare to obtain visible excretion on IVP if the GFR is very low, it is generally not worth doing an IVP if the blood urea is over 70 mg/100 ml (assuming the patient is on a normal diet), unless a special technique is used in which a 'double dose' of the contrast medium is given by intravenous drip. This is known as drip infusion pyelogram (DIP). Pictures taken for up to 60 minutes afterwards. Detailed pictures of the renal pelvis, calyces, and ureters may be even obtained in advanced renal failure. The side effects of intravenous pyelography are few: some patients have sensitivity reactions with hypotension, rashes, asthma, etc after injection of the contrast medium: to prevent this, a test dose should always be given intravenously in a patient with an allergic history before the main dose of the contrast medium is administered. Patients with multiple myeloma are liable to develop acute renal failure after intravenous pyelography which should therefore *not be carried out* in multiple myeloma patients unless a water diuresis is simultaneously present.

This is because the anuria in these patients is probably caused by precipitation of myeloma proteins in blood vessels in the kidney and in the tubules due to the additive effects of dehydration for the IVP and the increased viscosity of the blood in myeloma.

Question If no renal function can be detected bilaterally on intravenous pyelography, the patient having a normal protein containing diet, what is the blood urea level likely to be?

Answer 1. Normal. See **4.16**.
2. Above 70 mg/100 ml. See **4.21**.
3. Don't know. See **4.17**.

4.21 Your answer – if the IVP shows no function, the blood urea is likely to be above 70 mg/100 ml.

You are correct. Now let us consider the findings on intravenous pyelography. Before the injection is given a plain X-ray of the abdomen is taken. From this the presence of both renal outlines can usually be made out and the kidneys measured; usually the long axis from the upper pole to the lower pole is measured and is found to measure 12 to 13.5 cm. In addition gross variations in the shape of the kidneys may be seen, as well as radio-opaque renal calculi. Atrophy of one or both kidneys may be due to chronic glomerulonephritis, chronic pyelonephritis and unilateral renal artery stenosis. Hypertrophy of one kidney occurs within six months of removal or destruction of the contralateral kidney. If both kidneys are very large, polycystic kidney disease or bilateral hydronephrosis should be suspected.

Question What is the normal size of the long axis of the kidneys as measured on IVP?

Answer 1. 17 cm. Go on to **4.22**.
2. 12 to 13.5 cm. Go on to **4.18**.

4.22 Your answer – the normal length of the long axis of the kidneys is 17 cm. You are wrong. The normal length is 12 to 13.5 cm. Read **4.21** again.

4.23 Your answer – aspirin causes a 'telescoped' urine deposit. A telescoped deposit consists of red cells, red cell casts, white cells, white cell casts and granular casts. Aspirin does not influence red cell excretion unless a bleeding tendency is induced by reason of hypoprothrombinaemia. Go back to **4.19** and read it again.

4.24 Your answer – the cast would lead to the conclusion that the kidneys were normal. You are wrong. The cast is a granular cast which is almost always a sign of renal disease. Read **4.6** again.

4.25 Your answer – the IVP shows polycystic kidney. You are correct. One of the common abnormalities which is demonstrable on an IVP is chronic pyelonephritis, in which there is distortion of the pyramids often associated with irregular thinning of the cortex (see Fig. 4.25a).

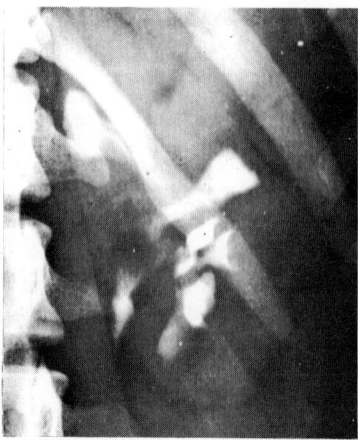
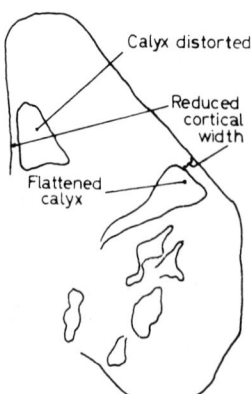

Fig. 4.25a

In contrast in ischaemic renal disease there is irregularity of the cortical depth but the underlying pyramids are normal in shape; the pyramids are distorted in chronic pyelonephritis.

Sometimes one kidney opacifies before the other; this may be purely an artefact but it may indicate urinary tract obstruction or unilateral non-obstructive renal disease. The sequence of changes in the IVP in obstruction of the renal pathways is as follows:

(1) Generalised flattening of the renal pyramids, all being equally affected. Look at Figs. 4.25b 1—4.

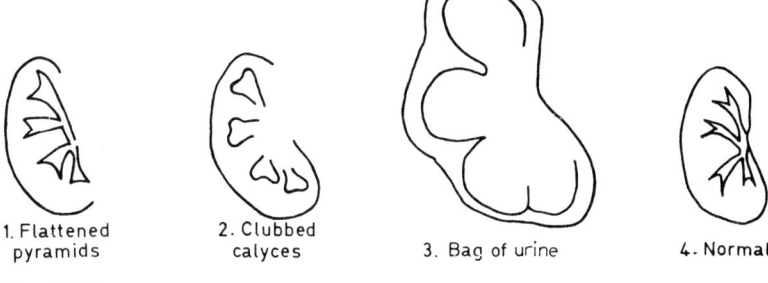

Fig. 4.25b

(2) Clubbing of calyces — the pyramids are compressed into becoming a depression on the calyces, rather than an elevation projecting into the calyx. The entire cortex becomes thinner.

(3) The entire kidney becomes a thin bag with a huge dilated pelvicalyceal system and very narrow cortex, rapidly deteriorating in function and showing no excretion on IVP.

Question If two pyramids are shown to be flattened and distorted, with thinning of the overlying cortex, the remainder being normal, what is the likely diagnosis?

Answer 1. Obstructive disease of urinary pathways. Go on to **4.29**.
       2. Pyelonephritis. Go on to **4.30**.
       3. Ischaemic disease. Go on to **4.31**.

4.26 Your answer — the IVP is normal.

You are wrong. Look at the IVP's in **4.18** again, then answer the question correctly, paying attention to the general configuration of the calyces.

4.27 Your answer — the IVP shows a hypernephroma.

You are wrong. A hypernephroma gives a more localised abnormality unless it is infiltrating the entire kidney when the IVP is unlikely to be densely radio-opaque. Read **4.18** again and choose the correct answer.

4.28 Your answer – vesico-ureteric reflux occurs in pyelonephritis.

You are correct, although it must be pointed out that many normal people have vesico-ureteric reflux but one cannot say whether they will develop pyelonephritis in the future.

Renal stones are often seen in X-ray examinations of the kidneys. They are composed of various types of calcium phosphate and calcium oxalate combinations, rendering the majority radio-opaque. Very large stones which fill the renal pelvis are called staghorn calculi, but there are often smaller stones in the renal pelvis whose intra-renal position can only be determined by several oblique views during urography. Cystine stones are radio-opaque as are some urate stones. The majority of urate stones are radiotranslucent and may be identified as

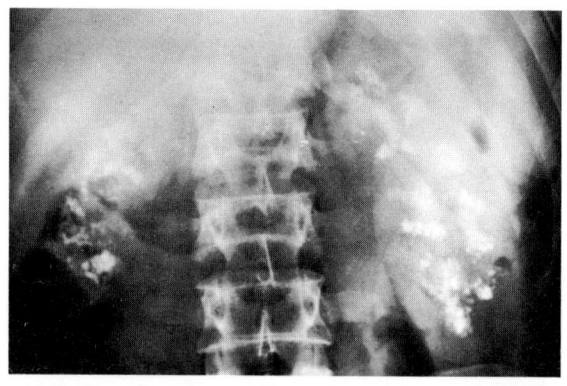

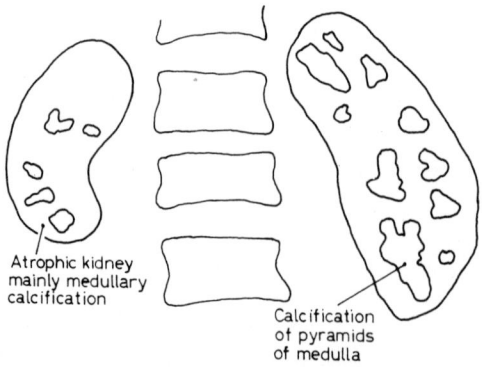

Fig. 4.28

filling defects on the IVP. Calcification scattered through the renal cortex and medulla is termed nephrocalcinosis. Nephrocalcinosis commonly occurs in hypercalcaemia due to vitamin D intoxication, sarcoidosis, hyperparathyroidism, and renal tubular acidosis, to mention a few of the commoner conditions. Fig. 4.28 shows a typical example of nephrocalcinosis. Occasionally, one sees renal calculi scattered through the papillary areas of the medulla; IVP discloses grape like clusters of distended collecting ducts in which there may be calculi. This condition is known as medullary sponge kidney and is a rare developmental anomaly.

Question Are cystine stones radio-opaque?

Answer 1. Yes. Go on to **4.36**.
2. No. Go on to **4.35**.

4.29 Your answer – if 2 of the pyramids are distorted under a localised area of cortical thinning the patient has obstructive disease of the urinary pathways.

You are not correct. In obstructive disease all the pyramids are flattened, not just 2, and the cortical thinning is not patchy and localised. Read **4.25** again.

4.30 Your answer – localised distortion of pyramids and overlying cortex is most likely to be due to chronic pyelonephritis.

You are correct. In about half the cases of chronic pyelonephritis vesico-ureteric reflux is present, i.e. urine passes from the bladder retrogradely up one or both ureters on micturition. This is obviously important from the point of view of the aetiology and pathogenesis of chronic pyelonephritis. Occasionally, in a patient who has a bladder full of opaque dye but none visible in the ureters 40 minutes after the injection of contrast medium during an IVP, reflux from bladder to ureters can be shown on micturition. Usually, however, it is necessary to place contrast medium in the bladder via a catheter to demonstrate vesico-ureteric reflux in the micturating cystogram. This procedure is done with a full sterile technique but there is the ever-present risk of introducing organisms capable of causing acute pyelonephritis because of the instrumentation procedure. Micturating cystography has shown that vesico-ureteric reflux is by no means constant in any one patient, varying from time to time, thus vitiating much of the theoretical benefit one would expect to accrue from the surgical correction of vesico-ureteric reflux in pyelonephritis. Reflux is common in children with pyelonephritis.

Question In what condition does vesico-ureteric reflux occur?

Answer 1. Pyelonephritis. Go on to **4.28**.
2. Hydronephrosis. Go on to **4.32**.
3. Don't know. Go on to **4.34**.

4.31 Your answer – if 2 of the pyramids are distorted with a localised overlying area of cortical thinning there is ischaemic kidney disease present.

You are only partly correct. In pyelonephritis there is frequently some vascular disease, but in pure vascular disease the pyramids under areas of cortical thinning are not distorted. Go on to **4.30**.

4.32 Your answer – vesico-ureteric reflux occurs in hydronephrosis.

Vesico-ureteric reflux can occur in hydronephrosis as well as in normal people, but it is mainly of importance in the aetiology of pyelonephritis. Read **4.30** again.

4.33 Your answer – the hydronephrosis and hydroureter of pregnancy are hormonal in origin.

You are correct.

Now let us consider retrograde pyelograms. Retrograde pyelograms require that the patient be cystoscoped and ureteric catheters inserted into the ureters; radio-opaque material is then injected through the catheters to fill the renal pelvis. The size and shape of the renal pelvis can be seen very clearly on retrograde pyelograms irrespective of the state of renal function. The disadvantages of retrograde pyelography are:

(1) Infection may be introduced by cystoscopy and ureteric catheterisation resulting in pyelitis, pyelonephritis, and cystitis.

(2) Cystoscopy is often painful, unless spinal or general anaesthesia is used. Local anaesthesia has more champions amongst urologists than among their patients.

(3) Some authorities, notably Hamburger of Paris, advise against retrograde pyelography in acute renal failure, although we have seen no ill effects from its occasional use in our anuric patients.

Careful retrograde pyelographic examination will show details of all the calyces, provided the patient is positioned carefully. It should be borne in mind that the pyelographic contrast media sink to the lowest position in the renal pelvis due to their high density compared with urine, and the patient will need positioning to show all the groups of calyces. If over-distention of the calyces is carried out, contrast medium will be seen leaking back through the kidney substance into the renal veins and renal lymphatics; this is known as pyelo-venous and pyelo-lymphatic back flow and is of no clinical significance.

The main indications for retrograde pyelograms are urological.

(1) Diagnosis of obstruction to ureters and pelvic-calyceal system.
(2) Stones in kidney or ureters.
(3) Tumours.
(4) Pyelonephritis and necrotising papillitis.
(5) Investigation of non-functioning kidney.
(6) Anuria.

Further consideration of this important method of examination of the renal tract will not be made here; it is dealt with fully in textbooks of urological surgery.

Question If a patient has anuria which may be due to ureteric obstruction by stones, which investigation would you carry out to establish the diagnosis?

Answer 1. Intravenous pyelography. Go on to **4.37**.
2. Retrograde pyelography. Go on to **4.40**.

4.34 Your answer – I don't know in what condition vesico-ureteric reflux occurs. In a small proportion of normal people reflux of urine from bladder to ureters occurs, but this occurs in a high percentage (50 per cent) in some published series of pyelonephritis. If organisms gain entry to the bladder in a person with vesico-ureteric reflux, the infection can readily reach the pelvis of the kidneys through the reflux of infected urine, and so cause pyelitis and pyelonephritis. Read **4.30** more carefully and answer the question again.

4.35 Your answer – cystine stones are not radio-opaque.
You are wrong. Cystine stones are radio-opaque although few physicians realise this. Go back and read **4.28** properly.

4.36 Your answer – cystine stones are radio-opaque.
You are correct. Hydronephrosis may occur without obvious obstruction to the urinary pathways; in pregnancy hydronephrosis and hydroureter are the rule and the resultant urinary stasis may be partly responsible for the frequency of urinary tract infections in pregnancy. The hydronephrosis and hydroureters may persist for up to six months after the end of pregnancy. The cause of the hydronephrosis in pregnancy is probably hormonal, this being suggested by experiments in which rats given progestogenic substances developed hydronephrosis. The hydronephrosis of pregnancy is unlikely to be due to mechanical obstruction of the ureters because the ureteric dilatation commences before the uterus is large enough to cause ureteric obstruction. Intravenous pyelography should be avoided in pregnancy wherever possible because of the possible dangers of irradiation to the foetus.

In diabetes insipidus of pituitary origin hydronephrosis sometimes occurs for unknown reasons; this should not be confused with *renal* diabetes insipidus following hydronephrosis, where the diabetes insipidus is due to damage to the concentration mechanism caused *by* the hydronephrosis or associated pyelonephritis.

Duplex ureters are a common developmental anomaly often diagnosed by intravenous pyelography and frequently associated with urinary tract infections and hypertension. This will be discussed later in the chapter on congenital anomalies.

Question Why does hydronephrosis develop in pregnancy?

Answer 1. Hormonal causes. Go on to **4.33**.
2. Obstruction of ureters by the gravid uterus. Go on to **4.39**.

4.37 Your answer − IVP would establish if the patient had anuria due to stone impacted in the ureter.

You are wrong. IVP should never be carried out in the anuric subject for the contrast medium cannot be excreted. Read **4.33** again without day-dreaming.

4.38 Your answer − the transfemoral route is the safer.

You are correct. Several types of renal artery stenosis are demonstrable on renal arteriography. There may be an atheromatous plaque at the commencement of the renal artery, occluding the mouth of the artery where it enters the aorta; there may be a fibroelastic constriction close to the aorta or anywhere on the renal artery; and there is frequently a post-stenotic dilatation. In young people the renal artery is sometimes seen to have a beaded appearance due to fibromuscular hyperplasia running along the entire length of the renal artery; this anomaly is sometimes bilateral. Fig. 4.38 illustrates an atheromatous renal artery stenosis. Look at the state of the aorta from which the renal artery opens − it is irregular due to the atheroma present.

Renal artery occlusion may rarely be caused by an embolus in sub-acute bacterial endocarditis or by a detached mural thrombus following myocardial infarction; if the occlusion is complete, the renal artery does not fill distal to the obstruction.

In hypernephromas the blood vessels of the neoplasm can usually be seen clearly: this appearance is diagnostic. In contrast, innocent cysts appear on all films to be quite devoid of vascularity; unfortunately, the occasional hyperne-

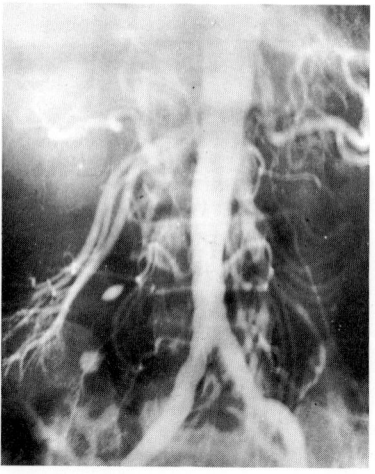

Fig. 4.38

phroma has no tumour vessel filling, so that absence of vascularity does not rule out neoplasm absolutely.

Question What does a beaded appearance of the renal artery in a young person suggest?

Answer 1. Atheroma. Go on to **4.43**.
2. Fibro-muscular hyperplasia. Go on to **4.44**.

4.39 Your answer – the hydronephrosis of pregnancy is caused by obstruction of the ureters by the gravid uterus.

You are wrong, in that it is unlikely that there is any ureteric obstruction. The ureters dilate long before the uterus is enlarged, and it has been shown in rats that administration of progestogens causes hydronephrosis, suggesting that female sex hormones are responsible for the dilatation of the uterus.

Now answer the question at the end of **4.36** correctly.

4.40 Your answer – retrograde pyelography would demonstrate the cause of anuria due to ureteric blockage by stones.

You are correct. Often the passage of a catheter up the affected ureter releases a gush of urine when the stone is pushed back into the distended portion of the ureter proximal to the obstruction. Usually the other kidney is non-functioning due to long standing disease which may not necessarily be calculous in type.

Renal arteriograms are a valuable diagnostic investigation. The technique as usually practised today is known as transfemoral renal arteriography: it is carried out by passing a catheter through the femoral artery and up into the aorta up to the mouths of the renal arteries into which injections of contrast medium can be given selectively. The main bug-bear of the earlier techniques of renal arteriography by transaortic puncture through the lumbar region was the occurrence of dissection of the aortic coats. This complication is virtually unknown in the transfemoral route of approach where the main danger is a femoral haematoma. Occasional patients develop anuria due to tubular necrosis after aortography by any route, and it is an investigation which should not be undertaken lightly. The principal indications for renal arteriograms are:

(1) Hypertension in patients below 35 or above 55 years of age. In the older age group of patients a high proportion will be found to have renal artery stenosis, but so will a large proportion of normotensive elderly people.

(2) Renal tumours. Tumour vessels can be seen in most hypernephromas.

(3) Renal cysts. These appear as an avascular shadow unless malignant.

(4) Pyelonephritis and hypertension. In chronic pyelonephritis there is a moth-eaten appearance due to patchy ischaemia of the cortex.

(5) Visualisation of renal arteries before operation (i.e., for relief of hydronephrosis caused by aberrant renal arteries).

There are three principal phases to be looked for on a renal arteriogram.

(1) *The arterial phase*, in which the entire arterial tree is visible from the main renal arteries to the cortical arterioles.

(2) *Nephrogram phase*, in which the blush of kidney tissue is clearly visible indicating filling of the capillaries and tubules.

(3) *Venous phase*. This phase is more difficult to distinguish and occurs when the venous channels are filling. It is rarely seen on routine examinations.

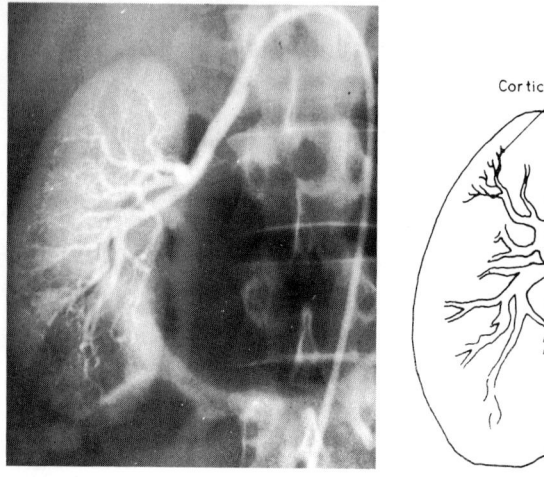

Fig. 4.40(a)

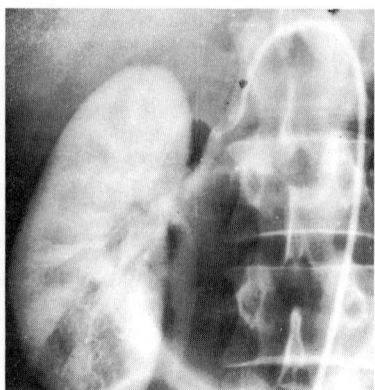

Fig. 4.40(b)

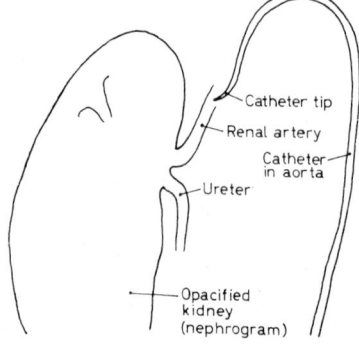

The first two phases are shown in Fig. 4.40 a & b. Look at the photographs and drawings.
Now answer the question.

Question Is retrograde renal arteriography through the femoral arteries safer than the lumbar transaortic method?

Answer 1. Yes. Go on to **4.38**.
2. No. Go on to **4.41**.
3. Don't know. Go on to **4.42**.

4.41 Your answer – retrograde percutaneous transfemoral renal arteriography is not safer than transaortic puncture.
You are wrong. Read **4.40** again.

4.42 Your answer – I don't know which is safer, the lumbar transaortic method or retrograde transfemoral renal arteriography.
The transaortic method involves putting a needle through the aortic wall. If the needle point moves back into one of the coats of the aortic wall during the injection, dissection of the aorta can result. This is very unlikely to happen with a catheter passed up from the femoral artery into the aorta. Now answer the question at the end of **4.40** again.

4.43 Your answer – a beaded appearance of the renal artery in a young person suggests atheroma.
It does not. A beaded appearance is not due to atheroma which gives a very irregular appearance, but to fibro-muscular hyperplasia. Answer the question at the end of **4.38** correctly.

4.44 Your answer – the beaded appearance of the renal arteries is due to fibromuscular hyperplasia.
You are correct. The next major type of renal investigation is renal biopsy. Renal biopsy has become widely used in the past 20 years and has resulted in considerable advances in our knowledge of the natural history of renal disease. In addition, it is a valuable diagnostic tool in the individual patient. There are two types of renal biopsy – percutaneous and open surgical biopsy.
(1) *Percutaneous:* this method can be done in a hospital ward. The patient lies prone. Local anaesthesia is used; the site of the biopsy is over the renal angle, below the 12th rib lateral to the erector spinae muscles. The site of the kidney is located with a thin lumbar puncture needle, the hub of the neddle moving cephalad with inspiration when the tip of the needle is in the kidney; the biopsy itself, commonly a Franklin modified Vim-Silverman needle (see Fig. 4.44) is then inserted and the biopsy taken. The complications of percutaneous biopsy are:

(a) Haemorrhage, early or delayed.
(b) Pain.
(c) Infection.
(d) Damage to one of the adjacent organs: the liver is the commonest organ biopsied in error, but colon, duodenum, adrenal, spleen and pancreas may be damaged.

Some physicians use image intensifyer X-ray machines during biopsy to locate the lower pole of the kidney and avoid complications (a) and (d) as well as to increase the chances of getting a successful biopsy.

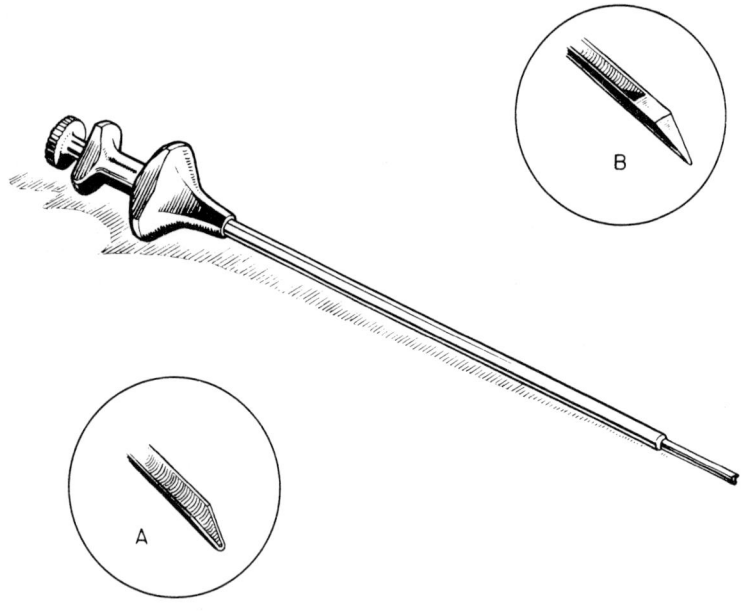

A: Cutting prong tips before modification
B: Tips after modification; note bevelled tip filled with silver solder (Franklin modification)

Fig. 4.44

(2) *Open surgical biopsy:* this is a more formidable surgical procedure but the actual site of biopsy can be selected by inspection, and bleeding from the kidney can be stopped by standard techniques of surgical haemostasis before the wound is sutured. Usually a general anaesthetic is used, but some physicians expose the kidney under local anaesthesia and then use a modified Vim-Silverman needle to take the biopsy rather than the standard surgical wedge.

Question Which type of renal biopsy is least likely to lead to biopsy of the wrong organ?
Answer 1. Percutaneous. Go on to **4.45**.
2. Open surgical biopsy. Go on to **4.46**.

4.45 Your answer – percutaneous renal biopsy is less likely to lead to biopsy of the wrong organ.

Percutaneous biopsy of the kidney is a blind procedure: the method of identifying kidney position is through respiratory movements of the kidney but this movement is also produced by liver and stomach. The position of the kidney should always be checked on an IVP before the biopsy. Other methods of determining the position of the kidney include:

(1) Biopsy on the X-ray table after IVP using a reference grid marked on the skin to help localise the kidney position.

(2) Radioactive mercurial diuretics can be given before the biopsy and the position of the kidneys assessed by their radioactivity.

(3) Ultrasonic methods may be used to detect kidney position.

It is now obvious therefore that inspection of the kidney at open surgical operation will result in fewer biopsies of the wrong organ than percutaneous biopsy. Go back and answer the question at the end of **4.44** correctly.

4.46 Your answer – open biopsy of the kidney results in fewer biopsies of the wrong organ. You are correct. Percutaneous renal biopsy is a blind procedure, and an IVP or tomograms of the kidney position should always be consulted before the biopsy is done. There are sophisticated methods of finding the kidney position in percutaneous renal biopsy:

(1) Using a reference grid on the skin at the time of IVP to correlate the position of the kidneys with skin marks and biopsying the patient on the X-ray table immediately afterwards.

(2) Giving intravenous radioactive mercurials and assessing the kidney position by means of their radioactivity.

(3) Ultrasonic echo sounding (similar to that used in detecting flaws in metals) can outline the position and depth of the kidneys.

The main argument in favour of open surgical biopsy is the safety of the procedure from the point of view of adequate haemostasis. In percutaneous biopsy, bleeding is common after biopsy, but is rarely serious. On the whole, percutaneous biopsy is the more convenient of the two methods and further discussion will be limited to the percutaneous technique.

The indications for percutaneous biopsy are:

(1) *Anuria*. In patients who are anuric and in whom there is no obstruction of the urinary pathways, biopsy should be carried out after the second dialysis to determine if there is any justification in dialysing any further. If acute tubular

necrosis is found on biopsy, dialysis should be continued in the knowledge that within the next few weeks recovery is likely. If oligo-anuric acute nephritis, cortical necrosis or renal infarction is found there is little point in dialysing for more than 50 days unless the patient is considered for a chronic haemodialytic programme or for renal transplantation.

Question What condition could you diagnose by renal biopsy in an anuric patient in which you could be confident of ultimate renal recovery.

Answer 1. Acute tubular necrosis. Go on to **4.48**.
2. Acute glomerulonephritis. Go on to **4.50**.
3. Total renal infarction. Go on to **4.47**.
4. Cortical necrosis. Go on to **4.52**.

4.47 Your answer – patients with total renal infarction can be confidently expected to recover from anuria. You are wrong. If both kidneys are totally infarcted or one is infarcted and the other absent or diseased, recovery is not possible. Read **4.46** again.

4.48 Your answer – in acute tubular necrosis the patient should recover from the anuria if properly managed.

You are correct. Now let us return to the indications for renal biopsy.

(1) **Anuria** – already discussed.

(2) **Nephrotic syndrome.** There are many causes of nephrotic syndrome, which are discussed later, in the chapter on nephrotic syndrome. Renal biopsy is particularly valuable in the diagnosis of all causes of nephrotic syndrome including membrano-proliferative (mesangio-capillary) glomerulonephritis, lipoid nephrosis without light microscopic change, amyloid, diabetes, systemic lupus erythematosus, focal glomerulonephritis, renal vein thrombosis, congestive heart failure, malignant hypertension, renal artery stenosis, quartan malaria, mercurial diuretics, troxidone, penicillamine, potassium chlorate, and other drugs.

(3) **Investigation of asymptomatic proteinuria.** Patients are frequently found to have proteinuria (which is not orthostatic or postural) on medical examination for life insurance. Renal biopsy is likely to lead to the correct diagnosis, which may be chronic glomerulonephritis, pyelonephritis, systemic lupus erythematosus, membranous glomerulonephritis, or focal glomerulonephritis; occasionally nothing abnormal is demonstrated.

(4) **Investigating the natural history of a disease.** This is purely a research procedure but it has yielded valuable information in our understanding of several renal diseases, notably lupus erythematosus, diabetes and glomerulonephritis.

Question In a patient with nephrotic syndrome is it possible to make a diagnosis of systemic lupus erythematosus by renal biopsy?

Answer 1. Yes. Go on to **4.49**.
2. No, Go on to **4.53**.
3. Don't know. Go on to **4.55**.

4.49 Your answer — it is possible to make a diagnosis of systemic lupus erythematosus by means of renal biopsy in a patient presenting with nephrotic syndrome.

You are correct. Renal biopsy should only be carried out if the following conditions can be met.

(1) No bleeding tendency should be present.

(2) Hypertension should be controlled so that the diastolic blood pressure is below 110 mm Hg.

(3) Both kidneys should be functioning. A biopsy by the percutaneous route should *never* be carried out on a solitary functioning kidney.

(4) No renal tumour, tuberculosis or pyonephrosis is suspected.

(5) Some investigators will not biopsy a uraemic or hypertensive patient because of the dangers of bleeding. If the hypertension is controlled this is a less likely cause of concern, but in uraemia there is frequently a bleeding tendency which may require dialysis before the biopsy, to prevent bleeding later.

No biopsy should be attempted without IVP and/or tomograms of both kidneys and 2 pints of blood should be cross matched first in case of bleeding. After the biopsy there is always danger of bleeding and 'clot colic' may result due to clots in the renal pelvis and ureter. Frank haematuria occurs in 10 per cent of patients so that unless the patient is anuric he should be given extra fluids orally to dilute the blood in the urine and prevent clot colic. His pulse and blood pressure should be recorded hourly for 24 hours to detect bleeding. Severe pain usually indicates a perirenal haematoma and pethidine may be needed for its control. Fatal bleeding usually occurs within 3 days of the biopsy. Percutaneous biopsies have a mortality of less than 1 per 1000. The success rate is about 95 per cent.

Question What does severe pain following a biopsy often indicate?

Answer 1. Perirenal bleeding. Go on to **4.57**.
2. Peritonitis. Go on to **4.58**.
3. Don't know. Go on to **4.59**.

4.50 Your answer — ultimate recovery can be expected in acute glomerulonephritis causing anuria.

You are probably wrong, if the anuria has persisted for longer than 7 weeks, the vast majority die although the occasional patient recovers. Read **4.46** again.

4.51 Your answer — the radioactive scintillogram defines the position and size of the kidneys.

Correct. Now read the following statements carefully. Pick the answers you think are correct with great care: an incorrect answer may disclose sufficient lack of understanding of basic points to require you to start working through the chapter again.

Statement 1 Granular casts indicate some renal abnormality.

Statement 2 Unmodified IVP should never be carried out with a blood urea level of 100 mg/100 ml.

Statement 3 Percutaneous renal biopsy is indicated in hypernephroma.

Answer
1. All statements are correct. Go on to **4.54**.
2. All statements are false. Go on to **4.56**.
3. 1 is correct, 2 and 3 are false. Go on to **4.60**.
4. 2 is correct, 1 and 3 are false. Go on to **4.62**.
5. 3 is correct, 1 and 2 are false. Go on to **4.63**.
6. 1 and 2 are correct, 3 is false. Go on to **4.64**.
7. 2 and 3 are correct, 1 is false. Go on to **4.65**.
8. 1 and 3 are correct, 2 is false. Go on to **4.66**.

4.52 Your answer – in cortical necrosis there will be recovery from anuria.

You are wrong; occasional patients survive renal cortical necrosis, but the overwhelming majority succumb. Read **4.46** again.

4.53 Your answer – renal biopsy cannot make the diagnosis of systemic lupus erythematosus in nephrotic syndrome.

You are wrong. Read **4.48** again paying particular attention to the nephrotic syndrome paragraph. Then answer the question correctly.

4.54 Your answer – all the statements are correct. You are wrong about statement 3, correct about 1 and 2. Percutaneous renal biopsy should never be done if a tumour is suspected lest the tumour cells be disseminated and implanted in the needle track. Go back to **4.49** and work on from there.

4.55 Your answer – I don't know if systemic lupus erythematosus can be diagnosed by renal biopsy in a case of nephrotic syndrome.

If you don't know you have not concentrated while you were reading **4.48**. Read it again properly. If you are being distracted either move to less distracting surroundings or stop reading. In no circumstances should you deceive yourself that you are learning when you are really wasting your time.

4.56 Your answer – all the statements are false. You are correct only with regard to statement no. 3. You are wrong about 1 and 2. Start at **4.1** again and work through the paragraphs. You have not as yet learned the contents well enough to proceed to the next chapter.

4.57 Your answer – severe pain after biopsy may indicate perirenal bleeding.

You are correct. A useful diagnostic method which is gaining popularity in the investigation of renal diseases is the radioactive scintillogram. This is based on the principle that radioactive materials which are selectively concentrated by the kidney such as ^{203}Hg chlormerhydrin or ^{131}I hippuran emit γ radiation which passes through the skin overlying the kidneys. This radiation can be detected by a probe moving rapidly over the back and converted by the use of appropriate amplifiers to vary the brightness of a bulb moving linearly over film, so that where the probe picks up much radioactivity the film will be exposed in the corresponding area and to a corresponding degree. If there is no radioactivity the film will not be exposed in that area. If the entire back over the renal areas is scanned after radioactive mercurial diuretics, the kidney size and shape will appear on the film in much the same manner as the thyroid outlines in a scinitllogram after ^{131}I is given. In the renal scintillogram (see Fig. 4.57) the position, shape of the kidneys, size and presence of tumours, cysts and infarcts can be determined with accuracy. Alternatively the gamma ray camera can be used to pick up the radioactive scintillations directly and rapidly. The major disadvantage of both methods at present is the high cost of the apparatus; if the apparatus is available it enables the urologist particularly to diagnose renal masses rapidly and safely without the dangers of aortography.

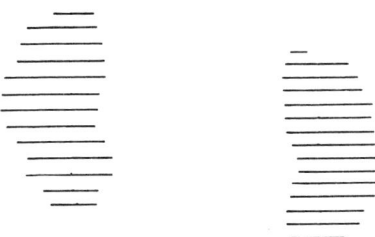

Fig. 4.57

Question Can a renal scintillogram define the position and size of the kidneys?

Answer 1. Yes. Go on to **4.51**.
2. No. Go on to **4.61**.

4.58 Your answer – pain indicates peritonitis. You are partly correct, but peritonitis rarely follows renal biopsy whereas bleeding is much more fequent. Read

4.49 again and answer the question correctly.

4.59 Your answer – I don't know what severe pain after a renal biopsy may indicate.

If you do not know you have not read **4.49** carefully. Read it again paying more attention. Don't forget that you can't day dream through a paragraph and expect to know its contents afterwards.

4.60 Your answer – 1 is correct; 2 and 3 are false.

You are wrong about statement 2. The IVP will not produce a renal shadow if the blood urea is above 100 mg/100 ml; moreover there may be some increase in the risk of doing an IVP if the patient is uraemic due to the delayed excretion of the potentially hazardous contrast medium. Now answer the question in **4.51** again.

4.61 Your answer – a renal scintillogram cannot define the position and size of the kidneys.

You are wrong. Read **4.57** again bearing in mind that the scintillogram will pick up γ rays from all renal tissues concentrating the radioactive mercurial compound.

4.62 Your answer – only statement 2 is correct.

You are wrong about granular casts. Work through the paragraphs from **4.1** until you think that you can answer the question in **4.51** correctly.

4.63 Your answer – statement 3 is correct. 1 and 2 are false.

You are quite wrong. You have retained none of the information you have been questioned about. Go back to **4.1** and work through the chapter again.

4.64 Your answer – statement 3 is false, the rest are true.

You are correct. You can now move on to the next chapter.

There are excellent colour illustrations of urine sediment stained by Sternheimer-Malbin technique in Blegen E., Enger E., Øystein W., Tidsskrift for Den norske laegeforening, 761, 1967.

Books for further reading are:
Hodson's chapter on Radiology of the Kidney in Black's Renal Disease, Blackwell, 1967, edited by D. A. K. Black.
Renal Radiology (Volume 5) of Urology Encyclopaedia. Springer, 1962.
Lippman, R. W. (1971). Urine and the Urinary Sediment. Springfield, Thomas.
Weller J. M. and Greene J. A. Examination of the urine, a programmed text.
    Appleton-Century-Croftes, New York, 1966.

4.65 Your answer — statement 1 is false, 2 and 3 are true.

Statement 1 is true and 3 is false. Start reading through the chapter again from **4.1**. Otherwise, you have so far wasted your time reading this chapter without remembering its contents.

4.66 Your answer — statement 2 only is false.

You are wrong. Only 3 is false. Read **4.20** again and work on through the chapter from there.

Time for this chapter: 55 minutes

Chapter 5
Glomerulonephritis

5.1 In this chapter the disease first discussed will be acute glomerulonephritis (AGN). In the classification of Longcope this is known as Type A and in the Ellis classification it is known as acute type I nephritis. Before going on to define the clinical features we shall first consider the aetiology of the disease. The majority of cases of AGN follow streptococcal infections commonly of the orophrynx but occasionally of the skin. The organism implicate in these infections is a Group A haemolytic streptococcus of a fairly circumscribed number of types. Type 12 is the commonest but infections with types 1, 4, 6, 23, and 49 (Red Lake) may also lead to the development of acute glomerulonephritis. It should be made clear that not all type 12 streptococci can cause nephritis, and that occasionally type 12 organisms may not cause haemolysis on a blood agar plate; thus the organisms may be missed in a routine laboratory if haemolytic colonies are being sought and the others ignored. This is possibly responsible for some of the group of AGN not preceded by an apparent haemolytic streptococcal infection, although there are grounds to suppose that some infections of viral origin may lead to AGN, such as mumps virus, Coxsackie virus and hepatitis virus, to name a few of the better documented virus causes.

Question What type of Group A haemolytic streptococci gives rise most frequently to acute glomerulonephritis?

Answer 1. Type 4. Go on to **5.2**.
2. Type 12. Go on to **5.3**.
3. Don't know. Go on to **5.4**.

5.2 Your answer – Type 4 infections give rise most frequently to AGN.

Wrong. Type 4 infections are frequently nephritogenic but type 12 is by far the commonest type to be found in AGN. Now answer the question at the end of **5.1** again correctly.

5.3 Your answer – type 12 causes AGN most frequently.

Good. The next point to be raised is how often does infection with a type 12 strain cause acute nephritis? The figures vary widely from epidemic to epidemic but the range 2 per cent to 30 per cent seems to cover most of the patients developing evidence of AGN after a type 12 infection. Obviously, the susceptibility of the patient must play some part, although the degree of nephrotoxicity of the type 12 organism may vary from one epidemic to the other. Many of these infections have been studied by Rammelkamp in epidemics affecting American servicemen.

He found that if there was microscopic haematuria at the height of the streptococcal infection about 1 in 4 developed acute nephritis later, whereas of those without red cells in the urine at the height of the infection only 1 in 20 developed acute nephritis. Acute nephritis follows a streptococcal infection within 10 days in most patients, whereas rheumatic fever has a much longer latent period – 18 days. In patients who develop high antistreptolysin titres after a type 12 infection, the incidence of AGN is greater than in those without high antibody titres.

Question A man of 23 is found to have microscopic haematuria at the height of a throat infection with type 12 streptococci. What are his chances of developing AGN within the next two or three weeks?

Answer 1. About 1 in 4. Go on to **5.5**.
2. About 1 in 20. Go on to **5.6**.

5.4 Your answer – I don't know what type of Group A haemolytic streptococci gives rise most frequently to AGN.

Well, you can't have been reading **5.1** with enough care. As you have just started this chapter you should be able to concentrate properly at this stage, so start reading **5.1** again and choose the correct answer next time.

5.5 Your answer – 1 in 4 patients with haematuria at the height of the infection develop subsequent acute glomerulonephritis.

Quite right. The pathogenesis of AGN has been the subject of many investigations. The major facts uncovered are as follows:

(1) Complement fraction C^1_3 falls to a very low level in AGN: this indicates that some immune reaction is occurring in which C^1_3 is used.

(2) Antibodies to renal tissue are found in the circulation in AGN.

(3) The antigen in acute post-streptococcal glomerulonephritis is a soluble protein which has been isolated from the cell wall of the β haemolytic streptococcus.

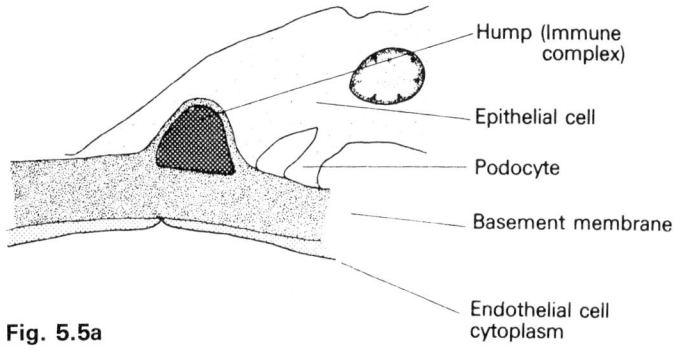

Fig. 5.5a

The combination antigen-complement-antibody takes place on the epithelial side of the basement membrane. These antigen-complement-antibody agregates appear as humps on electron microscopy. Look at figure 5.5a. Notice how the humps are discrete masses on the epithelial side of the glomerular basement membrane.

Now look at figure 5.5b. This is a glomerulus stained with fluorescent anti-IgG by Coon's technique. It shows a granular deposition of IgG, the common finding in acute post-streptococcal glomerulonephritis. The major animal studies dealing with the relationship of streptococci to AGN are:

(1) Cavelti and Cavelti produced glomerular lesions in rats by injections of

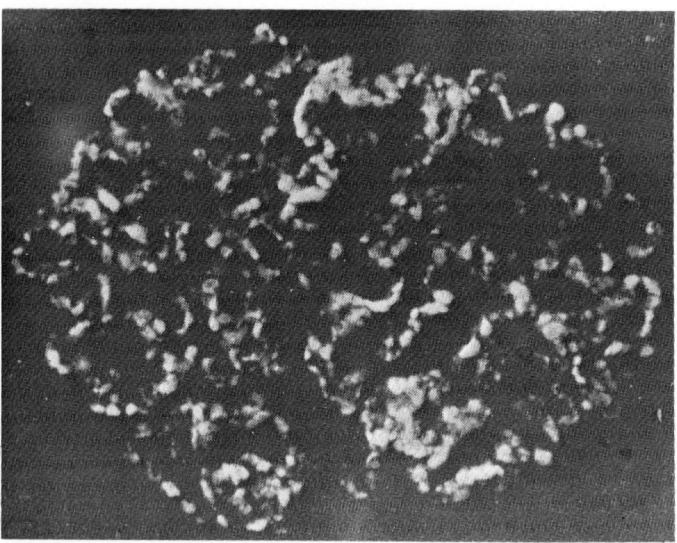

Fig. 5.5b

rat kidney homogenates mixed with killed Group A haemolytic streptococci: the streptococci were thought to render the rat kidney tissue 'auto-antigenic' and so antibodies were produced to kidney which attacked the recipient rat's kidneys.

(2) In mice, type 12 haemolytic streptococci were placed in intraperitoneal plastic diffusion chambers which permitted diffusion into the mice of soluble products only. Renal lesions developed 7 days after the inoculation and did not occur with other types of streptococci.

(3) Streptococcal proteins can be detected by fluorescent antibody tech-

niques in the renal glomeruli and tubules after intravenous injection of Group A streptococci.

Now answer the question.

Question Of what is the electron microscope hump on the epithelial side of the basement membrane composed?

Answer 1. Soluble streptococcal antigen. Go on to **5.7**.
2. Antigen-antibody-complement protein aggregate. Go on to **5.8**.

5.6 Your answer – 1 in 20 of the patients who develop microscopic haematuria at the height of the infection develop subsequent AGN.

You have misread the contents of **5.3**. Read it again and answer the question correctly.

5.7 Your answer – The hump consists of soluble streptococcal antigen. You are incorrect. It is likely that the streptococcal antigen has some antigenic properties similar to those of the glomerular basement membrane, so that the latter is the site of deposition of antibody-antigen-complement complex, the antibody being IgG most frequently. The humps consist of this complex. Now reread **5.5** again, and then answer the question after having digested the facts in the paragraph. Remember that you are still at the beginning of the chapter, and if you cannot concentrate, stop work and remove the distracting influences from the environment, or yourself from them.

5.8 Your answer – The hump consists of antigen-antibody-complement protein aggregates. You are correct. Now in acute glomerulonephritis, one of the striking features, as we shall see later, is the deposition of polymophonuclear leucocytes in the glomeruli. On electron microscopy the polymorphs are seen close to the basement membrane on the endothelial side, inside the capillary lumen. It is thought that the polymorphs are chemotactically attracted to the basement membrane, probably attracted by changes induced locally by antigen-antibody-complement complexes. This is an example of 'immune complex' glomerulonephritis. Lupus nephritis is also an 'immune complex' nephritis. In acute glomerulonephritis there is an increase in the excretion of fibrin-split products in the urine. Fibrin-split products come from fibrin or fibrinogen in the glomeruli, and in acute glomerulonephritis it is known that there is an increase in intraglomerular fibrin deposition. In some cases this may contribute to the production of renal failure.

There are also other types of antibody deposits detected in other forms of renal disease. The presence of anti-basement membrane antibodies is indicated by the appearance of smooth linear fluorescence in the glomeruli using the fluorescent antibody technique. The fluorescence outlines the capillary loops, the antibodies adhering to the outlining the basement membrane of the glomerular capillary loops. Look at figure 5.8 and compare it to figure 5.5a. Note the different patterns. Linear fluorescence occurs in several diseases; lipoid nephrosis (no light microscopic change); some cases of membranous glomerulonephritis, and in Goodpasture's syndrome. In Goodpasture's syndrome there are anti-basement-membrane antibodies which react with both pulmonary and glomerular basement membranes.

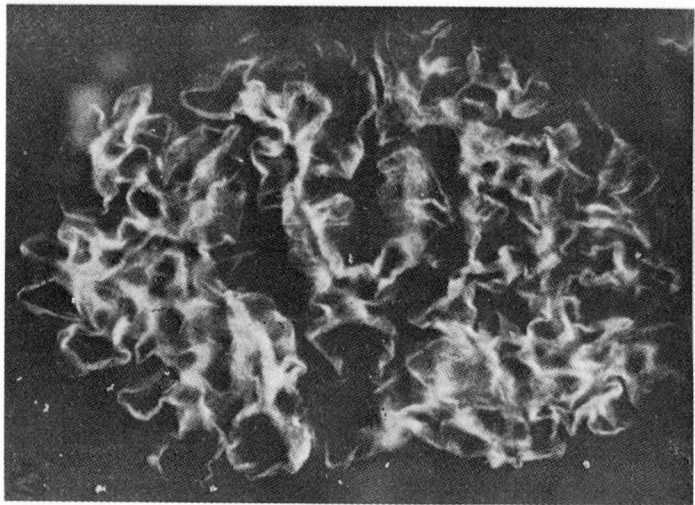

Fig. 5.8

Question Is AGN an immune-complex disease or an antiglomerular basement membrane (GBM) antibody disease.

Answer 1. Immune complex. Go on to **5.9**.
        2. Anti GBM. Go on to **5.10**.

5.9 Your answer – AGN is an immune complex disease. You are correct. Now answer the following question.

Question If you did not know whether a patient had acute nephritis or essential malignant hypertension and the serum complement C^1_3 level was found to be very low which of the two diagnoses would you choose?

Answer 1. Malignant hypertension. Go on to **5.11**.
        2. Acute nephritis. Go on to **5.12**.

5.10 Your answer — AGN is an anti GBM disease. Read **5.8** again.

5.11 Your answer — if complement C^1_3 concentration was low the patient would be more likely to have malignant hypertension. No. In AGN as well as in systemic lupus erythematosus (SLE) complement is consumed in an immunological reaction and so the plasma level of complement tends to be low in AGN and SLE. Now choose the correct answer to the question in **5.8**.

5.12 Your answer — if complement fraction C^1_3 is low, the more likely of the two diagnoses is AGN.

Good. Now we shall consider the pertinent facts about the pathology of AGN. First of all, it is a diffuse inflammatory disease involving *all* the glomeruli of both kidneys, as well as the tubules and interstitial tissues. It is important at the outset to realise that AGN may be predominantly a glomerulitis, a tubular nephritis or an interstitial nephritis; usually all three elements are involved, but the glomerular changes are so obvious and so striking that they receive most attention. Let us now examine the glomerular changes. (Look at Fig. 5.12.) The most obvious changes are (1) swelling of the glomerulus which completely fills Bowman's space. (2) The ischaemia of the capillary spaces, which contain few red cells. (3) Increased cellularity of the glomerulus. Endothelial cells are proliferated with swollen cytoplasm and there are numerous polymorphs in the glomerulus — these are rarely found in the normal glomerulus. (4) Mesangial cells are also increased. (5) The macula densa is infiltrated with polymorphs. Now answer the question.

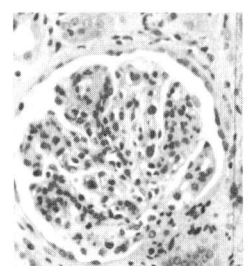 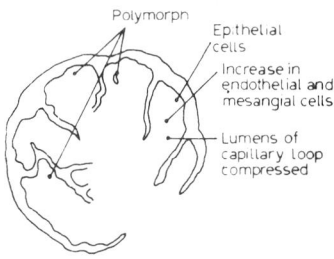

Fig. 5.12

Question Are polymorphs frequently found in the glomeruli in AGN?

Answer 1. Yes. Go on to **5.13**.
2. No. Go on to **5.14**.

5.13 Your answer – polymorphs are frequently found in the glomeruli in AGN. Correct.

The tubular changes of acute glomerulonephritis are less well recognised. In the proximal tubule there are many colloid droplets in the cytoplasm associated with the reabsorption of protein from the proximal tubule. Red blood cells are often found in the proximal tubular lumen. In the loops of Henle there are numerous casts of coagulated protein, the most frequent being red cell casts. In the distal tubule there are polymorphs in the macula densa, with a variety of casts in the lumen – hyaline casts, red cell casts, and haemoglobin casts. Some of the casts erode into the connective tissue surrounding the tubules, and a low-grade inflammatory response may result. In the interstitial tissues there may be an infiltration with polymorphs and lymphocytes, together with a slight separation of the tubules by oedema.

Question What type of cellular cast is commonest in the loop of Henle in AGN?

Answer 1. Red cell casts. Go on to **5.15**.
2. White cell casts. Go on to **5.16**.
3. Tubular cell casts. Go on to **5.17**.

5.14 Your answer – polymorphs are *not* found in the glomeruli of AGN.

One of the few conditions in which polymorphs are found in large numbers in the glomeruli is AGN. Some authorities go as far as stating that these polymorphs are a diagnostic feature in acute *post-streptococcal* glomerulonephritis. Now read **5.12** again and answer the question correctly.

5.15 Your answer – red cell casts are the commonest cast in AGN.

You are correct. We shall now go on to the natural history of AGN as reflected by the pathology of the disease. The majority of cases heal completely, but some continue into the phase of 'subacute glomerulonephritis', to use the classification of Volhard, or Rapidly Progressive Type I nephritis in the Ellis terminology. The clinical course of this will be dealt with in detail later, but at present suffice it to say that hypertension, oedema, proteinuria and microscopic haematuria continue until the patient dies of renal failure or hypertension in 6 to 18 months after the initial attack.

The kidneys are large and pale: histologically (see Fig. 5.15) there are epithelial crescents formed of proliferating capsular epithelial cells from Bowman's capsule which may obliterate a portion of or all of Bowman's space. This process occurs within 2 to 5 weeks of the onset of the acute attack; sometimes the entire glomerulus is crushed and the patient develops anuria if all are so affected. More commonly the crescents cause fibrosis of some glomeruli only, resulting in a loss of nephrons. The remaining tubules hypertrophy. Now answer the question.

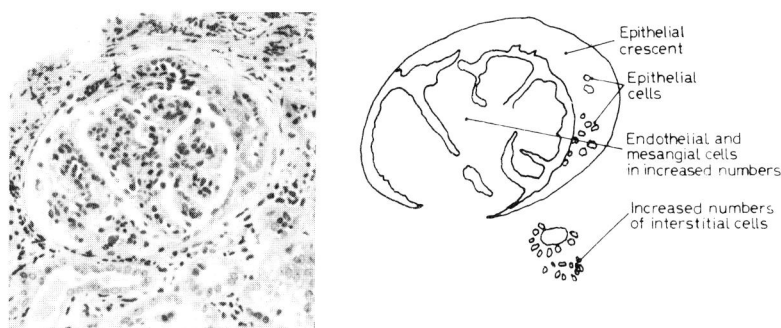

Fig. 5.15

Question What cells form the characteristic crescent in Bowman's space in subacute glomerulonephritis?

Answer 1. Endothelial cells. Go on to **5.18**.
2. Epithelial cells. Go on to **5.19**.
3. Capillaries. Go on to **5.20**.

5.16 Your answer – white cell casts are the commonest cast in AGN.

No. One of the characteristic features of the pathology of the tubular contents in AGN is the presence of red cells in the proximal tubule: in the loop of Henle and beyond the red cells become attached to casts made of precipitated protein, the two together forming red cell casts. Now answer the question in **5.13** properly.

5.17 Your answer – tubular cell casts are the commonest type of cast in AGN.

Red blood cells are prominent in the proximal tubular lumen and as they pass down into the distal tubule they become attached to the casts which are present, forming red cell casts. Tubular casts are *not* prominent in AGN. Now read **5.13** again.

5.18 Your answer – endothelial cells form the characteristic crescent of subacute glomerulonephritis.

Wrong. The crescent is formed from *epithelial* cells which line the parietal surface of Bowman's capsule. Now read **5.15** more carefully.

5.19 Your answer – the crescent is formed from epithelial cells.

You are correct. In some patients the disease tends to go on for years, sometimes with apparent healing and an asymptomatic stage which itself may last up to 20 or more years, to be followed inexorably by renal failure with or without hypertension. This is known as chronic glomerulonephritis or slowly progressive Type I nephritis of Ellis. Often there may be no clinical evidence of activity in the interim, but some patients have persistent proteinuria. These clinical details will be amplified later in the chapter and are intended to provide some facts with which to correlate the pathological findings. The kidneys are small and shrunken, with hyalinised, crowded glomeruli; some tubules are collapsed and other hypertrophied. The glomerular crescents are still present and progress until tiny tubules which form in the crescent become larger and surround the hyalinised glomerulus. Parts of the parietal basement membrane disappear. The hypertrophied tubules are often filled with casts. The interstitium if infiltrated with chronic inflammatory cells. The vessels are the seat of hypertensive change. A typical finding in chronic glomerulonephritis is shown in Fig. 5.19. Look at it and identify the structures.

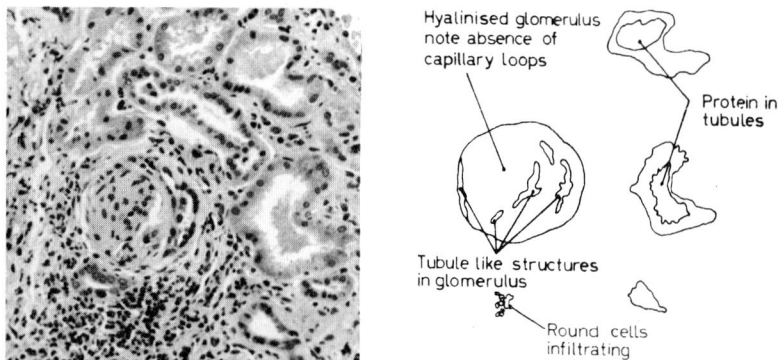

Fig. 5.19

Sometimes there are changes including thickening of the capillary basement membrane in the glomeruli as well as proliferation of glomerular epithelial and mesangical cells. This is known as membrano-proliferative glomerulonephritis, and it responds very poorly to therapy with immunosuppressive or corticosteroid drugs. There is also an associated fall in serum complement levels in many cases.

Question In membrano-proliferative glomerulonephritis with a low serum complement, would you expect an excellent response to immunosuppressive drugs?

Answer 1. No. Go on to **5.23**.
        2. Yes. Go onto **5.21**.
        3. Variable response. Go on to **5.22**.

5.20 Your answer – the crescent is formed from capillaries.
You have not been paying enough attention when reading **5.15**. Look at the figure in **5.15** and note the *epithelial* cells of the crescent coming from Bowman's capsule. Now answer the question at the end of **5.15** again.

5.21 Your answer. There will be a good response to treatment in membranoproliferative glomerulonephritis. No. The response to therapy is usually quite disappointing. You have not paid attention when you read **5.19**. Read it again.

5.22 Your answer. A variable response. You are guessing. Read **5.19** once again, and this time concentrate please.

5.23 Your answer – No. I would *not* expect a good response to immunosuppressive drugs.
You are correct. Let us now turn to the clinical features of AGN. The relationship to a preceding infection, (most frequently of the oropharynx) with Group A haemolytic streptococci of Types 12, 4, 49, 1 or 23 within the previous fortnight has been mentioned. The incidence is greatest between the ages of 3 and 7 but it can develop in children below the age of 2, in contrast to rheumatic fever which very rarely affects children under 2 years of age. Some adults get the disease, but the brunt of the attack falls on school age and pre-school youngsters. Males are affected twice as commonly as females. 80 per cent of the patients have a preceding upper respiratory tract infection, but a few have skin infections such as impetigo. A proportion of cases occur without any apparent preceding streptococcal infection and in one reported series the suggestion was made that the infection precipitating the attack of acute nephritis was viral in origin. It is difficult to be certain about the absence of a preceding streptococcal infection unless very strict care is taken to perform all the antibody tests (such as Antistreptolysin (ASO), antihyalurondose (AH), antistreptokinase (ASK)) repeatedly, as well as culture of the appropriate areas of the patient. It should be borne in mind that the ASO response is reduced by early treatment with antibiotics so that efficient therapy will tend to produce more misleading negative tests for preceding streptococcal infection. The latent period between infection and onset of major symptoms is 8 days in more than 50 per cent of patients, and rarely more than 2 weeks. If the patient is not having the initial attack but is suffering from an acute exacerbation of chronic nephritis, the latent period following exposure to the precipitating factor, be it viral or streptococcal, will be very short – within two or three days at most. The urine may contain red cells and some protein at the height of the fever of the oropharyngeal infection, but these often disappear only to reappear after the latent period.

Question If a man develops typical symptoms of acute nephritis one day after a sore throat, what is the likely diagnosis?

Answer 1. Acute exacerbation of chronic glomerulonephritis. Go on to **5.24**.
2. Acute glomerulonephritis. Go on to **5.25**.
2. Focal nephritis. Go on to **5.26**.

5.24 Your answer – if a man develops symptoms of acute nephritis the day following a sore throat, he probably has an exacerbation of chronic glomerulonephritis.

You are correct. Now let us examine the clinical features of acute glomerulonephritis, the acute Type 1 nephritis of Ellis. The cardinal features are haematuria, oedema, oliguria, hypertension, and proteinuria. There is no fever in an acute attack unless the patient is still suffering from the primary infection such as tonsillitis. The patient may well have forgotten the preceding infection during the latent period, and often goes to bed quite well only to waken the next day with a puffy face, some loin discomfort, and smoky or frankly bloody urine. The reason for the oedema of the face, which is strikingly noticeable periorbitally, is the absence of orthopnoea, which permits the patient to sleep flat, so that the face can become oedematous. In congestive heart failure there is usually sufficient orthopnoea to keep the patient's head propped up so the face is protected from oedema whilst the dependent parts such as the sacrum, genitals, and legs may be grossly distended by oedema fluid. The haematuria may be so mild as to go unnoticed but frequently the patient describes the urine as red, reddish brown, bloodstained, or – if slight haematuria is present – as smoky. The gross haematuria persists for a few days and then gradually disappears; microscopic haematuria may persist for much longer periods, (up to two years), before complete recovery takes place. Now answer the question.

Question Why do patients with acute nephritis develop facial oedema, although this is very uncommon in congestive heart failure?

Answer 1. Because the serum proteins are lower in acute nephritis. Go on to **5.27**.
2. Because the patients lie flat in acute nephritis. Go on to **5.28**.
3. Don't know. Go on to **5.29**.

5.25 Your answer – AGN is the probable diagnosis in a man who develops symptoms of acute nephritis the day after a sore throat.

The latent period between infection and the appearance of acute nephritis is about 8 to 10 days. If the patient has symptoms the day after a sore throat the diagnosis is more likely to be an exacerbation of chronic glomerulonephritis. Read **5.23** again more carefully.

5.26 Your answer – focal nephritis is the probable diagnosis in a man who develops symptoms of acute nephritis the day after a sore throat.

Focal nephritis develops more frequently at the height of an illness than the day after. The most likely diagnosis is an exacerbation of chronic glomerulonephritis. Read **5.23** again and answer the question correctly.

5.27 Your answer – facial oedema is more common in acute glomerulonephritis because the serum proteins are lower than in congestive heart failure.

No. This is not the cause of the facial oedema in acute nephritis as opposed to congestive heart failure. The obvious cause is the initial absence of orthopnoea, which permits the acute nephritic patient to sleep flat and so accumulate oedema fluid in the face. In congestive heart failure the patient is commonly orthopnoeic and so sleeps propped up; therefore, oedema fluid would drain out of the face. Now read **5.24** again and answer the question correctly.

5.28 Your answer – facial oedema is more common in acute nephritis than in congestive heart failure because in the former the patient is able to sleep lying flat.

You are correct. Now let us consider the hypertension which is common in acute glomerulonephritis. An elevation of the blood pressure occurred in the majority of Ellis's series; the usual diastolic pressure being 90 to 120 mm. The hypertension usually persists for at least one week, finally returning to normal gradually a few days *after* the patient has had a diuresis. In some patients (less than 1 in 20 of all patients affected by acute nephritis) the blood pressure remains elevated, proteinuria and microscopic haematuria persist and the patient enters the phase of subacute glomerulonephritis (rapidly Progressive Type 1 nephritis of Ellis). In others the patient's blood pressure returns to normal only to rise some years later with the onset of renal failure due to chronic glomerulonephritis. In from 5 to 10 per cent of patients suffering from acute glomerulonephritis, hypertensive encephalopathy develops, the clinical features being severe headache, vomiting, convulsions, hemiparesis, and other focal signs such as aphasia. There are associated mental abnormalities such as confusion, disorientation and coma. The child may develop hypertensive encephalopathy with a rise in diastolic blood pressure to 110 mm of mercury; the adult may develop diastolic blood pressure of 150–180 mm of mercury before the clinical features of encephalopathy supervene. In rats Byrom has shown that spasm of cerebral vessels occurs in hypertensive encephalopathy. The rise in blood pressure may give rise to signs of pulmonary oedema; basal crepitations are common in acute nephritis due to pulmonary congestion. The jugular venous pressure is commonly elevated; with peripheral oedema also present the clinical picture of congestive heart failure is present. It is possible that the congestive heart failure is frequently a manifestation of a toxic serous myocarditis rather than solely a result of hypertension, which is often mild.

Question Does the hypertension of acute nephritis usually subside to normal values before or after the diuresis which marks the end of the oliguric phase?

Answer 1. Before the end of the oliguric phase. Go on to **5.30**.
2. After the end of oliguric phase. Go on to **5.31**.

5.29 Your answer − I don't know why in acute nephritis facial oedema is common, but it is rare in congestive heart failure.

In acute nephritis the patient can lie flat, and gets oedema of the face. Read **5.24** again and try to answer the question correctly.

5.30 Your answer − the hypertension of acute nephritis usually subsides to normal values before the end of the oliguric phase.

You are wrong. Read **5.28** again then answer the question correctly.

5.31 Your answer − the hypertension of acute nephritis subsides after the end of the oliguric phase.

You are correct. The oedema of acute nephritis is probably due to salt and water retention; this occurs in any oliguric state in which intake of fluids and sodium salts is not controlled, and acute nephritis is no exception. Measurement of blood volume in acute nephritis has shown that hypervolaemia is present, the increase in blood volume being due to an increase in plasma volume, the red cell volume remaining constant. The hypertension of acute nephritis, together with toxic serous myocarditis result in death from heart failure in about 1 in 50 patients suffering from the disease. A similar number die of renal failure in the acute phase of acute nephritis. In these patients the oliguria persists or total anuria supervenes; the blood urea rises at a rate of 25 mg/100 ml per day. The majority of patients with total anuria succumb, although the occasional patient survives, diuresis supervening before the 49th day of anuria in these patients.

Question Is the increase in blood volume found in acute glomerulonephritis due to an increase in the number of red cells, an increase in plasma volume, or both?

Answer 1. Due to an increase in the number of red cells. Go on to **5.32**.
2. Due to an increase in plasma volume. Go on to **5.33**.
3. Due to an increase in both red cell and plasma volume. Go on to **5.34**.

5.32 Your answer − the increase in blood volume in acute glomerulonephritis is due to an increase in the number of red cells.

You are wrong. If you measure the plasma volume using Evans' blue and the red cell volume using ^{51}chromium tagged red cells, the plasma volume is found to be increased but the red cell volume is usually normal. Read **5.31** again.

5.33 Your answer − in acute nephritis the plasma volume is increased.

You are correct. Now answer the next question.

Question If a man with acute nephritis is anuric or severely oliguric for ten weeks is it likely that his kidneys will spontaneously recover?

Answer 1. Yes. Go on to **5.35**.
2. No. Go on to **5.36**.

5.34 Your answer – both red cell volume and plasma volume are increased.

No. Red cell volume remains normal but the plasma volume is increased in acute nephritis. Go back to **5.31** again.

5.35 Your answer – he is likely to recover after ten weeks of anuria or severe oliguria.

You are incorrect. It is more likely that his kidneys are irreversibly damaged. Go back to **5.31**, read it, then answer the question in **5.33** again.

5.36 Your answer – his kidneys are not likely to recover after ten weeks of anuria or severe oliguria.

You are quite right. The proteinuria in acute nephritis is variable. In some patients the glomerular leak of protein is over 5 g per day, leading to hypoproteinaemia in about 10 per cent of patients in Wilson's series. The occasional patient has developed acute nephritis with a total *absence* of proteinuria. The proteinuria in the majority of cases may persist for months; recovery may take place ultimately after proteinuria has persisted for one year. Microscopic examination of the urine in the acute stage of glomerulonephritis shows large numbers of red cells predominating together with red cell casts, white cells, white cell casts, and granular casts. The red cell casts are a diagnostic feature in making the differential diagnosis of glomerulonephritis. Occasionally the urine sediment contains more white cells than red cells, but this is exceptional. The urine osmolarity is usually over 400 mOsm/litre. The rise in blood urea is variable; in the majority of patients the blood urea rises to between 50 and 100 mg/100 ml; and in a small percentage values over 150 mg/100 ml occur, particularly in those with prolonged severe oliguria. The GFR is markedly reduced, but renal plasma flow is normal or increased. Tubular function is less impaired than glomerular function, as would be expected from the common histological appearance of a predominantly glomerular affection. As clinical recovery takes place the GFR increases gradually, although it may remain abnormal for months.

Question What type of cellular constituent is the commonest in the urine sediment in acute glomerulonephritis?

Answer 1. Red cells. Go on to **5.44**.
2. Red cell casts. Go on to **5.37**.
3. White cell casts. Go on to **5.38**.
4. Granular casts. Go on to **5.39**.
5. White cells. Go on to **5.40**.

5.37 Your answer – red cell casts are the commonest urinary sediment cellular finding in acute nephritis.

You are not quite correct. Red cell casts are very common and certainly indicate the presence of blood inside the renal tubules, and most commonly proximal to the loop of Henle, but red cells are always more plentiful than red cell casts. Go on to read **5.44**.

5.38 Your answer – white cell casts are most common in the urine of acute glomerulonephritis.

Sometimes white cells predominate in the urine, but this is unusual and, although white cell casts may be found, the usual finding is the red cell in large numbers. Go back and read **5.36** again.

5.39 Your answer – granular casts are the most common cellular constituents in the urine of acute nephritis.

Although granular casts are plentiful in the urine of acute nephritis, they are not the characteristic and diagnostic urinary finding. Red cells are much more striking. Read **5.36** again.

5.40 Your answer – white cells are the most common urinary constituents in acute glomerulonephritis.

You are partially correct in that white cells are found in the urine, but only very rarely are they more numerous than red blood cells which give the urine its striking reddish colour. Read **5.36** again and answer the question correctly.

5.41 Your answer – acute glomerulonephritis can occur even if the ASO titre is not elevated.

Good. Now let us consider the differential diagnosis of acute glomerulonephritis. First of all, focal nephritis. This is a common condition in which the haematuria occurs at the height of the infection and rapidly passes off.

Second, Henoch-Schönlein nephritis: this is associated with purpuric skin rashes, arthropathy, and intestinal colic with melaena, the renal features being haematuria with proteinuria.

Third, acute exacerbations of chronic glomerulonephritis are often confused with acute glomerulonephritis. The diagnosis can often be made on a history of a previous attack of nephritis, or previously documented albuminuria or hypertension found at a routine medical examination. An adequate history of earlier disease may be lacking and the diagnosis may be suggested by the onset of haematuria the day or two after an upper respiratory tract infection.

Fourth, nephrotic syndrome may be mistaken for acute nephritis with its oliguria and concentrated dark urine which may contain excessive numbers of red cells; there is facial swelling but the blood pressure is usually normal early in nephrotic syndrome caused by membranous glomerulonephritis.

Fifth, pyelonephritis may be associated with haematuria and may cause confusion with acute glomerulonephritis. Pyelonephritis is usually associated with fever, dysuria, and frequency, but acute nephritis may occasionally be associated with all these symptoms; even the presence of more white cells in the urine than red cells may occur in acute nephritis, although it is uncommon. The presence of organisms in the urine would suggest a urinary tract infection, although both pyelonephritis and acute glomerulonephritis may occur together. Malignant hypertension with haematuria and a raised blood pressure is sometimes confused with acute glomerulonephritis; and haematuria and hypertension due to polyarteritis nodosa may rarely cause confusion. Now answer the question below.

Question In acute glomerulonephritis, can there be occasionally more white cells than red cells in the urinary sediment?

Answer 1. Yes. Go on to **5.45**.
2. No. Go on to **5.42**.

5.42 Your answer – in acute glomerulonephritis there cannot be more white cells than red cells in the urinary deposit.

No. In occasional patients with acute glomerulonephritis the microscopic haematuria may be less striking than the large numbers of white cells in the urine. Now answer the question in **5.41** correctly.

5.43 Your answer – acute glomerulonephritis cannot occur in a patient whose ASO titre is not elevated during the illness.

The ASO titre may remain normal in any patient with acute glomerulonephritis for a variety of reasons:

(1) Acute glomerulonephritis may follow a non-streptococcal infection.
(2) The ASO titre is not invariably raised in infection with haemolytic streptococci.
(3) The ASO titre is frequently low if the patient is treated with antibiotics in the acute illness.

You can see therefore that you were wrong in the answer to the question in **5.44**. Go back and read **5.44** through once more.

5.44 Your answer – red cells are the commonest urinary cellular constituent in acute glomerulonephritis.

Good. The throat and any skin lesions should always be swabbed in acute glomerulonephritis in order to establish if β haemolytic streptococci are present; if the first culture is negative it should be repeated several times in order to increase the chance of obtaining a positive culture. Close contacts should also have throat swabs (e.g. members of family, fellow school children, army recruits). The ASO titre is frequently but not invariably elevated and as to elevation may be transient and is sometimes delayed for some weeks, it should be repeated several times if negative results are obtained. The use of antibiotics may suppress the antibody response so that the absence of a positive ASO titre does not exclude a streptococcal infection in patients receiving antibiotics. Anti NADase may be elevated, particularly after Type 12 infections. The haemoglobin level is depressed in about half the patients due to the increased plasma volume, but many patients have no anaemia at all. The anaemia is normochromic and normocytic and reverts rapidly to normal with diuresis. In a small number of patients with very high blood urea levels > 200 mg/100 ml, the anaemia is not dilutional in origin but is the common type of anaemia of renal failure. The leucocyte count is normal unless the patient is still suffering from the precipitating infection. The ESR is usually elevated unless congestive heart failure is present.

Question Can acute glomerulonephritis occur in a patient whose ASO titre is not elevated at any time during the illness?

Answer 1. Yes. Go on to **5.41**.
2. No. Go on to **5.43**.

5.45 Your answer – in acute glomerulonephritis there may occasionally be more white cells than red cells in the urinary deposit.

Correct. The treatment of the patient with acute glomerulonephritis can be divided into two parts:

(1) The treatment of the uncomplicated case.

(2) The treatment of the complications: hypertension, heart failure, and uraemia.

First of all, let us deal with the therapy of the uncomplicated case.

A. *Bed Rest*. During the acute illness it is customary to keep the patient at rest in bed, although the rationale of this is dubious. As soon as the haematuria has decreased and the patient feels well, there is little point in keeping the patient in bed at all.

B. *Restricted Fluid*. During the usual 1 to 2 weeks of oliguria the patient should be given restricted fluids, up to a total daily volume of 500 ml in addition to the volume of urine passed. The fluids should be glucose or fructose, 10 per cent, flavoured lightly with fruit juice. Fruit juices contain potassium and should therefore be used with caution in oliguric patients.

C. *Food*. Brod has advocated starvation initially in acute glomerulonephritis to reduce the number of complications by diminishing the immune response. Few patients can be persuaded to persist with this type of therapy. In the acute phase many patients have a poor appetite, but it is advisable to give them a 2000 Calorie low protein diet. If the patient is oedematous or has engorged neck veins the diet should contain very little sodium (10–20 mEq/day), and he should be dialysed to remove the excess extracellular fluid (ECF).

D. *Antibiotics.* The patient should be given penicillin 250,000 units 6 hourly intramuscularly to destroy any residual β haemolytic streptococci. Tetracycline is a drug that should be avoided: it tends to elevate the blood urea and if old may cause proximal tubular damage. Now answer the question below.

Question If a man with acute nephritis passes 250 ml of urine in a day what should his fluid intake be?

Answer 1. 250 ml. Go on to **5.47**.
2. 750 ml. Go on to **5.49**.
3. No fluids. Go on to **5.51**.

5.46 Your answer — use peritoneal dialysis to remove the excess fluid.

Correct. We have already mentioned the fact that about 4 per cent of patients with acute glomerulonephritis die in the acute phase according to Ellis' series: 5 per cent go on to develop subacute glomerulonephritis or rapidly progressive Type I nephritis, and 5 per cent develop chronic glomerulonephritis or slowly progressive Type I nephritis. Let us look at subacute glomerulonephritis. A typical history is as follows: a young man develops acute nephritis but instead of its clearing up in a week or two, he remains oedematous with persistent hypertension, persistent or intermittent haematuria and is anaemic. The blood urea is often elevated to 60–70 mg/100 ml. Death occurs from hypertension and renal failure in 6 to 18 months. Sometimes the patients develop nephrotic syndrome due to the gross proteinuria. Very occasionally patients recover from an apparent subacute glomerulonephritis after many months of microscopic haematuria and persistent proteinuria. The treatment of subacute glomerulonephritis is symptomatic: salt restriction and diuretics for the oedema, hypotensive agents for the hypertension, and oral antibiotics to prevent recurrence of streptococcal or other infection causing an anamnestic response. It is worthwhile giving both steroids and immunosuppressive drugs in subacute glomerulonephritis. These are dealt with more fully in Chapter 21. If the blood urea is low, i.e., below 100 mg/100 ml, then the patient can have a normal protein dietary intake; if nephrotic, he can have more protein in an effort to help restore his serum proteins to normal. If the blood urea is grossly elevated a low protein diet should be given. This will be discussed in Chapter 9 dealing with Chronic Renal Failure. Should renal failure occur to such a degree that renal function is unable to support life, chronic haemodialysis offers the best chance of survival.

Question A patient has persistent proteinuria, haematuria, hypertension, and oedema three months after acute nephritis. How long is he likely to survive the acute attack?

Answer 1. 5 years. Go on to **5.48**.
2. 6–18 months. Go on to **5.55**.
3. Indefinitely. Go on to **5.53**.

5.47 Your answer – give the patient 250 ml of fluid a day.

The fluid requirement of an apyrexial adult is about 500 ml a day more than the loss in the urine. So if he passes 250 ml in the urine, he should be given 250 + 500 ml = 750 ml. Now answer the question in **5.45** correctly after reading the paragraph once again.

5.48 Your answer – the patient will survive five years.

You are guessing, and that is no way to learn anything. Read **5.46** again, paying attention this time. If you can't concentrate due to external distractions, stop reading now unless you can move to less distracting surroundings. If there are no distractions try and read **5.46** again.

5.49 Your answer – 750 ml of fluid should be given.

Good. Now we can discuss the treatment of the complications.

(1) Hypertension. If the hypertension is mild, i.e. diastolic BP below 110 mm of mercury in the adult, it should not be treated unless the patient has the clinical features of left ventricular failure. If the hypertension is causing attacks of pulmonary oedema or if the patient has hypertensive encephalopathy, the hypertension should be treated vigorously. (a) Venesection of 500 ml; (b) intramuscular pentolinium (Ansolysen) should be given in increasing dosage in 2.5 mg increments every hour, until the diastolic blood pressure has been brought down to the safer levels of 110–115 mm of mercury, I.M. reserpine 4 mg or I.V. diazoxide is preferred by some.

(2) Heart failure should be treated by digitalising the patient; venesection and hypotensive drugs should be used if hypertension is causing left ventricular failure. If the patient is grossly overhydrated due to mismanagement (i.e. by free access to fluids during oliguria) peritoneal dialysis using 4.5 per cent glucose in the fluid will remove several litres of excess fluid in a few hours. It is worthwhile giving 1000 mg of furosamide intravenously over 10 hours in a drip infusion to produce some diuresis to an oliguric patient suffering from acute nephritis.

(3) Anuria or severe persistent oliguria. In a small proportion of patients the urine volume remains at less than 250 ml a day and in a few total anuria occurs. Persistent oliguria is treated by the following regimen:

(a) Oral fluid intake of (500 ml + total volume of urine passed per day) as 10 per cent glucose or Hycal (Beecham's).

(b) 2000 calorie diet containing 10–20 mEq of sodium, 3 g of nitrogen, chosen to contain the daily requirements of the essential amino acids in natural protein form, with the carbohydrate polymer, Caloreen added to provide further calories.

(c) Anabolic steroids, i.e. norethandrolone 25 mg daily.

Dialysis should be undertaken when indicated. The treatment of acute renal failure by conservative measures and dialytic methods will be dealt with in detail in Chapter 8. Now answer the following question.

Question A patient is sent to you suffering from acute nephritis with oliguria and has been subjected elsewhere to a misguided regimen of fluid intake so that he is oedematous and has distended neck veins. How can you remove the excessive fluid quickly.

Answer 1. Use peritoneal dialysis. Go on to **5.46**.
          2. Restrict oral fluid totally. Go on to **5.50**.
          3. Don't know. Go on to **5.52**.

5.50 Your answer — restrict oral fluids if the patient has oedema and neck vein congestion.

This will not remove fluid rapidly. Peritoneal dialysis will take off 3 to 4 litres in 12 hours if necessary. Read **5.49** again.

5.51 Your answer — no fluids should be given the patient.

No. Let us take the daily insensible water loss at 1 litre, if the patient is apyrexial. The water of metabolism produced by the patient's katabolism will be somewhere in the region of 400 ml to 500 ml. Thus the patient will need 500 to 600 ml of fluid a day if he passes no urine. If he passes urine, then the fluid volume of that will have to be added to the oral intake. Our patient will have to have 500 + 250 ml = 750 ml of fluid orally per day. Now read **5.45** and answer the question again.

5.52 Your answer — I don't know how to manage a patient with oedema and oliguria.

The answer to this question has been discussed in **5.49**. Read it again paying more attention to the text, and then answer the question correctly.

5.53 Your answer — the patient will survive indefinitely.

You are partly correct. This is only true, however, if chronic haemodialysis can be carried out, or if renal transplantation is successful, (and at present this appears to be a 50–50 chance in the *best* hands). Read **5.46** again and then aswer the question correctly.

5.54 Your answer — only statement 2 is true.

You are partly correct but statement 1 is also true. Start at **5.1** again and work through to **5.45**. Then answer the question correctly at the end of **5.70**. Your knowledge of acute glomerulonephritis is defective.

5.55 Your answer — the patient will be dead in 6–18 months.

Correct. Now we can consider chronic glomerulonephritis. In the majority of cases in hospital practice there is no history of an earlier attack of acute nephritis, and our knowledge of the natural history of chronic glomerulonephritis is to a great extent dependent on long term studies of acute nephritis such as have been done at the London Hospital by Ellis and Wilson. They have shown that only a small proportion of patients with acute nephritis develop chronic glomerulonephritis, roughly 1 in 10 at the most. It should be remembered that all hospital series are biased by a disproportionate number of complicated cases, so that the true incidence of chronic glomerulonephritis is probably a good deal lower than that just described. The clinical presentations of chronic glomerulonephritis are:

(1) An apparent recovery from an attack of acute nephritis, often with a persistence of proteinuria. After a variable period – up to 20 years – hypertension and renal failure supervene.

(2) Symptomless proteinuria: this is frequently discovered at medical examinations for insurance purposes.

(3) Nephrotic syndrome. It has been suggested that about half the patients who develop chronic glomerulonephritis pass through a nephrotic phase with hypoalbuminaemia, oedema, and massive proteinuria. The modern classifications of nephrotic syndrome and the Ellis classification are dealt with in the Chapter 6, Nephrotic Syndrome.

(4) Hypertension may be the presenting feature, either benign or malignant in type.

(5) Renal failure developing without prior evidence of renal disease. These patients have the symptoms and signs of uraemia – nausea, vomiting, hiccough, fatigue, anaemia with dyspnoea and cardiac failure, pruritus, pericarditis, bloody diarrhoea, and nocturia. Often the only symptom that can be discovered before the onset of uraemia is nocturia for a period of months or years.

Question What proportion of patients with chronic glomerulonephritis pass through a nephrotic phase?

Answer 1. About a quarter. Go on to **5.58**.
2. About half. Go on to **5.57**.
3. All the patients. Go on to **5.59**.

5.56 Before leaving the subject it is worth recommending some further reading:

Addis T. (1948) Glomerular Nephritis. New York Macmillan.
Cameron J. S. Brit. Med. Journ. 1972, **4**, 87, is well worth reading.
Wardle E. N. & Uldall P. R. Brit. Med. Journ. 1972, 4, 135, gives an up to date account research into fibrin split products in nephritis.
Ellis A. (1942) Lancet **1**, 72.
Earle D. P. & Seegal D. (1957) Natural history of glomerular nephritis. J. Chron. Dis. **5**, 3.
Hunsicker *et al.*, New Eng. J. Med. (1972) **287**, 835 deals with complement in nephritis.
Jennings R. B. & Earle D. P. (1961) Post-streptococcal glomerulonephritis. J. clin. Invest. **40**, 1525.

Rammelcamp C. H. (1962) Aetiology of glomerulonephritis, in Black D. A. K. (ed.) Renal Disease, p. 173. Blackwell Scientific Publications, Oxford.

Wilson C. (1962) The natural history of nephritis, in Black D. A. K. (ed.) Renal Disease, p. 188. Blackwell Scientific Publications, Oxford.

Schwartz's, and Relman's chapters in Strauss M. B. & Welt L. G. (eds.) (1971) Diseases of the Kidney. Churchill, London. 2nd edition.

Wannamaker L. New Eng. J. Med. 1970 **282**, 78.

Brown, J. J. et al. 1970. Brit. Med. J. I., 253.

Thiel, G. et al. 1970. Nephron 7, 67.

Now start the next chapter.

5.57 Your answer – about half the patients with chronic glomerulonephritis develop nephrotic syndrome.

Good. The prognosis of chronic glomerulonephritis is variable, principally because the date of the commencement of the disease process is unknown. The length of duration of symptoms of the disease varies from 1 to 40 years. The laboratory findings in a case of chronic glomerulonephritis include the following:

Casts – granular casts, broad granular and waxy renal failure casts, microscopic haematuria, excessive white cell excretion; there are oval fat bodies in the patients with nephrotic syndrome. Proteinuria is virtually always present, in variable amounts, usually (but not always) tending to fall from the 10–15 g/day encountered in the nephrotic phase to the 1–2 g/day commonly encountered in renal failure. The urinary osmolarity on water deprivation or Pitressin administration progressively diminishes as the disease progresses, ultimately being no higher than that of the plasma, (equivalent to an SG of 1010). The blood urea is elevated after the GFR has fallen to 25 ml/min and rises progressively to 450–600 mg/100 ml before death; this rise in blood urea is associated with an increasing acidosis, the plasma pH falling to levels of 7.1–7.20 when the GFR is 2–3 ml/min; this is accompanied by a decrease in total plasma CO_2 to 10–12 mMols/1 and a build up of organic acids, sulphate, and phosphate in the plasma. As the GFR falls the remaining living nephrons undergo osmotic diuresis, and at this stage loss of sodium into the urine may become very important, causing 'salt-wasting' or 'salt-losing' nephritis. The common causes of salt-losing nephritis are (1) chronic renal failure of any cause (2) pyelonephritis (3) Addison's disease. In chronic glomerulo-nephritis the salt loss has to be carefully measured because many patients lose so much salt that they suffer extracellular fluid volume contraction, and the hypovolaemia may exacerbate the renal failure and cause deterioration in renal function of extra-renal origin. This can be treated by careful resalination giving 1 to 2 litres of 0.9% saline (155–310 mEq of Na) because in addition to having a renal salt leak most chronic glomerulonephritics cannot excrete large amounts of salt quickly and go rapidly from one extreme of salt depletion to the other of excessive salt repletion and oedema.

Question In a patient dying of renal failure due to chronic glomerulonephritis, what is the magnitude of the daily protein loss in the urine?

Answer 1. None. Go on to **5.62**.
2. 15 g/day. Go on to **5.65**.
3. 1–2 g/day. Go on to **5.69**.

5.58 Your answer – about one quarter develop nephrotic syndrome.
You are wrong. About half the patients with chronic glomerulonephritis pass through a nephrotic phase. Read **5.55** again.

5.59 Your answer – all the patients have a nephrotic phase.
No. Many patients present with proteinuria, hypertension, or renal failure without ever passing through a nephrotic phase. Read **5.55** again.

5.60 Your answer – the anaemia of chronic glomerulonephritis is hypochromic.
No. The typical anaemia of renal failure is normochromic. Read **5.69** again.

5.61 Your answer – 3 is true, 1 and 2 are false.
You are quite wrong on all the statements. Start at **5.1** and go through the entire chapter again. If you do not you are wasting your time. Do *not* go on to the next chapter.

5.62 Your answer – there is no protein loss in a patient dying of chronic glomerulonephritis.
The protein loss usually diminishes as renal failure progresses, but most patients pass 1–2 g each day. Read **5.57** again and then answer the question correctly.

5.63 Your answer – the anaemia of chronic glomerulonephritis is normochromic.
You are correct. The serum proteins in chronic glomerulonephritis are altered in the nephrotic phase where the serum albumin is constantly depressed below 3g/100 ml; α_2 and β globulins are often elevated. When the patient's renal condition further deteriorates and the massive albuminuria of the nephrotic phase diminishes, the serum albumin rises to between 3 and 4 g/100 ml. The serum cholesterol level, which may have been as high as 600–800 mg/100 ml during the nephrotic phase, falls with the return of the serum albumin to normal levels. The concentration of plasma inorganic phosphorus climbs with progressing renal insufficiency to heights of 10–15 mg/100 ml. The serum calcium is depressed during the nephrotic phase of the disease, due to the fact that half the serum calcium is bound to albumin and hypoalbuminaemia is the rule in nephrotic syndrome. The serum calcium levels are frequently but inconstantly depressed in advanced chronic glomerulonephritis. In the presence of osteomalacia due to renal

failure, the serum calcium tends to be depressed, whereas in renal failure with predominant hyperparathyroidism Stanbury has shown that the serum calcium is often normal or elevated. In all forms of renal bone disease, the serum alkaline phosphatase is frequently but not invariably elevated.

Question A patient with chronic glomerulonephritis develops bone disease as a result of chronic renal failure and the following values are found:

Serum calcium − 6.8 mg/100 ml.
Serum inorganic phosphorus − 12.0 mg/100 ml.
Blood urea − 280 mg/100 ml.
Serum alkaline phosphatase − 36 KA units/100 ml.

What is the most likely type of bone disease here?

Answer 1. Hyperparathyroidism. Go on to **5.64**.
2. Osteomalacia. Go on to **5.67**.

5.64 Your answer − hyperparathyroidism is the most likely bone disease here.
No. In renal hyperparathyroidism the serum calcium is usually higher − normal or elevated.

5.65 Your answer − 15 g of proteinuria daily occurs in renal failure of chronic glomerulonephritis.
No. Such a large protein loss is uncommon in advanced renal failure. Go back and read **5.57** again. Then answer the question correctly.

5.66 Your answer − the anaemia of chronic glomerulonephritis is megaloblastic.
No. In chronic renal failure the commonest form of anaemia is not megaloblastic but is normochromic and normocytic. Read **5.69** again and answer the question correctly.

5.67 Your answer − osteomalacia is present.
You are correct. The treatment of chronic glomerulonephritis is: (1) control of the hypertension with suitable hypotensive agents such as guanethidine or α methyldopa: these should be given cautiously because of their cumulative effect in chronic renal failure. (2) Treatment of anaemia by blood transfusion. (3) Use of corticosteroids and immunosuppressives to halt or reverse the disease. These are dealt in Chapter 21 in more detail, but proliferative glomerulonephritis and membranous g-n respond sometimes to this form of therapy, whereas lobular and membrano-proliferative types of chronic glomerulonephritis do badly. (4) Low protein diet. (5) Dialysis. These will be discussed in the chapter on Chronic Renal Failure. The differential diagnosis is (1) Hypertension − all other causes (2) chronic pyelonephritis which is a frequently complicating factor in all renal dis-

ease: the presence of a positive urine culture with the appropriate urine sediment of pus cells and a history of recurrent frequency and dysuria with IVP changes showing distorted scarred calyces with cortical thinning over the affected calyces would favour a diagnosis of chronic pyelonephritis. Even microscopic or frank haematuria may occur in pyelonephritis but red cell casts are usually absent from the urine in this condition. (3) All causes of nephrotic syndrome. These are discussed in Chapter 6 on Nephrotic Syndrome. (4) Polyarteritis nodosa has the features of hypertension and renal failure, but there is often an arthropathy and a neuropathy to distinguish it from renal failure due to chronic glomerulonephritis. Now answer the question.

Question In a patient with renal failure, the urine sediment contains many pus cells per high power field, and grows E. coli on culture. There is a history of recurrent frequency and dysuria. What is the diagnosis?

Answer 1. Chronic glomerulonephritis. Go on to **5.68**.
2. Chronic pyelonephritis. Go on to **5.70**.
3. Nephrotic Syndrome. Go on to **5.72**.

5.68 Your answer – the patient has chronic glomerulonephritis.
You may be correct but on the data given the only obvious diagnosis is chronic pyelonephritis. Read **5.67** again and answer the question correctly.

5.69 Your answer – 1 to 2 g of protein are lost in the urine daily in advanced renal failure.
Good. The anaemia of chronic glomerulonephritis is usually normochromic and normocytic with a mean corpuscular haemoglobin concentration of 32 to 34. The haemoglobin gradually falls to below 5 g per cent unless the patient is transfused or treated by dialytic methods. The cause of the anaemia is similar to that in other conditions causing chronic renal failure and is partly due to an increase in haemolysis and partly due to a decreased output of red blood cells from the marrow. Renal erythropoietin is essential for normal haemoglobin synthesis, and its plasma concentration is found to be very low in advanced chronic glomerulonephritis. As the patient becomes anaemic he develops dyspnoea and ultimately heart failure. When the terminal phase is reached the patient develops thrombocytopenia and a bleeding diathesis due to inhibition of the various platelet and plasma factors (particularly Factor 7), responsible for normal blood coagulation. These abnormalities result in purpura and ecchymosis with bleeding of the gums, sordes, bloody diarrhoea, and haematemesis so common in renal failure. The leucocyte count is usually increased, with an increase in polymorphonuclear leucocytes, and the ESR is invariably elevated in the absence of congestive heart failure.

Question In chronic glomerulonephritis, what type of anaemia is common?

Answer 1. Hypochromic. Go on to **5.60**.

2. Normochromic. Go on to **5.63**.
   3. Megaloblastic. Go on to **5.66**.

5.70 Your answer – the diagnosis is chronic pyelonephritis.

Good. Now answer the questions after reading the statements below. Think carefully before you pick the answer: an incorrect answer may send you back to the beginning of the chapter again.

Statement 1 Type 12 haemolytic streptococci are the organisms most frequently responsible for acute glomerulonephritis.

Statement 2 In subacute glomerulonephritis death usually occurs within 6 to 18 months of the onset of the disease.

Statement 3 Proteinuria never occurs in chronic glomerulonephritis.

Answers
1. All the statements are true. Go on to **5.71**.
2. All the statements are false. Go on to **5.74**.
3. Statements 1 and 3 only are true and 2 false. Go on to **5.73**.
4. Statements 1 and 2 are true and 3 false. Go on to **5.75**.
5. Statements 2 and 3 are true and 1 false. Go on to **5.76**.
6. Statement 1 is true, 2 and 3 are false. Go on to **5.77**.
7. Statement 2 is true, 1 and 3 are false. Go on to **5.54**.
8. Statement 3 is true, 1 and 2 are false. Go on to **5.61**.

5.71 Your answer – all the statements are true.

You are partly right, but proteinuria is virtually constant in chronic glomerulonephritis. Go back to **5.57** and work on from there.

5.72 Your answer – the diagnosis is the nephrotic syndrome.

You are wrong. None of the features of the nephrotic syndrome have been mentioned. Pay more attention and read **5.67** again carefully. Then answer the question correctly.

5.73 Your answer – statement 2 is false.

You are only partly correct. Statement 1 and 2 are true but 3 is false. Start at **5.45** and work back from there.

5.74 Your answer – all the statements are false.

No. Statement 3 is the only false one. Start at the beginning of the chapter and work on. You have remembered little of what you have just read. Do not proceed to the next chapter until you have consolidated your knowledge of this one.

5.75 Your answer – statement 3 is false.

Good. You can now go on to **5.56**.

5.76 Your answer – statement 1 is false, 2 and 3 are true.

You are partly correct. Only 3 is false. Start at **5.1** and work on until you come to **5.45**, then go on to answer the question in **5.70** again.

5.77 Your answer – only statement 1 is true.

You are partly right but 2 is also true. Go back to **5.45** and read through from there.

Time for this chapter: 45 minutes

Chapter 6
Nephrotic syndrome

6.1 The nephrotic syndrome is a clinical and biochemical complex caused by many diseases; it is not a disease sui generis. It is, however, convenient to consider the features of the nephrotic syndrome which are shared in common by the many diseases which may present clinically as the nephrotic syndrome. The nephrotic syndrome consists of the following features: peripheral oedema, massive proteinuria, and hypoproteinaemia. Usually but not constantly, there is also hypercholesterolaemia. The oedema is caused by the hypoalbuminaemia; usually the serum albumin is depressed below 3 g/100 ml and sometimes as low as 0.5 g/100 ml; oedema develops almost constantly if the serum albumin is below 2 g/100 ml unless diuretics are used. The *total* serum globulin concentrations are frequently lowered, with often an elevation of α_2 and β globulins. The hypoalbuminaemia is caused by the protein loss in the urine; the extent of this protein loss is variable, a minimum of 3.5 g/1.73 m² of body surface per day being suggested by Schreiner. In the British Medical Research Council trial of steroids in the nephrotic syndrome, a proteinuria of 5 g per day was the minimum value acceptable for inclusion. Some authorities include the excretion of oval fat bodies in the urine in the description of the main features of nephrotic syndrome.

Question If a man has peripheral oedema, serum albumin of 1.8 g/100 ml and proteinuria of 0.5 g/24 hours, is the diagnosis of nephrotic syndrome tenable?

Answer 1. Yes. Go on to **6.3**.
2. No. Go on to **6.5**.
3. Don't know. Go on to **6.7**.

6.2 You should not be reading this paragraph if you are following the instructions at the end of **6.1**.

6.3 Your answer – the diagnosis of nephrotic syndrome is likely to be correct.
In the description of nephrotic syndrome in **6.1**, it was mentioned that proteinuria of at least 3.5–5.0 g/day had to be present before a diagnosis of nephrotic syndrome was acceptable. Your answer is therefore incorrect and indicates that you are not working properly. Read **6.1** again without allowing yourself to be distracted.

6.4 Your answer – differential protein clearance of macroglobulin being 100 per cent is compatible with 'no light microscopic change.'

You are not correct. The differential clearance of macroglobulin would be a very small percentage in nephrotic syndrome due to 'no light microscopic change' because there are fewer large pores than smaller pores in this condition; read **6.5** again and answer the question correctly.

6.5 Your answer – the diagnosis of nephrotic syndrome is not likely to be correct. Good. The maximum amount of protein lost per day in the urine in our experience is 51 g. The cause of the proteinuria, irrespective of the causal disease, is an increase in glomerular permeability. This may be considered to be due to a series of pores: in normal health these pores are too tiny to let albumin through in large amounts, but in nephrotic syndrome there are a large number of pores of varying size. The smaller proteins (such as albumin) can pass through smaller pores than the large proteins such as IgM and β lipoprotein. If there are more smaller pores than large pores in the diseased glomerulus the patient will lose more of the small proteins in the urine, i.e. the proteinuria will consist largely of albumin. If there are many large pores in the diseased glomerulus, the proteinuria will contain the larger protein molecules such as β lipoprotein, the macroglobulins, and complement, as well as the smaller protein molecules: the absolute amount of each protein excreted per day is governed by the serum level. It has been shown by Hardwicke and his colleagues in Birmingham that there is a correlation between the proportions of the various proteins lost in the urine in nephrotic syndrome and the histological cause of the disease. They have measured immunologically the urinary loss of the individual proteins in terms of the renal clearances, comparing the clearances of the individual proteins to that of the siderophilin, the latter being taken as 100 per cent. This ratio is known as the 'differential protein clearance.' If there are few large pores, the relative clearance of the macroglobulins compared to that of siderophilin will be low, say 5 per cent i.e., the differential protein clearance of macroglobulin is 5 per cent. If there are large numbers of large pores, the differential protein clearance of macroglobulin will be 100 per cent. In the nephrotic syndrome due to membranous glomerulonephritis the differential protein clearance is a very high per cent for the large molecular weight proteins. This is known as non-selective proteinuria. In nephrotic syndrome 'without light microscopic change,' differential protein clearance for large molecular weight proteins is a *small* percentage of siderophilin clearance. This is known as selective proteinuria. Now answer the question.

Question If the differential protein clearance of Gamma 1 macroglobulin is 100 per cent that of siderophilin is the patient likely to have nephrotic syndrome 'without light microscopic change?'

Answer 1. Yes. Go on to **6.4**.
2. No. Go on to **6.6**.
3. Don't know. Go on to **6.9**.

6.6 Your answer — the patient is *not* likely to have a 'no light microscopic change' type of nephrotic syndrome.

Good. The nephrotic syndrome is frequently associated with disordered lipid metabolism. The urine commonly contains oval fat bodies — these are free fatty globules in the urine — as well as fatty casts, and tubular cells containing fat globules. The plasma lipid pattern is abnormal in nephrotic syndrome, with an increase in total cholesterol, free cholesterol, phospholipids, and low density β lipoprotein. The cause of the hyperlipaemia is not known with certainty; there is a reciprocal relationship between hypoalbuminaemia and hyperlipaemia which has been the subject of conflicting animal experiments. Another view of the cause of hyperlipaemia is that it is associated with mobilisation of fat for energy purposes. Clinical data, as opposed to animal experiments, indicate a fairly good correlation between hypoalbuminaemia and hyperlipaemia in the majority of cases of nephrotic syndrome: but in lupus nephritis there are occasional cases in which the serum cholesterol is *not* elevated – the so-called 'pseudonephrotic' type of lupus nephritis. Schreiner has also noted normal cholesterol levels in patients with the nephrotic phase of acute glomerulonephritis. The prolonged hyperlipaemia of nephrotic syndrome is associated with an increased incidence of atheroma causing angina of effort and myocardial infarction if the coronary vessels are involved. The atheroma affecting the aorta may even cause renal artery stenosis by occluding the aortic opening of the renal arteries.

Question Is the serum cholesterol invariably elevated in nephrotic syndrome?

Answer 1. Yes. Go on to **6.8**.
         2. No. Go on to **6.10**.
         3. Don't know. Go on to **6.13**.

6.7 Your answer — I don't know if the diagnosis of nephrotic syndrome is correct.

The minimum amount of proteinuria which is found in nephrotic syndrome is 3.5 g/day; so this patient does not have nephrotic syndrome because his protein excretion is only 0.5 g/day. There was an adequate description in **6.1** of the amount of proteinuria in nephrotic syndrome. If you cannot remember it you are not learning satisfactorily. Go back over **6.1** again.

6.8 Your answer — the serum cholesterol is *always* increased in nephrotic syndrome.

No. In **6.6** it was indicated that the serum cholesterol was usually elevated in nephrotic syndrome but that lupus nephritis and acute glomerulonephritis sometimes caused exceptions to this rule. Your failure to retain this suggests that you have not been reading carefully enough. Go back over **6.6** again and answer the question after reading the paragraph.

6.9 Your answer – I don't know what this differential protein clearance indicates.

By differential protein clearance is meant the renal clearance of a protein 'X' compared to that of siderophilin: if the clearance of 'X' is one quarter of that of siderophilin, the differential protein clearance is 25 per cent.

In the case of a large protein such as a macroglobulin, with a molecular weight of 900,000, little will get through the small pores of the 'no light microscopic change' type of nephrotic syndrome, i.e., the differential protein clearance will be a very low percentage. In the membranous group of nephrotic syndrome, more large pores are present and these allow more of the larger proteins to get out so that the differential protein clearances of macroglobulin and siderophilin will be equal, i.e., 100 per cent. Now answer the question in **6.5** again.

6.10 Your answer – the serum cholesterol is *not* invariably elevated in nephrotic syndrome.

Correct. In nephrotic syndrome when oedema is increasing oliguria is usually present. The urine contains little sodium due to the increased secretion of aldosterone: the cause of the increased production of this hormone is probably hypovolaemia due to hypoproteinaemia. There is also a lowered plasma protein-bound-iodine level possibly due to a change in plasma proteins able to bind thyroid hormone rather than increased loss of thyroid hormone in the urine, although the evidence is controversial. Glycosuria occurs in nephrotic syndrome not necessarily due to diabetes mellitus but due to proximal tubular damage, probably by the large amounts of reabsorbed protein. The glycosuria is often present in trace amounts, with a normal blood sugar, and may require a period of up to *one minute* after application of the urine before the glucose oxidase stick (Clinistix) changes colour. Amino-aciduria is similarly a sign of proximal tubular damage.

Question If glycosuria is found in trace amounts in a nephrotic's urine is the patient sure to have diabetes mellitus?

Answer 1. No. Go on to **6.14**.
2. Yes. Go on to **6.11**.

6.11 Your answer – the patient is sure to have diabetes mellitus.

You are wrong because glycosuria commonly occurs in nondiabetics suffering from any other cause of nephrotic syndrome, presumably due to proximal tubular damage, i.e., a type of renal glycosuria. Go back and read **6.10** again before answering the question correctly.

6.12 Your answer – Membranous glomerulonephritis.

Good. The clinical features of membranous glomerulonephritis differ little from those of proliferative glomerulonephritis apart from the fact that in the latter disease there was a preceding nephritogenic streptococcal infection. The onset of oedema is often more sudden and striking in relation to an upper respiratory tract infection in proliferative glomerulonephritis whereas the onset in membranous glomerulonephritis is insidious, membrano-proliferative g-n may present as an acute nephrotic episode, or insidiously as nephrotic syndrome. Otherwise the lesions behave in a similar manner clinically. There is no hypertension in the majority of patients at the onset of membranous glomerulonephritis, but a sizeable minority *have* hypertension. Membranous glomerulonephritis proceeds inexorably with little chance of spontaneous remission until, after several years, renal failure supervenes. In proliferative glomerulonephritis there is an increased chance of the occasional patient undergoing spontaneous remission. Membranous glomerulonephritis has a remission rate of about 1 in 4 if cortico-steroids are used, and this improves to about 1 in 3 with the use of immunosuppressive drugs. In proliferative glomerulonephritis up to 50% of the patients will remit with steroid and immunosuppressive therapy. The urine in membranous glomerulonephritis contains few red cells: in proliferative glomerulonephritis it may contain many red cells, white cells and casts of all types. About half the patients with chronic proliferative glomerulonephritis go through a nephrotic phase. In proliferative glomerulonephritis the ASO titre is more often elevated than in membranous glomerulonephritis. The differential protein clearance of high molecular weight proteins is greater in membranous than in proliferative glomerulonephritis. In focal sclerosing glomerulonephritis the prognosis is particularly bad, a slow progression to renal failure being the rule, without response to steroids or immunosuppressive agents. In membranoproliferative (or the more accurate descriptive term – mesangio-capillary) glomerulonephritis there is often a lowered plasma complement (C^1_3) level due to its destruction by a nephritic factor referred to as C3NeF which have been demonstrated in the plasma of these patients. In the majority of cases the outlook is poor, but some cases respond to therapy with immunosuppressive drugs.

Patients with 'no light microscopic change' have the best prognosis, frequently remitting spontaneously or on therapy. Children commonly have this type of nephrotic syndrome and on immunosuppressive and steroid therapy 95% remit, but it is also frequent in adults, occurring in about 30 per cent of our series of nephrotic patients. The prognosis is much better in this group, but otherwise it is difficult to tell clinically which patient belongs to any of these pathological groups; hence the need for renal biopsy to assess the pathological picture.

Question Is there usually a history of streptococcal infection in membranous glomerulonephritis?

Answer 1. Yes. Go on to **6.15**.
    2. No. Go on to **6.17**.

6.13 Your answer – I don't know if the serum cholesterol is invariably elevated in nephrotic syndrome.

If you have been reading **6.6** carefully you would have learned that in both lupus nephritis and acute glomerulonephritis there are exceptions to the rule of elevation of the serum cholesterol in the nephrotic syndrome. Go back over **6.6** with greater care, avoiding distraction if you can.

6.14 Your answer – the patient is *not* certain to have diabetes mellitus.

Good. The next step is to consider each of the commoner causes of the nephrotic syndrome. First of all let us clear up some of the confusion caused by the fact that the Ellis classification of nephritis was a clinical rather than a histological classification.

Ellis Type II nephritis was a clinical picture of an insidious nephrotic syndrome with survival for years, 20 or more, but ultimately four out of five patients died of the disease or did not recover from it, where as one in five ultimately recovered; the disease was not associated with an elevated blood pressure or blood urea at first but over the course of years the patient developed hypertension and renal failure.

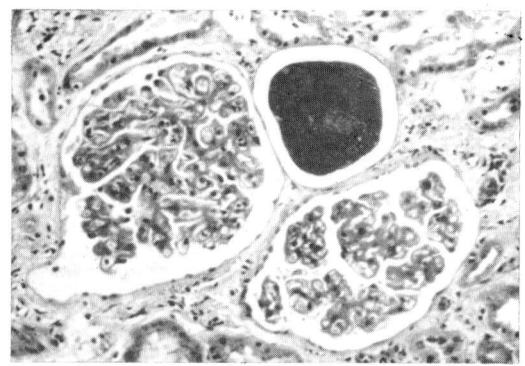

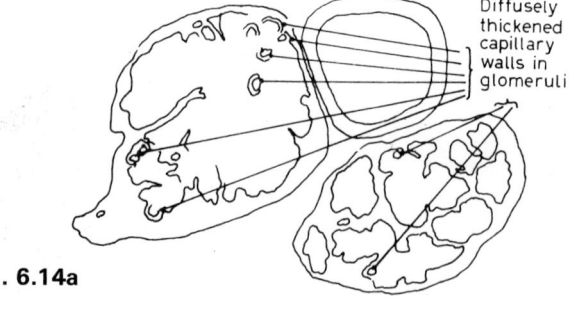

Fig. 6.14a

The Ellis classification of Type II nephritis nowadays is rarely used because the diagnosis of nephrotic syndrome is clarified by renal biopsy; that is, a pathological diagnosis is usually made. The majority of Ellis Type II nephritis patients have either a membranous or a proliferative glomerulonephritis i.e., a chronic form of glomerulonephritis, if they are adults. Some adults and the majority of children have 'no light microscopical change' visible in the kidney apart from proximal tubular changes due to protein in the tubule wall. There are constant changes in all patients with heavy proteinuria — on electron microscopy of the glomeruli the podocytes or foot processes of the epithelial cells are fused.

The appearance on light microscopy of the kidney in membranous glomerulophritis is shown in Fig. 6.14a.

The basement membranes of the glomerular capillaries are thickened in *all* glomeruli uniformly; the capillary lumens are obstructed and there may be lobulation of the tuft. There is always a slight increase in interstitial cells. In proliferative glomerulonephritis there is often an antecedent history of streptococcal infection and acute glomerulonephritis. The appearance of a typical biopsy is shown in Fig. 6.14b.

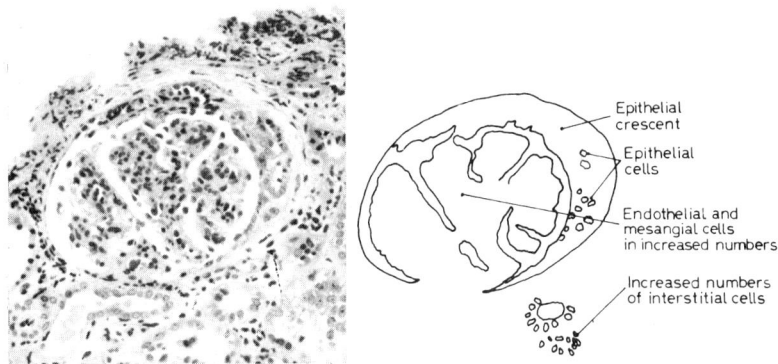

Fig. 6.14b

There is an increase in endothelial and epithelial cells; polymorphs and small round cells are present in the glomerulus: crescent formation or capsular tuft adhesions may be present. There are often irregular patchy thickenings of the basement membrane — quite easily distinguished from the uniformly thickened basement membrane of membranous glomerulonephritis. In membranoproliferative glomerulonephritis (synonyms mesangiocapillary or lobular glomerulonephritis) there is an increase in the mesangial tissues with a characteristic thickening of the capillary wall with a tramline or double or split appearance of the basement membrane. Look at Fig. 6.14c, overleaf.

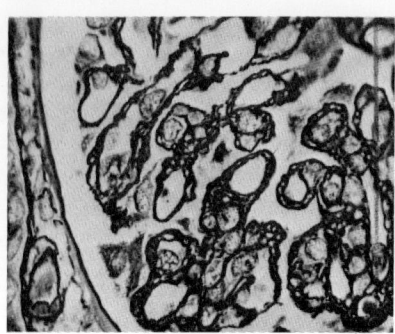
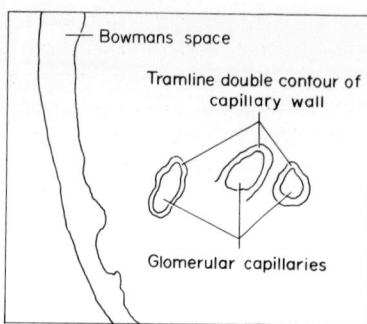

Fig. 6.14c

In focal sclerosing glomerulonephritis at first there may be so few changes that it is incorrectly diagnosed as minimal change glomerulonephritis, but later on there is sclerosis of segments of some glomeruli which may progress total obliteration of the glomeruli. Now answer the question.

Question What type of nephrotic syndrome has this biopsy appearance? (Fig. 6.14d)

Answer
1. Membranous.
   Go on to **6.12**.
2. Proliferative.
   Go on to **6.16**.
3. Membrano-proliferative.
   Go on to **6.18**.

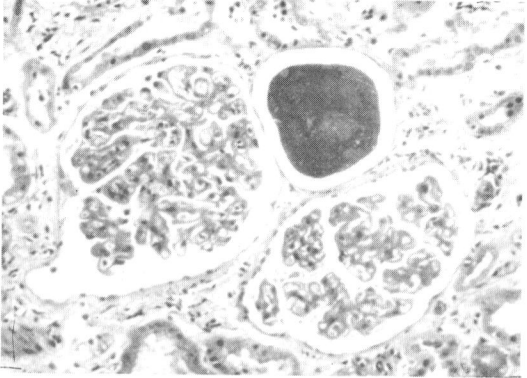

Fig. 6.14d

6.15 Your answer — there is usually a history of preceding streptococcal infection in membranous glomerulonephritis.

You are wrong: in membranous glomerulonephritis the onset of the disease is insidious — oedema of the feet and legs. Go back to **6.12** and read it again.

6.16 Your answer — proliferative glomerulonephritis.

You are wrong. Go back to **6.14** and look carefully at the figures, read the paragraph and choose the answer carefully.

6.17 Your answer — there is usually *no* history of preceding streptococcal infection in membranous glomerulonephritis.

Good. The next most common group of patients with nephrotic syndrome are diabetics with diabetic glomerulosclerosis or Kimmelstiel-Wilson syndrome. The pathological appearances of this disease are usually a diffuse glomerulo-sclerosis; in some patients nodules may be conspicuous; the so-called nodular form is not necessary for the development of nephrotic syndrome as Kark's group have shown in a painstaking model of clinical, histological and biochemical correlation of data. A biopsy of typical diffuse diabetic glomerulosclerosis is shown in Fig. 6.17.

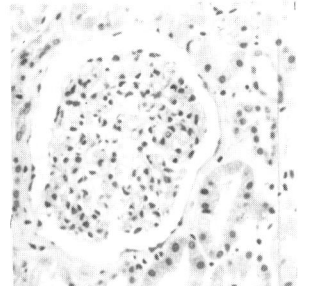 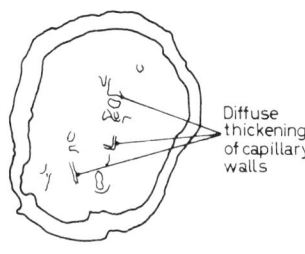

Fig. 6.17

The patient has usually, but not always, been diagnosed as suffering from diabetes mellitus several years before, usually about 10 to 15 years but sometimes much longer. The prognosis is poor: the average length of survival after the onset of nephrotic syndrome is three years, although it is by no means rare to see a diabetic who has had nephrotic syndrome for eight to ten or more years. The majority have hypertension, and nearly all have diabetic retinopathy with microaneurysms of the retina, and diabetic neuropathy. There is little definite correlation between adequacy of diabetic control and the onset of diabetic glomerulosclerosis. The causes of death are usually renal failure and/or hypertension and its complications. A point that should be remembered is that nephrotic urines if tested with 'Clinitest' tablets give a purplish colour due to protein which may be misinterpreted as indicating the absence of glycosuria. It is preferable to test nephrotic urines routinely with Clinistix, which is not affected by the protein content of the urine. However it is an elevated blood glucose level and diabetic glucose tolerance curve which are necessary in the diagnosis of diabetes mellitus rather than the presence of glucose in the urine alone.

Question How long is the average patient likely to survive after the onset of nephrotic syndrome caused by diabetic glomerulosclerosis?

Answer 1. Ten years. Go on to **6.20**.
        2. Three years. Go on to **6.22**.

6.18 Your answer – membrano-proliferative glomerulonephritis.

You are *not* correct. There is always a slight increase in cells in membranous glomerulonephritis but there are not enough cells here to justify the diagnosis you have made. Go back to **6.14** and look carefully at the figures before answering the question again.

6.19 Your answer – diabetic glucose tolerance tests in uraemia indicate diabetic renal disease.

No. In renal failure a diabetic glucose tolerance test is common and does not indicate long standing diabetes mellitus. Read **6.22** again.

6.20 Your answer – average length of survival in nephrotic syndrome due to diabetic glomerulosclerosis is ten years.

No. The average survival is three years after the diagnosis of nephrotic syndrome has been made. Read **6.17** again.

6.21 Your answer – it does not mean that the renal failure is always due to diabetes mellitus.

Correct. Now answer the next question.

Question Do patients with nodular diabetic glomerulosclerosis invariably develop nephrotic syndrome?

Answer 1. Yes. Go on to **6.23**.
2. No. Go on to **6.25**.

6.22 Your answer – survival is three years on the average.

Correct. Occasionally diabetics with diabetic glomerulosclerosis causing nephrotic syndrome have very mild diabetes, which may have escaped detection. In uraemia the glucose tolerance test is frequently diabetic in type; this complicates the picture, for uraemic hyperglycaemia may be misinterpreted as long-standing diabetes mellitus, and the aetiology of the nephrotic syndrome may be wrongly thought to be diabetic glomerulosclerosis. The absence of a diabetic retinopathy should always make one suspicious of the diagnosis of diabetic glomerulosclerosis, and one should assume this is incorrect if the fundus is normal.

Treatment of the diabetes is usually not particularly difficult in the nephrotic phase; and patients rarely have ketones in the urine. It is frequently forgotten that, although the majority of long-standing diabetics have diffuse diabetic glomerulosclerosis, only a small proportion develop nephrotic syndrome. In diabetic nodular glomerulosclerosis (the Kimmelstiel-Wilson syndrome), some patients do not pass through a protein losing phase and may present initially with chronic renal failure. Now answer the question.

Question If a glucose tolerance test shows a diabetic curve in a uraemic patient, is the uraemia always due to antecedent diabetic kidney disease?

Answer 1. Yes. Go on to **6.19**.
2. No. Go on to **6.21**.

6.23 Your answer – they invariably develop nephrotic syndrome. This is not correct: many patients with diabetic nodular glomerulosclerosis do not develop a nephrotic phase but pass into a stage of chronic renal failure without any apparent oedematous phase. Read **6.22** again and then answer the question in **6.21** again.

6.24 Your answer – the serum cholesterol is always elevated in SLE nephrotic syndrome.
You are wrong. In so-called pseudo-nephrotic syndrome the serum cholesterol is normal, not elevated. Go back and read **6.25**, then answer **6.27** again.

6.25 Your answer – they do *not* invariably develop nephrotic syndrome.
You are correct. Systemic lupus erythematosus is a common collagen disease, of unknown aetiology but with autoimmune features, which causes nephrotic syndrome. It is most frequent in females age 20 to 40, the female/male ratio being 4:1. About half the patients with systemic lupus erythematosus have renal disease. The histological features (see Fig. 6.25) are glomerulitis, thickening of the capillary loops (wire loop lesions), karyorrhexis, necrosis, haemotxylin bodies, and interstitial nephritis.

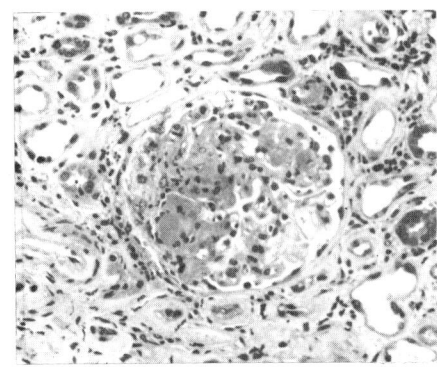
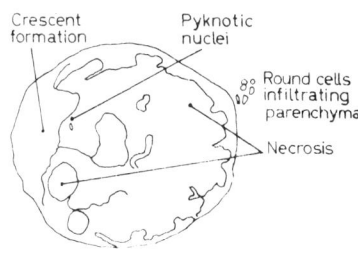

Fig. 6.25

The various types of lupus renal lesions are discussed in the Chapter 10 on Collagen Disease and the Kidney. Lupus nephrotic syndrome is fairly uncommon, probably accounting for *one in three of patients with renal involvement in SLE*. The immunological features are:

(1) IgG and complement are deposited in the glomerulus in granular form, as shown by fluorescent antibody staining.
(2) Antinuclear factor is present in the majority of patients with SLE.
(3) LE cell test is usually but not constantly positive.
(4) Increased incidence of anti-nuclear factor in relatives.

The diagnosis of systemic lupus in nephrotic syndrome is usually possible clinically and is based on the features of butterfly rash on the face, violaceous rash on the hands, thrombocytopenia, leucopenia, haemolytic anaemia, hepatosplenomegaly, polyarthritis, erythema multiforme, pleurisy, pericarditis, and mitral murmurs.

The urine contains a 'telescoped' deposit — red cells, white cells, red and white cell casts, granular casts, renal fail casts, fatty and waxy casts — as well as large amounts of protein, particularly albumin and IgG globulin. The Wasserman test often shows a biologic false positive reaction. The serum complement is low, as in acute glomerulonephritis. The serum cholesterol is *inconstantly* elevated, the other biochemical features being indistinguishable from any other type of nephrotic syndrome. Now answer the question.

Question How common is lupus nephrotic syndrome in patients with lupus renal involvement?

Answer 1. One in three. Go on to **6.27**.
       2. Don't know. Go on to **6.29**.

6.26 Your answer — the serum cholesterol is *not* invariably elevated in lupus nephrotic syndrome.
    Correct. Now answer the next question.

Question Is the level of the serum complement elevated, normal, or depressed in nephrotic syndrome due to lupus?

Answer 1. Elevated. Go on to **6.28**.
       2. Depressed. Go on to **6.31**.
       3. Normal. Go on to **6.33**.

6.27 Your answer — one in three has lupus nephrotic syndrome.
    Good. Now answer the next question.

Question Is the serum cholesterol invariably raised in nephrotic syndrome due to systemic lupus?

Answer 1. Yes. Go on to **6.24**.
       2. No. Go on to **6.26**.

6.28 Your answer — serum complement is elevated in lupus nephrotic syndrome.
    You are wrong. Read **6.25** and answer the question in **6.26** again. Remember that serum complement levels are depressed in systemic lupus and acute glomerulonephritis.

6.29 Your answer — I don't know how frequent lupus nephrotic syndrome is in lupus renal involvement.
    About one in three patients with renal involvement in lupus has the nephrotic syndrome. Go back and read **6.25**.

6.30 Your answer – the prognosis in 'pseudo-nephrotic' syndrome was thought to be a few months.

Good. It is now likely that this was an unnecessarily gloomy prognosis and the level of the serum cholesterol may be unrelated to the life prognosis of lupus nephrotic syndrome.

Another cause of nephrotic syndrome is amyloid disease. Amyloid disease may be: (1) Primary or (2) Secondary to a number of diseases such as chronic suppuration, chronic osteomyelitis, TB, lung abscess, bronchiectasis, Crohn's disease (regional enteritis), ulcerative colitis, rheumatoid arthritis, Hodgkins disease, actinomycosis, syphilis. (3) Multiple myeloma. We shall discuss these diseases in so far as they have bearing on renal involvement.

First of all let us consider *primary amyloidosis:* although some authorities (eg. Muehrcke) have found a rather low incidence of renal involvement (one in ten) in primary amyloidosis, others have found up to one in four have renal disease. The majority of primary amyloid cases seen in England are sporadic cases, but in the Near and Middle East familial amyloid is common; workers in Israel and in France have investigated familial Mediterranean fever and found a high incidence of nephrotic syndrome due to amyloid in this disease. In familial Mediterranean fever the patient is usually a Jew (most commonly of Oriental extraction), an Armenian or an Arab. The patients have recurrent febrile attacks, abdominal pain and peritonitis, polyarthritis and a constant massive proteinuria which causes nephrotic syndrome to develop. Death results from renal failure.

Question What is the cause of death in Familial Mediterranean Fever with amyloidosis of the kidneys?

Answer 1. Renal Failure. Go on to **6.36**.
2. Febrile attacks. Go on to **6.38**.
3. Don't know. Go on to **6.40**.

6.31 Your answer – serum complement is depressed in systemic lupus erythematosus.

You are correct. The prognosis of nephrotic syndrome due to lupus was thought at first to be worse in the so-called pseudo nephrotic group with death in a few months after diagnosis, whereas the patients in the high-cholesterol lupus nephrotic group had a much longer life expectancy, often measured in years: but this differentiation has been disputed. With high dosage steroid therapy (i.e. 60 to 100 mg Prednisone daily), there is a good chance of suppressing the disease or at least preventing progression in the majority of cases, but some patients deteriorate despite therapy. The treatment of all types of lupus nephritis is discussed in the Chapter 10 on Collagen Diseases and the Kidney.

Question What was the life prognosis of the 'pseudo-nephrotic group' of lupus nephrotic syndrome once thought to be, although this is now dubious?

Answer 1. A few months. Go on to **6.30**.
2. Several years. Go on to **6.32**.
3. Same as lupus nephrotic syndrome with a high cholesterol. Go on to **6.34**.

6.32 Your answer – the prognosis in pseudo-nephrotic syndrome of lupus was though to be several years.

No. At first the prognosis of the 'pseudo-nephrotic group' with a low serum cholesterol was thought to be a few months only, but some subsequent work has suggested that the prognosis in this disease does not differ from that of lupus nephritis with high serum cholesterol. Go on to **6.30**.

6.33 Your answer – serum complement level is normal in SLE nephrotic syndrome.

The level of serum complement is depressed in both acute glomerulonephritis and systemic lupus erythematosus. Read through **6.25** again before answering the question in **6.26** again.

6.34 Your answer – the prognosis was thought to be the same as in lupus nephrotic syndrome with a high serum cholesterol.

At first it was thought that patients with a low serum cholesterol died within a few months, whereas the high cholesterol group had a better prognosis but this now seems to be unlikely, and it is possible that the level of the serum cholesterol is not related to the prognosis in nephrotic syndrome due to SLE. Go on to read **6.30**.

6.35 Your answer – primary amyloid deposits do *not* always stain with Congo Red.

Correct. Renal amyloid involvement usually presents as proteinuria which may persist for years without any other clinical sign; in some patients the albuminuria becomes massive and the patient develops nephrotic syndrome. Uraemia may supervene without a nephrotic phase occurring, and ultimately renal failure usually develops in patients with amyloid nephrotic syndrome. Renal vien thrombosis is a common complicating factor in renal amyloid disease, being characterised by rapidly progressive renal failure or a nephrotic picture. Generally the blood pressure in patients with renal amyloid remains normal. The ESR and total serum globulin are elevated, but the anaemia of renal failure is often absent. The diagnosis of amyloid disease of the kidneys is made by percutaneous renal biopsy; the presence of a positive Congo Red test suggests that the patient has amyloid disease but does not necessarily mean that he has renal involvement.

Question If a patient with renal amyloid disease suddenly develops a rapidly progressive renal failure, what complication has developed?

Answer 1. Nephrotic syndrome. Go on to **6.39**.

2. Renal vein thrombosis. Go on to **6.41**.
3. Don't know. Go on to **6.43**.

6.36 Your answer – death is usually due to renal failure.

Correct. Secondary amyloid, due to suppuration and many other diseases (some of which were stated in the preceding paragraph), involves the kidneys in at least three quarters of the patients with this disease. In myeloma there is renal amyloidosis in 3 per cent of patients. The histological picture of amyloidosis of the kidneys is shown in Fig. 6.36. There is a deposition of a fibrillary material which

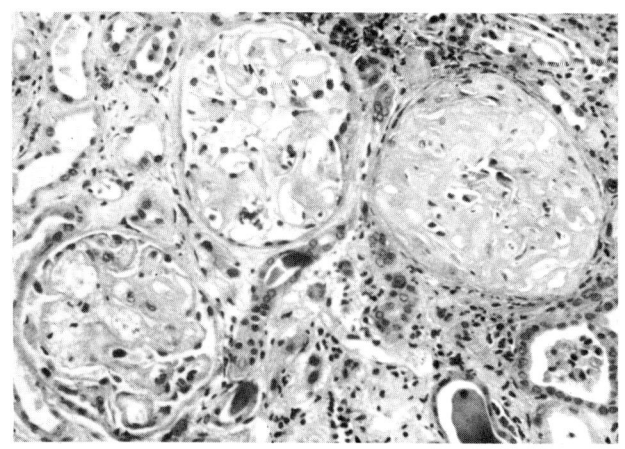

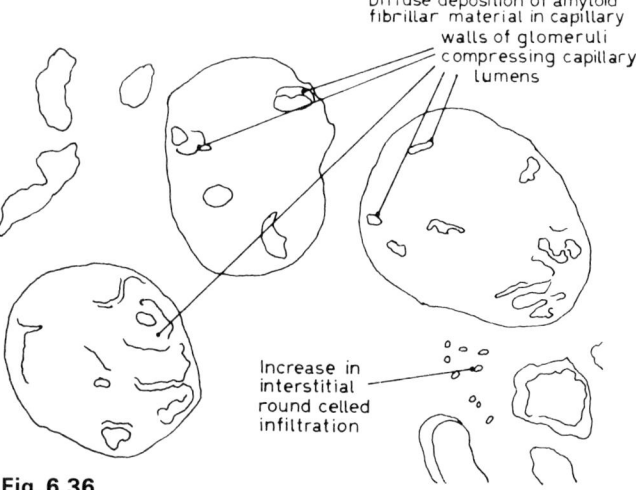

Fig. 6.36

stains red with Congo Red in secondary amyloid: primary amyloid often does not stain in this way. The amyloid is laid down in the walls of capillaries gradually encroaching until it occludes the capillary lumen; finally the glomeruli are replaced by amyloid tissue. The amyloid tissue has been shown by fluorescein-labelling to contain γ globulin.

Question Do primary amyloid deposits always stain red with Congo Red?

Answer 1. Yes. Go on to **6.37**.
2. No. Go on to **6.35**.

6.37 Your answer – primary amyloid deposits always stain red with Congo Red.
No. Secondary amyloid usually stains red, but primary amyloid stains unpredictably with Congo Red. Go back and read **6.36** again.

6.38 Your answer – the cause of death in familial Mediterranean fever with renal amyloidosis is febrile attacks.
No. The cause of death in patients with renal amyloidosis is usually renal failure. Go back and answer the question in **6.30** correctly after reading the paragraph again.

6.39 Your answer – rapidly progressing renal failure of sudden onset in amyloid disease is caused by nephrotic syndrome.
You are incorrect in that the nephrotic syndrome of renal amyloid does not usually progress rapidly with renal failure of sudden onset. Renal failure is insidious in its onset and very slow in its development in nephrotic syndrome of renal amyloid. Renal amyloid may be complicated with renal vein thrombosis in which there is a rapidly progressive renal failure or nephrotic syndrome. Now answer the question in **6.35** again.

6.40 Your answer – I don't know what is the cause of death in familial Mediterranean fever with renal amyloidosis.
The cause of death in renal amyloidosis of any cause is usually renal failure, unless the disease process causing the amyloid is itself fatal. In familial Mediterranean fever the amyloid is 'primary' in type i.e. the aetiology is unknown, and the patients frequently die of renal failure. Now go back and answer the question in **6.30** again.

6.41 Your answer – renal vein thrombosis is responsible for the rapid onset of renal failure in amyloid disease.
You are correct. There are many other causes of nephrotic syndrome, which are seen less frequently than those already described. *Congestive heart failure* is usually associated with proteinuria which occasionally reaches 15–20 g/day,

although more common proteinuria of only 1–2 g/day is found. The mechanism of the albuminuria is not certain but may be

(1) Relative renal anoxia damaging the glomeruli.
(2) Higher pressure in the renal veins, causing an increase glomerular permeability.
(3) Mercurial diuretics, being given for the treatment of congestive heart failure, have themselves been implicated as the cause of nephrotic syndrome, and the use of teething powders containing inorganic mercury compounds is associated with the development of nephrotic syndrome in infants.

Question How much proteinuria per day is usually found in patients with congestive heart failure?

Answer 1. 1–2 g/24 hours. Go on to **6.42**.
2. 15–20 g/24 hours. Go on to **6.45**.
3. Don't know. Go on to **6.49**.

6.42 Your answer – the usual amount of proteinuria in congestive heart failure is 1–2 g/day.

Good. Renal vein thrombosis is a cause of nephrotic syndrome. The factors which are known to be precipitating causes of renal vein thrombosis are:

(1) Neoplasm. The site of the growth may be remote, as in carcinoma of stomach or pancreas; occasionally the inferior vena cave is directly involved in secondary neoplasm of the liver, with a hard irregular liver with tender nodules; or hypernephroma tissue growing down the renal vein and so invading the inferior vena cava.
(2) Amyloid disease.
(3) Trauma, sometimes at operation, to the renal veins or inferior vena cava.
(4) Spontaneous renal vein thrombosis is a common complication of nephrotic syndrome irrespective of aetiology. This may well be due to the elevated fibrinogen levels which are found in nephrotic syndrome, with an increase in the number of platelets and an elevation of Factor 5 and Factor 8 concentrations. They are presumably partly responsible for the increased clotting tendency seen in nephrotic syndrome.
(5) Indwelling cannulae in the inferior vena cava.

The diagnosis of inferior vena caval obstruction can often be made by the presence of large anastomotic vessels coursing up the abdominal wall, anastomosing the inferior with the superior venae cava.

Question If a man with nephrotic syndrome is found to have an enlarged, hard, irregular liver with tender lumps on it, what do you consider the most likely diagnosis?

Answer 1. Renal vein thrombosis, following secondary neoplasm of the liver. Go on to **6.44**.
2. Secondary deposits in liver. Go on to **6.46**.
3. Amyloidosis of the liver. Go on to **6.48**.
4. Don't know. Go on to **6.51**.

6.43 Your answer – I don't know what causes the rapidly progressive renal failure in amyloid disease.

Amyloid involvement of the kidneys is a slowly progressive disease of the kidneys; the sudden onset of a rapidly progressing renal failure is associated with the complication of renal vein thrombosis; now read **6.39** again before you answer the question.

6.44 Your answer – the diagnosis is secondary neoplasm in liver with renal vein thrombosis.

Good. The clinical manifestations of renal vein thrombosis may be grouped into two separate syndromes.

(1) Nephrotic syndrome.

(2) Rapidly progressive renal failure with haematuria and venous infarction of the kidney.

The nephrotic group may have obvious evidence of secondary neoplasm or obstruction of the inferior vena cava, with an otherwise unremarkable nephrotic syndrome. Look at Fig. 6.44a. This is an infrared photograph showing anastamotic veins on the abdomen of a man with inferior vena caval thrombosis and nephrotic syndrome. There may be stigmata of amyloid disease or of the diseases predis-

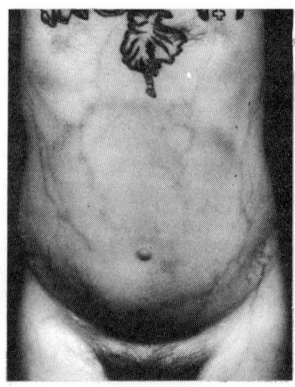

Fig. 6.44a

posing to amyloid disease. Remember that amyloid disease is associated with thrombosis of the renal *venules* in the kidney, although sometimes the renal veins themselves are involved. Often there are no clinical features to differentiate this from any other type of nephrotic syndrome. The diagnostic features on renal biopsy are disputed, but the most frequent changes are:

(1) Interstitial oedema.
(2) Basement membrane thickening in glomeruli.
(3) Margination of leucocytes i.e., leucocytes lie close to the capillary wall and not in the center of the capillary lumen.

Diagnosis of inferior vena caval obstruction by venography is itself adequate to suggest that a nephrotic patient has renal vein thrombosis. Venography sometimes shows that the inferior vena cava is patent but that the normal impression in the radio-opaque column caused by blood streaming in from the renal veins may be absent. This is shown in Fig. 6.44b & c.

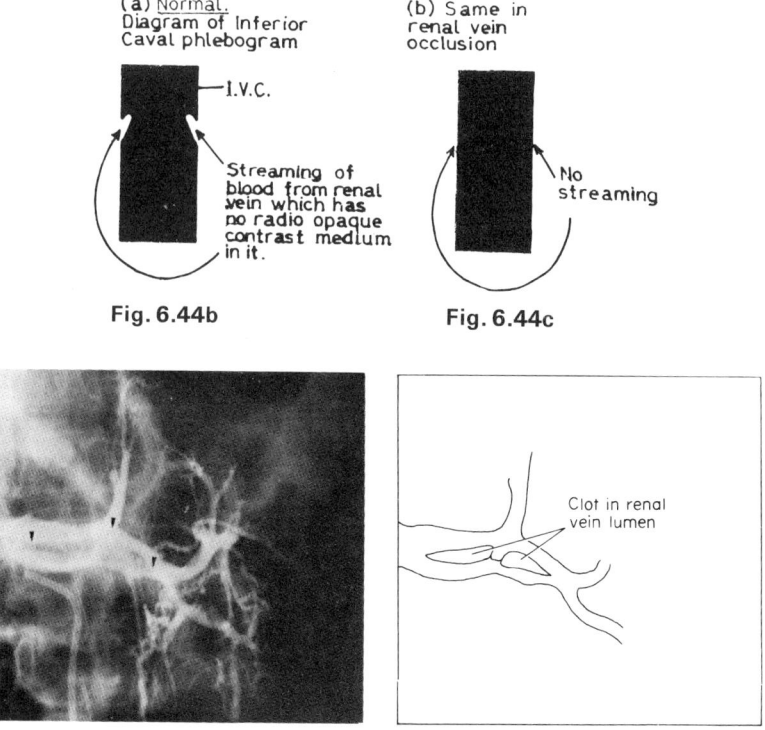

Fig. 6.44b

Fig. 6.44c

Fig. 6.44d

Streaming may also be absent in advanced renal disease where the renal blood flow is markedly reduced. In other cases selective renal phlebography may show actual translucency in the renal veins where a clot is present (6.44d), or may show absence of venous filling in areas of clotting.

The treatment of renal vein thrombosis is with anticoagulants; the symptomatic treatment of the nephrotic syndrome will be dealt with later.

Question Would you be prepared to accept a diagnosis of renal vein thrombosis if the patient had a patent inferior vena cava and evidence of vigorous streaming from the renal veins?

Answer 1. Yes. Go on to **6.52**.
2. No. Go on to **6.50**.
3. Don't know. Go on to **6.54**.

6.45 Your answer — 15—20 g/day of protein are commonly lost in the urine day in congestive heart failure.

You are correct in that 15—20 g of protein are occasionally lost in the urine in some patients with congestive heart failure, and this amount of protein loss can lead to hypo-proteinaemia and the nephrotic syndrome. Protein loss of this magnitude is rare in congestive heart failure; usually the amount of protein lost is 1—2 g/day in with congestive heart failure. Now answer the question in **6.41** again.

6.46 Your answer — secondary deposits in the liver.

You are correct in that the irregular, hard, nodular liver is probably affected by secondary neoplasm, but the nephrotic syndrome requires explanation: neneprotic syndrome can be caused by renal vein thrombosis which itself may be associated with neoplasm. The bulk of the new growth in the liever is a common cause of inferior vena caval obstruction and renal vein thrombosis. Now answer the question in **6.42** again.

6.47 Your answer — there is no protein loss in the urine in congestive heart failure.

This is not correct. Proteinuria is common in congestive heart failure, usually fairly small in amount — between 1—2 g/day. Occasionally this proteinuria is massive and gives rise to the nephrotic syndrome. Now read **6.41** again and answer the question correctly.

6.48 Your answer — amyloidosis of the liver.

You are wrong. Amyloidosis of the liver gives a smoothy enlarged liver which may be associated with renal vein thrombosis. An irregular hard liver with tender nodules is characteristic of a liver with secondary deposits in it. Now read **6.42** again.

6.49 Your answer — I don't know how much proteinuria there is usually in congestive heart failure.

The amount of protein usually excreted in the urine in congestive heart failure is about 1–2 g/day; the reason for this proteinuria is not known with absolute certainty but it may well be due to an increase in the pressure in the renal veins in congestive heart failure, or to the impairment of blood supply to the kidneys. Occasionally, the loss of protein in the urine is massive and leads to the development of nephrotic syndrome. Now read **6.41** more carefully. Try to concentrate and do not 'scan' the lines. Speed reading should be avoided.

6.50 Your answer — I would not be prepared to accept the diagnosis as renal vein thrombosis.

Good. Malignant hypertension can rise to massive proteinuria, and it is the probable cause of the proteinuria in renal artery stenosis which is itself a cause of nephrotic syndrome. There are many other causes of nephrotic syndrome, many of them associated with toxic substances, — drugs or organisms. Mercurial diuretics and mercury teething powders have been implicated as causes of the nephrotic syndrome in adults and children respectively; but there is no proof that the administration of mercury compounds is the cause of nephrotic syndrome and not just coincidentally related. Thus nephrotic syndrome occurs in adults with congestive heart failure who have not received mercurials; and nephrotic syndrome is not particularly rare in children not receiving mercurial diuretics. Similarly syphilis has been shown to be a cause of the nephrotic syndrome, with remission of the nephrotic picture after treatment of the syphilis. Malaria is an important and common cause of the nephrotic syndrome in countries where quartan malaria is endemic. In Nigeria it has been shown that malaria is the most common cause of the nephrotic syndrome, and if the malarial infestation is controlled, a large proportion of cases recover competely. The disease is an immune complex disease caused by damage to the basement membrane and capillary loops, by an immune complex consisting of the antigen of P. malariae, antibody of IgC and IgM, and complement. The diagnosis can be made with certainty by the use of immunofluorescent studies on renal biopsy specimens with antibodies to P.malariae. There is a scattered granular fluorescence typical of immune complex disease. Treatment is by means of diuretics, sodium restriction and antimalarial drugs. Recovery is to be expected unless renal failure has developed. On the other hand, Tridione (troxidone) and potassium perchlorate can certainly cause nephrotic syndrome in man, and penicillamine administration has also produced nephrotic syndrome. Finally, there is a group of inherited nephrotic disease which may appear in infancy in the first year or two of life and is associated with a rapidly progressive fatal course; other types appear in adult life and may persist for years.

Question What is the prognosis in inherited nephrotic syndrome in infancy?

Answer 1. Rapidly progressive fatal course. Go on to **6.53**.
2. Persist for years. Go on to **6.55**.
3. Don't know. Go on to **6.57**.

6.51 Your answer – I don't know what the diagnosis is.

In **6.42** you have read that secondary neoplasm of the liver can give a hard irregular liver with tender nodules and that hepatic secondary deposits may be associated with renal vein thrombosis. Now answer the question in **6.42** correctly.

6.52 Your answer – I would accept the diagnosis of renal vein thrombosis in the presence of streaming.

You are incorrect to accept the diagnosis in the presence of apparently good evidence of blood flowing through the renal veins. Read **6.44** again and answer the question correctly.

6.53 Your answer – inherited infantile nephrotic syndrome has a rapidly progressive fatal course.

Correct. The treatment of nephrotic syndrome, irrespective of cause, is primarily symptomatic: the first aim is to make the patient free of oedema and this can be achieved in almost all patients. The second aim, attainable in a smaller proportion of patients, is the suppression of cure of the primary disease. First the symptomatic therapy of oedema removal will be considered: this is carried out by removal of sodium from the body by means of diuretics, restriction of sodium intake by a low salt diet, and increase in the plasma oncotic pressure by intravenous albumin and dextrans. The diuretics used are thiazide diuretics such as chlorothiazide, which is given in a dosage of 2 g daily together with oral potassium supplements such as slow K 30 mEq/day. Aldactone A (spironolactone) is given in addition if the response to chlorothiazide is inadequate, the dose used being 25 mg q.d.s. Occasional patients require the more powerful oral diuretics such as ethacrynic acid or frusemide (Lasix). Furosemide or frusemide (Lasix) is to be preferred to ethacrynic acid (*Edacrin*) because the latter is known to be a cause of acute renal failure, and is therefore best avoided in patients with pre-existing renal disease. Mercurial diuretics may be employed occasionally, but these are very infrequently required. There is little point in attempting to remove sodium from the body by diuretics unless the sodium intake is controlled by a low salt diet containing not more than 20 mEq of sodium a day.

Question What dose of chlorothiazide would you give a patient with nephrotic oedema?

Answer 1. 25 mg four times a day. Go on to **6.58**.
2. 2.0 g/day. Go on to **6.56**.

6.54 I don't know whether the diagnosis of renal vein thrombosis is correct or not. If you don't know, you have not read **6.44** with enough care. Streaming is a sign of blood flowing from the renal veins into the inferior vena cava. If it is present it is unlikely that there is an occlusion of the renal veins adequate to cause nephrotic syndrome. Now read **6.44** again (to make sure you have not missed any other facts), before you answer the question again.

6.55 You answer – inherited nephrotic syndrome in infancy persists for years.
You are wrong. In infantile inherited nephrotic syndrome the prognosis is bad, the majority of patients dying in a few months. The prognosis is better in the inherited nephrotic syndrome appearing in adults. Read **6.50** again.

6.56 Your answer – the dose of chlorothiazide is 2.0 g/day.
Correct. Now answer the next question.

Question Is there any need to restrict sodium intake in the diet of a patient with nephrotic oedema?

Answer 1. Yes. Go on to **6.61**.
2. No. Go on to **6.59**.
3. Dont' know. Go on to **6.63**.

6.57 Your answer – I don't know the prognosis in inherited nephrotic syndrome in infancy.
The prognosis is remarkably bad, death occurring in a few months. You should read **6.50** again before answering the question again.

6.58 Your answer – The dose of chlorothiazide for treatment of nephrotic oedema is 25 mg q.d.s. No. The dose of chlorothiazide in nephrotic syndrome is 1.0 g b.d. i.e. 2.0 g a day. You should be familiar with this dose. Go back and read **6.53** again.

6.59 Your answer – there is no need to restrict sodium intake in nephrotic patients with oedema.
No. The treatment of oedema is by removal of sodium from the body, so decreasing the extracellular fluid volume. This is accomplished by the use of diuretics which remove sodium in the urine; this is pointless if more sodium is freely poured into the body by unrestricted sodium intake. Thus it is necessary to restrict the intake of sodium and repeatedly deplete the patient of sodium by diuretics until the oedema has disappeared. Go back and answer the question in **6.56** correctly.

6.60 Your answer – an increase in urine protein excretion occurs.

You are correct. Further symptomatic methods of treating nephrotic syndrome to remove oedema are:

(1) Resin administration such as Katonium. This is a resin in the potassium and ammonium cycle and is given to remove sodium from the intestinal contents, exchanging potassium and ammonium for the sodium in the bowel. The dose of Katonium is 15 g t.d.s. The disadvantages are the fact that it tastes like finely powdered sand, and that electrolyte estimations need to be carried out weekly on patients taking resins to correct any serious electrolyte imbalance which may develop.

(2) Osmotic diuresis may be used, giving mannitol, 10 per cent, in a volume of 1 litre intravenously over 6 to 8 hours; in osmotic diuresis sodium is lost due to the increased volume of fluid moving rapidly down the tubule and passing the sites of sodium reabsorption too quickly for adequate sodium absorption to have taken place. Now answer the question.

Question Does Katonium remove sodium from the intestinal contents, or does it remove potassium?

Answer 1. Removes sodium. Go on to **6.65**.
        2. Removes potassium. Go on to **6.68**.
        3. Don't know. Go on to **6.70**.

6.61 Your answer – sodium restriction is necessary in the diet in nephrotic syndrome.

You are correct. The salt intake has to be low whether diuretics are being given or not, if the serum albumin is below 2.0 g/day, because the urine in these circumstances is virtually sodium free due to the secretion of excessive amounts of aldosterone in hypoproteinaemic conditions; most sodium absorbed from the food will thus be retained in the body in the absence of diuretics. Another approach to the subject and one occasionally employed is the elevation of the plasma oncotic pressure by intravenous albumin or intravenous dextran. The effect of these is to cause a diuresis with loss of the oedema fluid, but the effect is transient due to the rapid and *increased loss* of protein in the urine if plasma albumin concentration is increased. Dextran has a limited life before it is metabolised; it may also cause blockade of the reticulo-endothelial system and is best avoided. Perhaps the most useful aspect of intravenous infusions of plasma albumin is that they raise the morale of the chronically ill patient who sees the oedema disappearing, albeit transiently, after a long period of unsuccessful diuretic and dietary therapy.

Question What is the effect on urinary protein loss of giving plasma albumin intravenously to increase the plasma oncotic pressure?

Answer 1. No effect. Go on to **6.64**.
        2. Increase urinary protein excretion. Go on to **6.60**.

3. Decrease urinary protein excretion. Go on to **6.62**.
4. Don't know. Go on to **6.66**.

6.62 Your answer — there is a decrease in urinary protein.
No. The reason for this is as follows:
Plasma albumin clearance, like any other clearance, is expressed by the formula
$C = UV/P$ where C = clearance of plasma in ml/min.
U = urinary albumin concentration.
V = volume of urine formed per minute.
P = plasma concentration of albumin.

Now if 'P' is elevated by infusing albumin, then if C is to remain constant UV must increase i.e., albumin excretion rate must increase. Now answer the question in **6.61** correctly.

6.63 Your answer — I don't know if it is necessary to restrict sodium intake in nephrotic oedema.

The purpose of removing sodium from a patient by diuretics is to reduce the extracellular fluid volume. This can be done by using diuretics to actively remove sodium from the body, but there is little point in doing this unless the intake of sodium is controlled carefully to prevent as much sodium being absorbed from the diet as is being lost in the urine. Now answer the question in **6.56** again.

6.64 Your answer — there is no effect on the urinary proteins.

No. The plasma protein concentration increase will increase the urinary protein loss. You will understand this better if you consider that if plasma albumin clearance ($C = UV/P$) remains constant, then elevation of 'P' i.e., plasma albumin concentrations will result in an increase in UV i.e., the urinary albumin excretion per minute.

Now answer the question in **6.61** correctly.

6.65 Your answer — katonium removes sodium from the intestinal gut.

Good. Peritoneal dialysis may be required to remove resistant oedema. Very rarely Southey's tubes may be needed. Usually, however, more basic therapy is used to suppress possible unkown immune inflammatory and allergic factors important in the pathogenesis of nephrotic syndrome. The most important of the drugs used are the cortico-steroids, such as prednisone. Prednisone in a dose of 30–60 mg/day will affect a cure in a high percentage of patients with lipoid nephrosis of children or 'no light microscopic change' of adults, and in those in whom prednisone does not work, or in whom relapse occurs immunosuppressive drugs such as chlorambucil, azothiaprine (Imuran) or cyclophosphamide will usually cause a remission in 95 per cent of patients with this type of disease. In about half the patients with membranous glomerulonephritis a similar response can be found using steroid and immunosuppressive drugs in combination, and in 1 in 3 of those with proliferative glomerulonephritis. In membrano-proliferative glomerulonephritis, and in the patient with lobular mesangial thickening and some cell proliferation, about 1 in 20 respond favourably to these drugs. Severe lupus nephritis can often be suppressed by high dosage of steroids; the subject of steroid therapy of Lupus nephritis will be considered in Chapter 10 on 'Collagen Diseases and the Kidney'. Steroids are contra-indicated in the treatment of amyloid disease of the kidney, there being some evidence that the renal lesions in some cases of amyloid disease deteriorate more rapidly when cortico-steroids are given. In secondary amyloid disease the renal lesion may improve if the cause, such as osteomyelitis, is cured; nevertheless, if the renal amyloid is far advanced so that renal failure has supervened, there is no likelihood of improvement in the renal condition despite cure of the primary disease. There is no curative therapy for primary amyloid disease involving the kidneys. Now answer the question.

Question Has Prednisone treatment in a dosage of 30–60 mg/day any effect on proteinuria in patients with nephrotic syndrome without light microscopic change?

Answer 1. Yes. Go on to **6.67**.
2. No. Go on to **6.69**.
3. Don't know. Go on to **6.91**.

6.66 Your answer – I don't know what the effect is on urinary albumin loss.

The answer to this question will be more easily understood if you bear in mind the fact that albumin clearance is $C = UV/P$, where C = clearance of plasma in ml/min.

U = urine volume.
P = plasma albumin concentration.

If the plasma albumin concentration is elevated, the *clearance* remaining constnat, then UV i.e., albumin excretion per minute, must also increase. Now read **6.61** and answer the question correctly this time.

6.67 Your answer – Prednisone reduces the proteinuria in the 'no light microscopic change' type of nephrotic syndrome.

Good. ACTH has often been advised in the therapy of nephrotic syndrome and it occasionally will prove effective in a dose of 40 units daily when prednisone (60 mg daily) is not found to be effective. There is no curative therapy for nephrotic syndrome due to diabetic glomerulosclerosis; the only treatment indicated is control of the diabetes and removal of oedema by the methods previously described. Renal vein thrombosis causing nephrotic syndrome is an indication for anticoagulant therapy in the *first few days* after onset. Well established nephrotic syndrome due to renal vein thrombosis is *not* an indication for starting anticoagulant therapy unless pain is present due to extension of the venous thrombosis. In drug induced nephrotic syndrome the offending drug should be withdrawn at once, as soon as its possible rôle is realised.

Question A man of 47 with long standing diabetes is found to have nephrotic syndrome and becomes free of oedema on diuretic therapy. A renal biopsy confirms the diagnosis of diabetic glomerulosclerosis. His diabetes is found to be poorly controlled, with blood sugars of about 300 mg/100 ml consistently. What further treatment is indicated?

Answer 1. None. Go on to **6.72**.
2. Better control of diabetes. Go on to **6.74**.
3. Don't know. Go on to **6.76**.

6.68 Your answer – Katonium removes potassium from the intestinal contents.
No. Katonium is in the potassium and ammonium cycles, and removes sodium from the gut in exchange for potassium and ammonium ions. Now read **6.60** again.

6.69 Your answer – prednisone has no effect on proteinuria in 'no light microscopic change' nephrotic syndrome.
You are partly correct in that prednisone has no effect on some patients with no light microscopic change visible histologically, but the majority of patients show some response by reduction in, or total disappearance of, proteinuria. Now answer the question again after reading through **6.65** again.

6.70 Your answer – I don't know what Katonium removes.
Katonium has potassium and ammonium ions in it which are exchanged for sodium ions in the gut. Now read **6.60** again, then answer the question again.

6.71 Your answer – the patient is not likely to recover from membranous glomerulonephritis.
You are correct. Diabetic glomerulosclerosis causing nephrotic syndrome has an average life prognosis of three years, but many patients survive up to ten years. Lupus nephritis causing nephrotic syndrome has a variable prognosis but the unduly pessimistic three months prognosis of the so-called pseudo-nephrosis of SLE is disputed; the life span of 'high cholesterol' lupus nephritis on steroid therapy is at least three years providing the disease was not too advanced when corticosteroid therapy was commenced.

Renal vein thrombosis has a very poor prognosis if associated with neoplasm or amyloid but the nephrotic patient with post-traumatic or spontaneous renal vein thrombosis and nephrotic syndrome may recover completely although some remain oedematous for years.

Question What is the average duration of life in nephrotic syndrome due to diabetic glomerulosclerosis?

Answer 1. A normal life span. Go on to **6.75**.

2. Three years. Go on to **6.79**.
3. Don't know. Go on to **6.77**.

6.72 Your answer – no treatment is indicated.

No. Blood sugar levels consistently about 300 mg/100 ml indicate that the patient is not properly controlled. The only therapy for diabetic glomerulosclerosis apart from symptomatic control of oedema is adequate control of the blood sugar levels in the hope that adequate diabetic control will reduce the rate of progression of the diabetic complications. There is no evidence that adequate control of the diabetes will have any effect on the rate of progress of diabetic glomerulosclerosis, but it is in any case sound advice that diabetes should be well controlled. Now read **6.67** again and answer the question correctly.

6.73 Your answer – he is likely to recover from membranous glomerulonephritis.

No. Few patients recover from membranous glomerulonephritis, which is a chronic disease. Go back to **6.74** and read it carefully before you answer the question again.

6.74 Your answer – better control of the diabetes.

This is correct although there is little proof that adequate control of diabetes will reduce the rate of deterioration of diabetic glomerulosclerosis. The prognosis of nephrotic syndrome will now be discussed.

First and foremost the lack of a large number of series of studies of nephrotics in which the clinical and histological appearances are known, is responsible for the chaotic state of the literature. There are exceptions to this, notably Kark's group in Chicago and Earle's group in the same city, but generally the follow ups are for a short period of time and there is no clinicopathological study comparable to that of Sir Arthur Ellis' clinical study. Bearing this in mind the prognosis of each of the types of nephrotic syndrome will now be considered.

(a) 'No light microscopical change' – the prognosis in many patients is excellent, with spontaneous remission or drug induced remission, in 95 per cent of patients. There is some suggestion that those who do not recover may develop membranous glomerulonephritis later.

(b) Membranous glomerulonephritis – this rarely remits spontaneously but 1 in 4 remit with steroid treatment. The majority of patients do not recover from the disease. It may persist for ten to twenty years before renal failure and hypertension supervene. This is the group which most closely corresponds with Ellis's type 2 nephritis.

(c) Proliferative glomerulonephritis: – the prognosis in this disease depends upon the type of proliferative glomerulonephritis. If there are many crescents and the patient has the clinical features of subacute glomerulonephritis, there is only a slender chance of recovery, and death will ensue within 18 months. If the picture is that of the nephrotic phase of chronic glomerulonephritis, death will occur ultimately but may be postponed for even several years. If the proliferative glomerulonephritis is part of an acute nephritis, a sizeable proportion of patients will recover from the disease completely. The various forms of proliferative glomerulonephritis have been classified by Churg, Habib and White into

1. Diffuse proliferative glomerulonephritis of post streptococcal origin, usually transient.
2. Mesangial proliferation in which there is a slight increase in mesangial cells and mesangial thickening.
3. Focal sclerosing glomerulonephritis which may start as so-called minimal change and eventually develop into a sclerotic segment of some glomeruli which may eventually obliterate entire glomeruli.
4. Diffuse glomerulonephritis with crescents which are predominantly small.
5. Membrano-proliferative or mesangiocapillary or lobular glomerulonephritis where there is both mesangial proliferation and sclerosis together with diffuse thickening of the capillary walls. This is very easily recognised if silver staining is used, when the splitting of the basement membrane is obvious.

The prognosis in focal sclerosing glomerulonephritis is bad, and many patients die of renal failure in a matter of a few years. There is usually no response to any known therapy. Mesangiocapillary (membranoproliferative) G.N. most often does not respond to treatment, although I have had some success, including arrest of the disease for 3 years, using cyclophosphamide. In pure mesangial proliferation, remission is the rule with steroids.

Question Do the majority of patients with membranous glomerulonephritis have a spontaneous remission with recovery from the disease?

Answer 1. Yes. Go on to **6.73**.
2. No. Go on to **6.71**.
3. Don't know. Go on to **6.78**.

6.75 Your answer – diabetic nephropathy is associated with a normal life span.
Nephrotic syndrome associated with diabetic nephropathy has a bad prognosis, the average survival being about three years. If you consider the histological lesions associated with Kimmelstiel-Wilson syndrome, you will realise that there is progressive impairment of the capillary blood flow due to the encroachment on the lumen of the nodular masses of mucopolysaccharide material characteristic of the disease. Now answer the question correctly at the end of **6.71**.

6.76 Your answer – I don't know what treatment is indicated.
Diabetic glomerulosclerosis is treated symptomatically by control of oedema and control of the diabetic state. In this case the diabetes is badly controlled, with blood sugars around 300 mg/100 ml. There are two purposes in controlling the blood sugar levels; reducing the rate of development of the renal complications and

blood sugar avoiding the development or exacerbation of other diabetic complications. Now answer the question in **6.67** correctly.

6.77 Your answer – I don't know the prognosis in nephrotic syndrome due to diabetes.

You have not been concentrating properly; the prognosis is poor in this disease, and the average length of survival is three years only. When you consider the extent of the damage to the capillaries in this disease caused by the encroachment on the capillary lumen of the nodular masses of mucopolysaccharide, it is not remarkable that the average length of survival is only three years. Now read **6.71** carefully before you answer the question.

6.78 Your answer – I don't know the prognosis in membranous glomerulonephritis.

The prognosis in this disease is bad for recovery but is compatible with several years of life. Go back and read **6.74** more carefully. You are not concentrating hard enough. Don't attempt to 'scan' or 'speed read' the paragraphs, or you may miss vital information.

6.79 The life span in this disease is three years.

Correct. The next point to be discussed is the differential diagnosis of the nephrotic syndrome. There is little difficulty in making a diagnosis of the nephrotic syndrome if adequate biochemical aid is available. On clinical grounds alone there is occasional confusion with congestive heart failure because of the simultaneous presence of oedema and proteinuria, but the presence of neck vein engorgement indicates the presence of heart failure rather than nephrotic syndrome, although this does not exclude the rare combination of the two diseases which is diagnosed by combined clinical and biochemical means. Cirrhosis of the liver is also often confused by the beginner because of the presence of massive oedema in the absence of neck vein congestion, but the absence of proteinuria excludes the diagnosis of nephrotic syndrome. Sometimes nephrotic syndrome is diagnosed erroneously in acute glomerulonephritis because of the presence of oedema and proteinura, and it is true that occasionally in acute nephritis the proteinuria is so massive that a diagnosis of nephrotic syndrome due to acute nephritis is substantiated, but this diagnosis should not be made without adequate biochemical evidence. From time to time a patient with myxoedema is thought to be suffering from the nephrotic syndrome, but the absence of proteinuria soon rules out the diagnosis. Now answer the question.

Question In a patient with oedema and proteinuria on clinical testing who is found to have the following biochemical features; serum albumin 4.0 g/100 ml, daily urinary protein 1.5 g/day, would you accept a diagnosis of nephrotic syndrome?

Answer 1. Yes. Go on to **6.81**.
2. No. Go on to **6.83**.
3. Don't know. Go on to **6.85**.

6.80 You answer − lupus erythematosus.
   No. Hepatosplenomegaly occurs in SLE but it is the chronic osteomyelitis which points to secondary amyloid disease. Read **6.83** again before answering the question correctly.

6.81 Your answer − I would be prepared to make a diagnosis of nephrotic syndrome.
   No. The patient has too low a protein loss for this diagnosis to be accepted and no hypoalbuminaemia. Read **6.79** again and then answer the question correctly.

6.82 Your answer − amyloid disease.
   You are correct. Now answer the next question.

Question A patient with nephrotic syndrome has a history of acute nephritis five years earlier. Which of the following three diagnoses is the most likely cause of his nephrotic syndrome?

Answer 1. Proliferative glomerulonephritis. Go on to **6.86**.
2. No light microscopical change. Go on to **6.88**.
3. Don't know. Go on to **6.90**.

6.83 Your answer − he has not got nephrotic syndrome.
   Correct. The differential diagnosis of the various causes of the nephrotic syndrome is frequently impossible on clinical grounds. A history of diabetes would favour a diagnosis of diabetic glomerulosclerosis but the presence of glycosuria is by itself misleading, for glycosuria, with a normal blood sugar level is frequently found in nephrotic syndrome due to any cause. A history of acute nephritis or of hypertension would indicate that the patient had proliferative glomerulonephritis causing nephrotic syndrome. The stigmata of butterfly skin rash on the face, pyrexia, hepatosplenomegaly, pleurisy, pericarditis, and polyarthritis suggest the nephrotic syndrome is caused by systemic lupus erythematosus with lupus glomerulonephritis. Dilated veins on the lower abdomen would favour a diagnosis of renal vein thrombosis. Hepatosplenomegaly, diarrhoea, and a chronic suppurative lesion would suggest secondary amyloid disease. It should be remembered, however, that the majority of patients with nephrotic syndrome are without distinguishing features. Now answer the question.

Question What is the likely cause of nephrotic syndrome in a man who has chronic osteomyelitis and hepatosplenomegaly?

Answer 1. Lupus erythematosus. Go on to **6.80**.

2. Amyloid disease. Go on to **6.82**.
3. Don't know. Go on to **6.84**.

6.84 Your answer – I don't know the cause of nephrotic syndrome in this case.
The presence of a chronic suppurative lesion such as chronic osteomyelitis suggests that secondary amyloid disease may be present, and the hepatosplenomegaly would support this: Read **6.83** with more care.

6.85 Your answer – I don't know if the diagnosis of nephrotic syndrome is acceptable.
The diagnosis of the nephrotic syndrome is a combined clinical and biochemical exercise, and in the example you have just been given the patient has not got the requisite hypoproteinaemia, and his proteinuria is not massive. He therefore has not got nephrotic syndrome. Now read **6.79** again and answer the question correctly.

6.86 You answer – proliferative glomerulonephritis.
You are correct. Now look carefully at the three statements which follow:
Statement 1 In nephrotic syndrome, the daily urine protein excretion is less than 1 g.

Statement 2 Membranous glomerulonephritis usually does not recover spontaneously.

Statement 3 Renal vein thrombosis is often associated with amyloid disease.
Before you pick the answers remember than an incorrect choice may send you back to the beginning of the chapter.

Answer 1. All the statements are true. Go on to **6.87**.
2. All the statements are false. Go on to **6.89**.
3. Statement 1 is true, 2 and 3 are false. Go on to **6.92**.
4. Statement 2 is true, 1 and 3 are false. Go on to **6.93**.
5. Statement 3 is true, 1 and 2 are false. Go on to **6.94**.
6. Statements 1 and 2 are true, 3 is false. Go on to **6.95**.
7. Statements 1 and 3 are true, 2 is false. Go on to **6.96**.
8. Statements 2 and 3 are true, 1 is false. Go on to **6.97**.

6.87 Your answer – all the statements are true.
You are correct about 2 and 3 but you have missed the point about the massive proteinuria present in nephrotic syndrome. Go back to **6.1** and read through to **6.10** inclusive. Then answer **6.86** again.

6.88 Your answer – no light microscopic change.
This is incorrect because there is no history of preceding acute glomerulo-

nephritis in the majority of cases of nephrotic syndrome with no light microscopic change. Read **6.83** again and then answer the question in **6.82** correctly.

6.89 Your answer – all the statements are false.

You are correct about statement 1 only. Go back to **6.44** and read the chapter through from there.

6.90 Your answer – I don't know the cause of nephrotic syndrome in this case.

A past history of acute glomerulonephritis is suggestive of proliferative glomerulonephritis being the cause of nephrotic syndrome. Read **6.83** carefully then answer the question in **6.83** again.

6.91 Your answer – I don't know if prednisone has any effect on proteinuria.

Prednisone reduces the amount of the proteinuria in many cases of nephrotic syndrome without histological (i.e., light microscopical) change. Read **6.65** again and then answer the question correctly.

6.92 Your answer – statement 1 is true, 2 and 3 are false.

You are quite wrong on all three statements. Go back to the beginning of the chapter and read it through again.

6.93 Your answer – statement 2 is true; 1 and 3 are false.

You are correct about 2 and 1 but wrong about 3. Go back to **6.71** and read on from there.

6.94 Your answer – statement 3 is true, 1 and 2 are false.

You are correct about statements 3 and 1, but wrong about statement 2. Read on from **6.44** to **6.71** and answer the question in **6.86** again, correctly this time.

6.95 Your answer – statements 1 and 2 are true, 3 is false.

You are wrong about statements 1 and 3. Read from **6.1** to **6.44** and then from **6.71** onwards.

6.96 Your answer – statements 1 and 3 are true, 2 is false.

You are correct about statement 3 only. Go back and work through from **6.1** to **6.71**, then answer **6.86** again.

6.97 Your answer – statements 2 and 3 are true, 1 is false.

You are correct. You have now finished this chapter, but before leaving the subject you may wish to read more on the subject of nephrotic syndrome:

Reviews of nephrotic syndrome
Cameron, J. S. 1971 J. Royal Coll. Physicians **5**, 282.
Kark R. M. et al. (1958) Ann. int. Med. **49**, 751.

Schreiner G. E. (1963) in Strauss M. B. & Welt L. G. (eds.) Diseases of the Kidney. Churchill, London.

Churg, J. et al. 1970 Lancet I, 1299.

Diabetic nephropathy

Gellman D. D. et al. (1959) Medicine **38**, 321.

Lupus nephritis

Muehrcke R. C. et al. (1957) Medicine **36**, 1; (1964) J. lab. clin. Med. **64**, 888.

Simenhoff M. L. & Merrill J. P. Nephron **1**, 308.

Amyloid of kidneys

Barclay G. P. T. et al (1960) Quart. J. Med. **29**, 137.

General

British Med. J. 1970 **2** 58. Leading article.

Hayslett J. P. et al 1969. New Eng. J. Med. **281**, 181.

Berger, J. et al. in Advances in Nephrology Vol. 1 edited by Hamburger Crosnier & Maxwell Year Book Publishers 1971.

Time for this chapter: 25 minutes

Chapter 7
Pyelonephritis

7.1 Infections of the urinary tract are fairly easily diagnosed in the acute attack but more difficult to diagnose in the chronic state. The relationship between acute and chronic pyelonephritis is ill-defined and at present the diagnosis of chronic pyelonephritis is frequently one of the most difficult in the entire spectrum of renal disease.

Acute pyelonephritis is a disease which occurs frequently, and affects all age groups. It is commoner in females; in adults between 20 and 40 years old, 10 females are affected for every male. The predisposing causes are (1) the short female urethra; the male urethra is longer and more tortuous than the female so that ascending organisms find it easier to reach the female bladder. (2) The female urethra is frequently subject to trauma in sexual intercourse and childbirth. (3) The female urethral meatus is more readily contaminated with faeces than is the male urethra.

The organisms which most commonly cause acute pyelonephritis are Escherichia coli, Proteus, B. pyocyaneus, Aerobacter, enterococci and staphylococci. E. coli is the commonest organism in patients who have *not* had genito-urinary operations, simple instrumentation, or urinary tract obstruction, while the other organisms are found in those patients who have had surgical interference. Now answer the question.

Question Is acute pyelonephritis commoner in males than in females?

Answer 1. Yes. Go on to **7.3**.
2. No. Go on to **7.4**.

7.2 Your answer – E. coli is commonly responsible for acute pyelonephritis in non-obstructed and non-instrumented patients.

Correct. Beeson has shown that the NH_4 liberated from urea splitters in pyelonephritis can inhibit complement's activity and lead to a decreased resistance to micro-organisms. The factors predisposing to acute pyelonephritis are (1) Obstruction of urinary pathways whether due to stricture of urethra, prostatic obstruction, ureteric stone, stricture, neoplasm or periureteric fibrosis. (2) Sexual trauma in females. (3) Urinary stasis in pregnancy. Hydroureters and hydronephrosis occur early in pregnancy and may last up to six months after pregnancy has terminated. The urinary stasis which occurs is one of the factors responsible for the frequent urinary tract infections in pregnancy. 30 to 40 per cent of pregnant patients who are found to have bacteriuria subsequently develop acute pyelonephritis. (4) Renal calculi. 50 per cent of patients with renal stones have infected urine; it is very difficult to eradicate urinary tract infection in the presence of unrelieved obstruction or of stones. (5) Metabolic factors; (a) Diabetes mellitus is associated with an increased incidence of urinary tract infections, particularly dramatic being the very severe acute pyelonephritis associated with necrosis of the renal papillary tissue — necrotising papillitis. This will be discussed in more detail later, but suffice it to state here that this is a very severe type of pyelonephritis, steadily progressive and frequently fatal. (b) Hypokalaemia and hypercalcaemia are frequently associated with renal tract infections. (c) Phenacetin abuse, common in Scandinavia but occurring sporadically elsewhere, can lead to necrotising papillitis or to a less dramatic but equally lethal pyelonephritis. Now answer the question.

Question What type of renal tract disease is associated with phenacetin addiction?

Answer 1. Acute pyelonephritis. Go on to **7.5**.
2. Necrotising papillitis. Go on to **7.7**.
3. Renal stone. Go on to **7.9**.

7.3 Your answer — acute pyelonephritis is commoner in males than in females. No. The reverse is true. The reasons are given in **7.1**. Go back and read **7.1** and then answer the question.

7.4 Your answer — acute pyelonephritis is commoner in females than in males. You are correct. Now answer the next question.

Question What is the commonest organism responsible for acute pyelonephritis in patients who have *not* had surgical intervention or obstruction?

Answer 1. E. coli. Go on to **7.2**.
2. Proteus. Go on to **7.6**.
3. Don't know. Go on to **7.8**.

7.5 Your answer — phenacetin causes acute pyelonephritis.
You are partly correct in that phenacetin is associated with necrotising papillitis which is a very acute form of acute pyelonephritis. Now go on to answer the question in **7.7**.

7.6 Your answer — acute pyelonephritis in non-obstructed and non-instrumented patients is caused by Proteus.
You are incorrect. Read **7.1** again and then answer the question in **7.4**.

7.7 Your answer – renal papillary necrosis is due to phenacetin.
Correct. Now answer the following question.

Question Why is urinary tract infection so common in the pregnant woman?
Answer 1. Endocrine factors. Go on to **7.10**.
2. Dilated urinary tract with urinary stasis. Go on to **7.11**.
3. Don't know. Go on to **7.12**.

7.8 Your answer – I don't know the organism responsible for acute pyelonephritis.
Read **7.1** and concentrate on what you are reading. Then answer the question in **7.4** again.

7.9 Your answer – renal stones are associated with phenacetin addiction.
You are wrong. Phenacetin is associated with acute necrotising papillitis. Read **7.2** again.

7.10 Your answer – endocrine factors are the cause of the urinary tract infection in pregnancy.
You are partly correct in that high levels of progestogens are responsible for the urinary tract dilatation, which is the actual factor thought to be the cause of the urinary tract infections. Answer the question again after reading section **7.2**.

7.11 Your answer – urinary tract infections during pregnancy are frequent due to urinary stasis associated with dilated urinary tracts.
Good. The pathology of acute pyelonephritis will now be described. The pelvic mucosa is congested, and the urine in the pelvis may be blood stained or purulent. Sectioning the kidney reveals small abscesses scattered throughout the cortex with linear abscesses in the medulla. Some of the abscesses are confluent wedges, the base being cortical and the apex being in the medulla. Histological examination shows micro-abscesses in the renal parenchyma with polymorphonuclear leucocytes infiltrating the surrounding tubular tissue. Sometimes there is an alterative glomerulitis with polymorphs infiltrating the glomeruli. If the lesion is subacute the leucocyte infiltration becomes predominantly lymphocytic and plasma cell rather than polymorphonuclear in type. In chronic pyelonephritis organisms can rarely be seen histologically in the parenchyma, but fluorescent antibodies to some of the commoner bacterial antigens can be demonstrated to be present in the interstitium of the kidney. These patients may have a so-called non-bacterial pyelonephritis. The urine in acute pyelonephritis may be frankly blood-stained; more often it is cloudy due to large numbers of pus cells. If the unspun specimen is examined under the microscope there will be seen vast numbers of pus cells, white cell casts,

red cells, epithelial cells, and organisms; the last are very readily seen with phase contrast microscopy. The urine often smells ammoniacal if an ammonia producing organism such as Proteus is present. The pH is very high, sometimes above 8.4, due to bacterial action producing ammonia. Culture will yield an organism in the urine of all patients with acute pyelonephritis. In necrotising papillitis, the urine contains necrotic papillary tissue. To detect this tissue the urine should be strained through 'butter muslin' in suspected cases.

Question What type of cell infiltrates the renal parenchyma and forms micro-abscesses in acute pyelonephritis?

Answer 1. Polymorphs. Go on to **7.15**.
2. Lymphocytes. Go on to **7.13**.
3. Plasma cells. Go on to **7.14**.

7.12   Your answer – I don't know the reason for the frequency of urinary tract infections in pregnancy.

You should have remembered that there is urinary stasis in pregnancy caused by the presence of hydronephrosis and hydroureter which are themselves thought to be of endocrine origin. Now read **7.2** again before you answer the question again.

7.13   Your answer – the cell infiltrating the parenchyma is the lymphocyte.

No. The lymphocyte is present in more chronic forms of the disease. Read **7.11** again and answer the question correctly.

7.14   Your answer – the cell infiltrating the renal parenchyma is the plasma cell.

You are wrong. Plasma cells are found in subacute forms of the disease. Read **7.11** again and then answer the question correctly.

7.15   Your answer – the cell infiltrating the tubular parenchyma is the polymorphonuclear leucocyte.

Good. The clinical features of acute pyelonephritis are usually, but not always, characteristics. The patient, a young woman, develops malaise, fever, dull loin pains over the renal areas extending anteriorly, with dysuria, frequency and sometimes strangury. The urine smell may be complained of, or haematuria may be observed. The frequency of micturition may be so great that the patient has to pass urine every half hour, with severe pain accompanying the passage of the urine. The temperature may go up to 102°–103° with rigors. In children the onset may be heralded by convulsions, and pyrexia, with screaming on micturition in infants. All infants and children with pyrexia of unknown origin or convulsions should have the urine examined to exclude acute pyelonephritis. Sometimes an acute pyelonephritis in a child or adult is symptomless and is discovered on examination of the urine. In other children, nocturnal enuresis is the presenting symptom. On examination the typical adult is febrile, sweating, and with a toxaemia. The renal angles are tender to palpation. The urine has up to 3 g of protein per day in most cases. The blood pressure is normal. In infections of the renal parenchyma there is a readily measurable plasma antibody response to the bacterial antigen, whereas in cystitis and urethritis there is no measurable plasma antibody response. The blood urea is not usually elevated unless there is prior renal tract disease or the patient has severe disease such as necrotising papillitis, or in the occasional patient who presents with abdominal pain and vomiting, the latter leasing to an extrarenal blood urea elevation.

Question In a child with nocturnal enuresis should a urine culture be done routinely?

Answer 1. Yes. Go on to **7.17**.
        2. No. Go on to **7.18**.
        3. Don't know. Go on to **7.16**.

7.16 Your answer − I don't know if the urine should be cultured in enuresis.

You have not concentrated when you read **7.11**. Read it again and answer the question correctly. Don't day dream when you are reading, and avoid distractions if you can.

7.17 Your answer − a urine culture *should* be done in children with nocturnal enuresis.

Good. This is essential to exclude asymptomatic pyelonephritis. Now answer the next question.

Question In acute pyelonephritis is renal angle tenderness often found?

Answer 1. Yes. Go on to **7.20**.
        2. No. Go on to **7.19**.

7.18 Your answer − a routine urine culture should not be done in a child with nocturnal enuresis.

Your are wrong. A child with nocturnal enuresis may have a urinary tract infection. Read **7.15** again, more carefully this time, and answer the question.

7.19 Your answer − there is *no* real angle tenderness in acute pyelonephritis.

You are wrong. One of the few physical signs of acute pyelonephritis is renal angle tenderness. Go back and read **7.11** again then answer the question in **7.10** again.

7.20 Your answer − there *is* renal angle tenderness in acute pyelonephritis.

Good. The white cell count is elevated with a polymorphonuclear leucocytosis, which rapidly subsides with response of the disease to treatment, although organisms may still be present in the urine. The symptoms of acute pyelonephritis usually last for 3 or 4 days; the increased excretion in pus cells in the urine may persist for a few days or weeks. The antibiotic used in acute pyelonephritis should be that to which the organism is sensitive. In practice if the patient has had no instrumentation or urinary tract obstruction, and a rod shaped organism is visible on microscopy of the urine, it is often wise to begin sulphonamide therapy using sulphafurazole 2 g, every 4–6 hours with alkalinisation of the urine. Should culture fail to show the expected E. coli sensitive to sulphonamides, the appropriate antibiotic should be substituted. If the symptoms pass off but the urine culture remains positive *the patient is not cured*. Every effort should be made to treat any obstruction in the renal tract, for infections are often impossible to eradicate in the presence of obstruction or stone. Urinary tract calculi should also be removed if they are associated with an apparently ineradicable infection. Bacteriuria may indicate an active infection of the renal parenchyma or at least a predisposition to an attack of acute pyelonephritis. Thus in a large series of pregnant women Kass found that of those with bacteriuria who were treated with antibiotics, none developed clinical acute pyelonephritis whereas of those untreated with bacteriuria, 40 per cent developed acute pyelonephritis later in pregnancy. In children recurrent urinary tract infections are often associated with reflux of urine from the bladder up the ureters on micturition (vesico-ureteric reflux).

Question Would you be satisfied with the treatment of a patient with acute pyelonephritis who has relief of symptoms but whose urine on culture continues to yield a growth of E. coli?

Answer 1. Yes. Go on to **7.23**.
2. No. Go on to **7.21**.

7.21 Your answer – I would not be content with relieving a patient's symptoms of acute pyelonephritis if there was a persistent bacteriuria.

Correct. The interpretation of what is to be considered a significant bacteriuria has been simplified by the technique of colony counting using various urine dilutions. A count of 100,000 organisms/ml or more in an early morning urine specimen is considered significant of urinary tract infection. Counts of 10,000 or less/ml are usually due to contaminants. *Thus there is no need to pass catheters to obtain a urine specimen which is adequate for bacteriological examination.* Cleansing of the genitals with suitable antiseptics and collection of a mid-stream specimen are sufficient. Contaminants from the urethra rarely give a colony count exceeding 10,000 organisms/ml and almost always less than 100,000/ml. These figures only apply to urine which is passed in the early morning, i.e., fairly concentrated urine which has either been cultured at once or has been refrigerated at 4°C whilst awaiting culture. Urine kept at room temperature is an excellent culture medium and organisms multiply so rapidly that no conclusions can be drawn from counting the number of colonies per ml on a pour-plate of diluted urine if the urine has not been kept at 4°C to inhibit growth of organisms. Now answer the question.

Question A mid-stream specimen of urine contains 5,000 organisms ml on colony count. Is this a significant bacteriuria?

Answer 1. No. Contaminants only. Go on to **7.22**.
2. Yes. Significant bacteriuria. Go on to **7.24**.

7.22 Your answer – 5,000 organisms/ml represents contaminants only.

Good. The easiest way of reducing the incidence of acute pyelonephritis is to prevent it by avoiding urinary tract instrumentation as far as possible. *Never pass a catheter if it is not absolutely necessary.* The former obstetrical and gynaecological preference for catheter specimens of the urine is obsolete: mid-stream specimens are adequate for most bacteriological purposes. In the best hands catheterisation is associated with a 2 per cent incidence of urinary tract infection even with scrupulous aseptic precautions. Similarly cystoscopy should be avoided unless there is no alternative. If instrumentation of the genito-urinary tract is to be carried out it must be done under conditions of scrupulous sterility. Catheters should not be left in the bladder draining into a simple bottle. The wooden spigot which fits into a catheter should be placed in the museum and not in the end of a catheter. In those cases where continuous drainage is needed the catheter should be attached to a sterile plastic bag. Antibiotic therapy of pregnant women having significant bacteriuria has been shown to prevent pyelonephritis, and similarly *all* patients with significant bacteriuria should receive antibiotics before they develop recurrent pyelonephritis, which may ultimately lead to chronic pyelonephritis and renal failure. The precise relationship between chronic pyelonephritis and recurrent attacks of acute pyelonephritis or persistent bacteriuria is at present ill defined. Surgical intervention (to relieve obstruction or renal stones) may be needed to obtain a permanent cure of urinary tract infection. Pyelonephritis associated with vesico-ureteric reflux of infected urine (from the bladder up the ureter) is not necessarily an indication for reimplantation of the ureters, because reflux may clear up spontaneously, particularly as affected children grow older. In adults chronic pyelonephritis in the presence of vesico-ureteric reflux is an indication for reimplantation of the ureter in the bladder in such a manner as to prevent reflux. This is done by inserting the ureter obliquely through the muscle of the bladder wall, and is designed to prevent reflux of urine from the bladder to the urine when the pressure in the bladder rises when micturition takes place.

Question Is there any need for doing routine catheterisation to obtain specimens for urine culture?

Answer 1. Yes. Go on to **7.29**.
2. No. Go on to **7.25**.

7.23 Your answer – I would be satisfied with relief of symptoms in spite of persistent bacteriuria.

You should not be so content with your ineffectual treatment. Remember that anyone with a persistent bacteruria may have an active pyelonephritis or be liable to develop an active pyelonephritis. Read **7.20** again and choose the correct answer.

7.24 Your answer – 5,000 organisms/ml is a significant bacteriuria.

No. A figure of < 10,000/ml is usually due to contaminants. From 10,000–100,000 organisms/ml is suspicious and should be repeated; over 100,000/ml is a significant bacteriuria. Read **7.21** again and answer the question correctly.

7.25 Your answer – there is no need for catheterisation to obtain specimens for urine culture.

Good. The therapy of acute pyelonephritis is basically similar to that of an acute infection anywhere in the body; this involves giving the antibiotic to which the organisms are sensitive in adequate amounts to obtain high tissue levels. Acute pyelonephritis is a tissue infection. The early idea that acute pyelonephritis was a *urinary* infection and that therefore antibiotics had only to be given in a dosage sufficient to yield high *urinary* concentrations is probably erroneous because the dose of antibiotics given on this basis is inadequate to kill organisms in the kidney parenchyma, (although Stamey and his colleagues argue that medullary tissue and urine concentrations of antibiotics are comparable). 85 per cent of recurrent urinary tract infections in the female represent infections with new organisms.

There is some evidence that organisms can persist as protoplasts forms in the kidney tissues, and be responsible for relapse rather than the bacteriostatic effect of simple sulphonamides. They require special hyperosmotic media for culture and are resistant to the penicillins but not to the tetracyclines and erythromycin.

Sulphonamides will often be the chemotherapeutic agents of choice particularly in coliform infections. It should be remembered that adequate hydration is essential with urinary outputs of at least 2 litres a day, for this not only keeps the sulphonamide crystals dissolved but it has been demonstrated by Epstein that water diuresis itself favourably influences urinary tract infections. If the organisms are not sensitive to sulphonamides the appropriate antibiotic should be selected. A mixture of sulphonamide and trimethoprim is known as Septrin or Bactrim and has a bactericidal effect. It is very useful in the therapy of pyelonephritis, but in advanced renal failure it may be retained in the body with elevated serum levels and may cause skin rashes. Streptomycin, tetracyclines, colistin, and kanamycin are contraindicated in the presence of azotaemia unless the dosage is modified (see Chapter 20). Sometimes the organisms isolated constantly reappear after therapy with adequate dosage of antibiotics to which they are sensitive according to in vitro tests although many of the infections are reinfections with new organisms; even if apparently the same organism is isolated phage typing may show that is in fact a new organism. Bear in mind that sometimes E. coli is isolated as microcolonies which grew out after 72 hours, i.e. when the plates would normally have been thrown out as sterile. Microcolonies are tiny, atypical colonies of E. coli. In these circumstamces, long term antibiotic therapy can be undertaken.

An alternative form of antibacterial therapy for use when the infection is due to organisms resistant to antibiotics is to make the urine extremely acid by giving oral methionine in very large doses — up to 16—18 g/day. This is dangerous in advanced renal failure (GFR < 10 to 15 ml/min) because of nitrogen content of methionine which is catabolised to urea. This causes nausea, vomiting, and diarrhoea in some people, but the urine may become sterile on this treatment when no other type of therapy has succeeded.

In the acute attack of pyelonephritis it is customary to give alkalinising medication, such as sodium citrate or sodium bicarbonate to relieve dysuria. In the presence of renal failure, potassium salts should be avoided. Now answer the question.

Question Where is it important to get an adequate concentration of antibiotic in acute pyelonephritis?

Answer 1. Kidney tissues. Go on to **7.28**.
2. Urine. Go on to **7.27**.
3. Don't know. Go on to **7.37**.

7.26 Your answer — the renal parenchyma is infiltrated with lymphocytes and plasma cells.

You are correct. The clinical features of chronic pyelonephritis are not clear cut. The disease may be associated with the following clinical pictures:

(1) Typical history of recurrent urinary tract infections: recurrent fever, dysuria, loin pain, and positive urine culture with pyuria. There may be an obvious cause for the recurrent attacks such as renal tract obstruction, stone, hydronephrosis, or in-dwelling catheters, or, occasionally, familial pyelonephritis. In addition there may be the factors of hypokalaemia, nephrocalcinosis, gout, chronic analgesic ingestion, vesico ureteric reflux, and irradiation of the kidneys.

(2) Hypertension. Weiss and Parker found that chronic pyelonephritis was very commonly associated with hypertension and thought it was the cause of the majority of cases of renal hypertension. The X-ray changes of chronic pyelonephritis have been described in Chapter 4. In the presence of unilateral chronic pyelonephritis hypertension may occasionally be improved by removal of the small, contracted pyelonephritic kidney.

(3) Renal failure. Renal failure of insidious onset may be the presenting feature of chronic pyelonephritis. Because the process progresses very slowly, the patient may present with renal osteomalacia or renal hyperparathyroidism. Many female patients have had a urinary tract infection earlier in life, most commonly in early marriage, in pregnancy, or at its termination, and this can hardly be

relied on as positive proof that the cause of their chronic renal failure is chronic pyelonephritis.

Question Does chronic pyelonephritis commonly present as renal hypertension?

Answer 1. Yes. Go on to **7.32**.
2. No. Go on to **7.34**.

7.27 Your answer – it is important that the antibiotic concentration should be adequate in the urine.

Acute pyelonephritis is a renal infection with the kidney parenchyma being involved rather than simply an infection of the urine. However, you are correct in the view of Stamey et al., who think that urinary levels are important because they reflect medullary tissue levels of antibiotics. They are at present in a minority in this view. Now read **7.25** again and answer the question correctly.

7.28 Your answer – it is important to secure adequate kidney tissue concentration of antibiotics in the therapy of acute pyelonephritis.

You are correct. There are various types of recurrent acute or subacute pyelonephritis in which there is frequently an obvious underlying cause – such as recurrent instrumentation, indwelling urinary catheters, urinary tract obstruction, vesico-ureteric reflux, renal or bladder calculi, or prolonged analgesic ingestion. The clinical features are of recurrent attacks of fever, loin pain, dysuria and frequency: some patients have no fever, others have constant dysuria or loin pain; positive urine cultures confirm the diagnosis. The distinction between the clinical picture of recurrent acute pyelonephritis, subacute pyelonephritis and chronic pyelonephritis is blurred. It should be clearly emphasised that our knowledge of chronic pyelonephritis is incomplete: we know little about its natural history and much of our knowledge of its pathology is based on autopsy studies. The importance of chronic pyelonephritis and much of the basic information about its pathological picture were described by Weiss and Parker. The pathological picture is as follows: the kidneys are usually small unless hydronephrosis is present. The surface is covered with U shaped scars, the cortex being narrow underneath the scars. Nodular areas of dilated tubules alternate with the scarred areas. The walls of the pelvis are reddened. The changes seen on microscopy (see Fig. 7.28) are: colloid casts within tubules, infiltration of lymphocytes and plasma cells in the renal parenchyma, and pelvic inflammatory change. There may be more acute activity as shown by the presence of pus cells in the tubules, and the renal parenchyma and glomeruli may be invaded by polymorphs as well as strangled by periglomerular fibrous tissue. The vessels are frequently involved with a chronic endarteritis which may cause vascular occlusion and result in infarcts with scarring of the kidney. The vascular changes of the frequently associated hypertension are also found in the kidney.

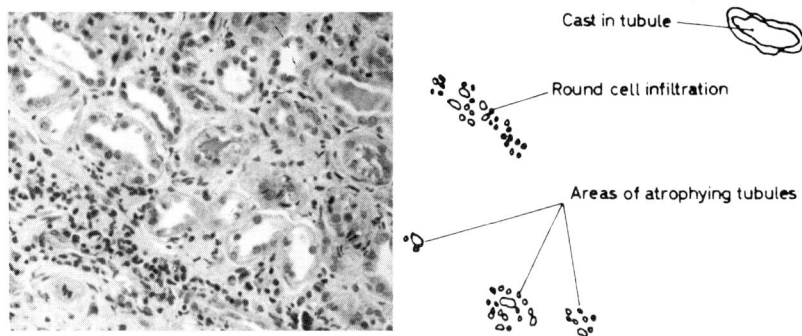

Fig. 7.28

Question What cells infiltrate the renal parenchyma in chronic pyelonephritis?
Answer 1. Lymphocytes and plasma cells. Go on to **7.26**.
2. Polymorphonuclear neutrophils. Go on to **7.36**.
3. Eosinophils. Go on to **7.30**.

7.29 Your answer — there is a need for routine catheterisation to obtain specimens intended for urine culture.

You are wrong. For the majority of routine urine cultures catheterisation is an unnecessary hazard, because of the chance of introducing organisms into the urinary pathways which may cause a pyelonephritis. Read **7.22** again with more care: then answer the question correctly.

7.30 Your answer — the cells infiltrating the renal parenchyma in chronic pyelonephritis are eosinophils.

No. The cells infiltrating the renal parenchyma are usually the cells characteristic of chronic inflammation, namely lymphocytes and plasma cells, although there are occasional areas with neutrophil polymorphs indicating acute inflammation. Now answer the question correctly after reading **7.28** again.

7.31 Your answer — chronic pyelonephritis is not likely to cause 20 g protein loss/day.

Correct. The functional changes induced by chronic pyelonephritis are primarily those of distal and collecting tubular dysfunction as well as generalised renal damage:

(1) *Impairment of urine concentrating ability:* this may result at worst in nephrogenic diabetes insipidus resistant to vasopressin. Milder lesions may cause a fall in Tm^cH_2O disproportionately greater than the reduction is GFR.

(2) *Impairment of acidification ability:* the urine pH may not fall below 5.3

on the Wrong and Davies ammonium chloride test. Ammonia excretion is reduced disproportionately to the general reduction in GFR. This acidification defect may give rise to a form of renal tubular acidosis.

(3) *Sodium retaining ability:* The extreme form of loss of ability to retain sodium gives rise to salt-losing nephritis, in which the salt loss is so great as to cause hypotension due to severe salt depletion, pigmentation, nausea and vomiting and ultimately death from salt loss. Minor degrees of a 'sodium leak' are common in chronic pyelonephritis and may require oral sodium chloride therapy.

Question Is chronic pyelonephritis a cause of inability to acidify the urine during an ammonium chloride test?

Answer 1. Yes. Go on to **7.38**.
2. No. Go on to **7.35**.
3. Don't know. Go on to **7.39**.

7.32 Your answer – chronic pyelonephritis commonly presents as renal hypertension.

Good. The diagnosis of chronic pyelonephritis may be obvious in the history of repeated or recurrent urinary tract infection, but in patients without these symptoms reliance has to be placed on investigations:

(1) Proteinuria may be absent but is usually present in amounts of up to 3 g/day (unless there is associated malignant hypertension or congestive heart failure, in which case the proteinuria may be heavier).

(2) Urine culture: this is frequently positive but not all patients have a bacteriuria: positive cultures occur in one quarter to one half of the patients with chronic pyelonephritis.

(3) Increase in white cell excretion in the urine. Pyuria is frequent but not constant in chronic pyelonephritis. Because of this lack of constancy in the white cell excretion in pyelonephritis the 'pyrexal' test was introduced. This is described in Chapter 4 which should be consulted for details (**4.19**). Because of the disadvantages of this test the prednisone test (see **4.19** if you have forgotten this) was introduced. Both these tests are by no means conclusive, and negative results do not absolutely exclude a diagnosis of chronic pyelonephritis. White cell casts by themselves are not pathognomonic of chronic pyelonephritis: they can be found in the urine in glomerulitis of many types.

(4) IVP. The changes on IVP due to chronic pyelonephritis may show irregularity of both kidneys, or one kidney may be smaller than the other. The cortex is irregularly thinned and the underlying pelvicalyceal pattern distorted.

Question If a patient is found to have a proteinuria of 20 g a day in the absence of congestive heart failure or malignant hypertension, would you consider that chronic pyelonephritis is the cause of the proteinuria?

Answer 1. Yes. Go on to **7.33**.
2. No. Go on to **7.31**.

7.33 Your answer — I would think that chronic pyelonephritis is the cause of proteinuria.

No. Chronic pyelonephritis rarely causes proteinuria of over 3 g per day. This was stated in **7.32**, the contents of which you have not absorbed adequately. Go back and read it, and then answer the question correctly.

7.34 Your answer — chronic pyelonephritis does *not* commonly present as renal hypertension.

You are wrong. It is a common cause of renal hypertension. Go back and read **7.26**.

7.35 Your answer — chronic pyelonephritis is *not* a cause of inability to acidify the urine.

You are wrong. Acidification ability is one of the distal tubular functions which is specifically disturbed in chronic pyelonephritis. You have not absorbed the information in **7.31**. Go back and read it again.

7.36 Your answer — the cells infiltrating the renal parenchyma are polymorphs.

You are correct in that there are often areas of polymorph infiltration indicating *activity* i.e., acute upon chronic pyelonephritis but most commonly the cells typical of chronic pyelonephritis are lymphocytes and plasma cells, i.e., the cells typical of *chronic inflammation*. Now answer the question at the end of **7.28** correctly.

7.37 Your answer — I don't know where it is important to get an adequate concentration of antibiotic in acute pyelonephritis.

Acute pyelonephritis is an infection of the kidney tissues primarily, so that it is important to have an adequate tissue concentration of antibiotic to kill the organisms in the renal parenchyma. The dose of antibiotic needed to attain adequate urinary concentrations of antibiotic is quite insufficient to achieve adequate tissue concentrations, although Stamey and colleagues doubt this view. Now read **7.25** again and answer the question correctly.

7.38 Your answer — chronic pyelonephritis causes impairment of urinary acidification.

Correct. The place of renal biopsy in the diagnosis of chronic pyelonephritis is controversial; pyelonephritis is a patchy disease, and the biopsy needle may fail to remove any affected tissue. On the other hand culture of renal tissue removed at biopsy may lead to identification of the organism responsible for the disease and so appropriate antibiotic measures can be started in patients whose urines are persistently sterile. It is wise to culture the tissue in special media to enable protoplast forms of organisms to grow. These do not grow on standard media and may therefore be missed. In advanced renal disease it is harder to obtain biopsy material due to the increased toughness of the kidney and the smaller target the kidneys present to the biopsy needle. The treatment of chronic pyelonephritis is divisible into antibiotic therapy and symptomatic treatment. The antibiotic therapy has already been discussed under acute pyelonephritis, and may be given as a long-term course of antibiotics over a period of years although this is of dubious efficacy. The symptomatic therapy includes cautious hypotensive drug treatment of hypertension if renal failure in present, and treatment of chronic renal failure generally (see Chapter 9). In particular Shohl's solution (which contains sodium citrate and citric acid) may be found very useful for two reasons:

(a) to provide extra sodium to remedy the sodium leak
(b) to correct the acidosis of renal failure.

In *unilateral* pyelonephritis in a patient with severe hypertension, the response to nephrectomy is disappointing in most cases, and the patient would be well advised to undertake hypotensive drug therapy for the hypertension rather than operation until the response to nephrectomy is more predictable in these patients.

Question A woman has *bilateral* chronic pyelonephritis with severe hypertension: one kidney in 12 cm in length and the other is 8 cm in length. Would you treat the hypertension with hypotensive drugs or remove the smaller kidney first?

Answer 1. Try hypotensive drugs first. Go on to **7.42**.
2. Nephrectomy first. Go on to **7.44**.

7.39 Your answer — I don't know if chronic pyelonephritis is associated with an inability to acidify the urine.

The ability to acidify the urine is one of the distal tubular functions damaged early in chronic pyelonephritis. You have not been concentrating when reading **7.31**. Go back and read it again, paying attention to the contents. Do not day dream.

7.40 Your answer — all the statements are false.

You are wrong about statements 1 and 2. Start at the beginning of the chapter and work through until **7.26**, then answer the question at the end of **7.42** again.

7.41 Your answer — statement 3 is true only.

You are completely wrong. Start at **7.1** and work through the chapter again, otherwise you will have been wasting your time.

7.42 Your answer — hypotensive drugs should be tried first.

You are correct. Before choosing the appropriate answers to the statements below think carefully. If your answer indicates that you have not absorbed the information in the chapter you may find that you have to read the chapter again from the beginning.

Statement 1 E coli is the commonest infecting organism in acute pyelonephritis in which there has been no surgical intervention or urinary tract obstruction.

Statement 2 In acute pyelonephritis in adults, dysuria is common.

Statement 3 Chronic pyelonephritis does not result in renal failure.

Answer 1. All the statements are true. Go on to **7.43**.
2. All the statements are false. Go on to **7.40**.
3. Only statement 1 is true, 2 and 3 are false. Go on to **7.45**.
4. Only statement 2 is true, 1 and 3 are false. Go on to **7.46**.
5. Only statement 3 is true, 1 and 2 are false. Go on to **7.41**.
6. Statement 1 is false, 2 and 3 are true. Go on to **7.47**.
7. Statement 2 is false, 1 and 3 are true. Go on to **7.48**.
8. Statement 3 is false, 1 and 2 are true. Go on to **7.49**.

7.43 Your answer – all the statements are true.

You are partly correct but statement 3 is false. Go back to **7.26** and then pick the correct answer.

7.44 Your answer – do a nephrectomy first.

No. The results from nephrectomy in unilateral pyelonephritis are occasionally spectacular but are more frequently disappointing. In bilateral pyelonephritis, even with one kidney more affected than the other, there is little indication for removing the smaller kidney before an extensive trial of hypotensive therapy. Now read **7.38** again and answer the question correctly.

7.45 Your answer – only statement 1 is true.

You are wrong about statement 2 only. Read on from **7.11** to **7.26** inclusive, then pick the correct answer to **7.42** again.

7.46 Your answer – statement 2 is true, the rest false.

You are wrong about statement 1. Read from **7.1** to **7.10** inclusive, then choose the correct answer in **7.42**.

7.47 Your answer – statement 1 is false, 2 and 3 are true.

You are correct about statement 2 only. Start at the beginning of the chapter and work through from **7.1** to **7.11**, and then go on to **7.26** and work on through from there.

7.48 Your answer – statement 2 is false, 1 and 3 are true.

You are correct about statement 1 only. Work through the chapter again from **7.11** and concentrate this time.

7.49 Your answer – statement 3 is false.

You are correct. References you may care to read before going on to the next chapter are:

Bengtsson, Ulla (1962) Acta med. Scand. Supplement, 388.

Brod J. (1962) Chronic pyelonephritis, in Black D. A. K. (ed.) Renal Disease, p. 279. Blackwell, Oxford.

Freedman L. R. (1971) in Strauss M. B. & Welt L. G. (eds.) 2nd edition Diseases of the Kidney. Churchill, London.

Stamey T. C. et al. (1965) Medicine **44**, 1.

Kleeman C. R. et al. (1960) Medicine **39**, 3.

Aoki S. et al. 1969 New Eng. J. Med. 281, 1375.

Lancet, leading article, 1970 **1**, 758.

A detailed monograph well worth reading is Quinn E. L. & Kass E. H. (eds.) (1960). Biology of Pyelonephritis. Little Brown, Boston.

Also up to date is Renal Infection and Renal Scarring. Edited by P. Kincaid–Smith & K. F. Fairley. Mercedes Press Melbourne 1971.

A book which has a very practical approach is Kunin, C. M. Detection, Prevention and Management of Urinary Tract infections. Lea & Febiger 1972.

Time for this chapter: 40 minutes

Chapter 8
Acute renal failure

8.1 Acute renal failure is a common medical emergency, being precipitated by many causes varying from surgical trauma to glomerulonephritis. Acute renal failure can be divided into the following groups:

(1) *Pre-renal or extra-renal*
(2) *Post-renal or obstructive*
(3) *Renal*

Let us first consider the *pre-renal group*. If the blood supply to the kidney is reduced a little, the urine volume may be somewhat reduced. Thus, in dog experiments, if the GFR is reduced up to 30 per cent the urine osmolarity increases; greater falls in GFR are associated with a fall in urine osmolality and urine volume, which decreases until oliguria is present, oliguria being defined as a urine volume of less than 400 ml/day. Renal parenchymal damage occurs when the renal plasma flow has fallen to 5 per cent of its normal value. Often it is impossible to ascertain on clinical findings if renal or extra-renal causes are responsible for acute renal failure, but measurement of urine sodium and urea concentrations if often helpful. If the urine sodium concentration is below 60 mEq/1 the patient has probably not got acute tubular necrosis, i.e., renal disease, causing his acute renal failure: acute tubular necrosis is usually associated with urinary sodium concentrations of over 70 mEq/1. Similarly, urinary urea concentration of 2 per cent or more suggests that extra-renal factors are responsible for acute renal failure; concentrations of urea below 2 per cent are more often associated with renal disease per se. Perlmutter has found that the ratio urinary urea concentration to plasma urea concentration is usually less than 10 in renal disease, and greater than 10 in renal failure due to extra-renal factors. It should be remembered that none of these methods based on sodium or urea concentration is reliable in 100 per cent of cases. Eliahou has used the ratio of urinary osmolarity to plasma osmolarity to differentiate pre-renal from renal failure. Osmolarity ratios of 1.4 or more would indicate pre-renal uraemia whereas 1.1 to 1.0 indicate renal parenchymal disease. In our hands this has proved useful but is not completely reliable. Before going on to consider the extra-renal causes of acute renal failure answer the question.

Question A woman of 34 is found to be severely oliguric. Her urinary osmolarity is 320 mOsm/1, urinary sodium concentration 100 mEq/1, urinary urea 400 mg/100 ml, blood urea 350 mg/100 ml, plasma osmolarity 320 mOsm/1. Would you consider her to be in acute renal failure because of renal or extra-renal causes?

Answer 1. Renal. Go on to **8.3**.
2. Extra-renal. Go on to **8.5**.
3. Don't know. Go on to **8.7**.

8.2 Your answer – rehydrate the patient with intravenous fluids.

Good. In only an occasional case is there any difficulty in determining if a case of acute renal failure is due to extra-renal causes; sometimes one is surprised to find patients with acute renal failure who turn out not to have kidney disease, but have obstruction to urinary pathways. The first clue to the presence of urinary tract obstruction is *total* anuria. In extra-renal and renal diseases causing anuria, the anuria is rarely absolute, urine volumes vary up to 250 to 300 ml per day and this is more correctly termed oliguria. If *no urine at all is passed*, the *diagnosis is likely to be obstruction of the urinary pathways*; occasionally, bilateral renal infarction or acute anuric glomerulonephritis are responsible. However even in bilateral obstructive disease some patients may continue to pass urine. The presence of absolute anuria is a good pointer to the diagnosis of absolute obstruction but its absence by no means excludes obstructive uropathy.

In *all* patients with severe oliguria of doubtful origin, cystoscopy should be performed: if nothing is found obstructing the bladder neck, bilateral ureteric catheterisation up to the renal pelvis should be carried out. The commoner causes of urinary tract obstruction are: urethral stricture, stone in urethra, prostatic hypertrophy, phimosis, carcinoma of prostate; bladder tumour involving both ureteric orifices or the only functioning ureteric orifice. The ureters may be obstructed by pressure from outside from a neoplasm of the cervix or body of the uterus or by periureteric fibrosis, or from the inside as in stone in the only functioning ureter, stricture, sulphonamide crystals, neoplasm of the ureter or renal pelvis. Occasionally anuria is due to necrotic lumps of renal papillae blocking the ureter in necrotising papillitis. It should be borne in mind that obstruction of one ureter rarely results in anuria unless the contralateral kidney is diseased or absent.

Question If a patient is totally anuric, i.e. urine volume nil/24 hours, which of the following diagnoses is probably correct?

Answer 1. Acute tubular necrosis. Go on to **8.4**.
2. Urinary pathway obstruction. Go on to **8.9**.
3. Renal infarction. Go on to **8.11**.

8.3 Your answer – she is in acute renal failure due to renal disease.

Very good. The pre-renal causes of acute renal failure can be grouped into those with a reduced blood volume causing a reduction the blood supply to the kidney, and those in whom the blood volume is normal but the cardiac output is low due to heart failure:

(1) Reduced blood volume: this may be due to diarrhoea of any cause but

particularly the severe diarrhoea of cholera, ulcerative colitis, and severe dysentry. Haemorrhage of sufficient rapidity to reduce the plasma volume can cause acute renal failure. Diabetic acidosis is also commonly complicated by renal failure. Vomiting also causes acute renal failure, particularly the vomiting of pyloric stenosis and that associated with obstruction of the small intestine just below the ampulla of Vater and duct of Wirsung. Sometimes post-operative suction on the upper alimentary tract results in the loss of large volumes of electrolyte-containing fluids silently and inconspicuously, leading to oligaemia and renal failure, unless fluid and electrolyte loss has been conscientiously replaced.

(2) Low cardiac output with normal blood volume occurs in severe myocardial infarction and in advanced mitral valve disease causing acute renal failure as a terminal event overshadowed by the low cardiac output.

The treatment of acute renal failure due to pre-renal uraemia is to correct the precipitating oligaemia and dehydration by adequate appropriate intravenous fluids (blood or saline) or to improve the cardiac output, depending on the aetiology. If there is the slightest possibility of an extra-renal factor it is certainly wise to give 400 mg of frusemide (furosemide or Lasix) in 200 ml or 5 per cent glucose over a period of 4 hours. This will promote a diuresis of at least 40 ml of urine per hour in extra-renal cases, and may prevent their progression to renal anuria. If it does not produce a diuresis, give another 1000 mg i.v. over 10 hours in a drip. Ethacrynic acid can also promote a diuresis in doses of 1 mg/kg body weight i.v. It has been soundly established that even in acute tubular necrosis some patients respond to diuretics such as frusemide or ethacrynic acid provided they are given early on in the course of the disease. Do not give more than 100 mg of lasix per hour because of the danger of temporary deafness developing. Now answer the question.

Question A patient suffering from cholera has a blood urea of 300 mg/100 ml and is severely oliguric and dehydrated. What treatment is indicated?

Answer 1. Replace the fluid lost with intravenous saline. Go on to **8.2**.
2. Restrict the fluid intake because of the oliguria. Go on to **8.6**.

8.4 Your answer – acute tubular necrosis is present.

You are probably incorrect because total anuria is present and this is commonly associated with urinary tract obstruction. Less commonly one finds total anuria in massive renal infarction and in acute anuric glomerulonephritis. Now read **8.2** again and answer the question correctly.

8.5 Your answer – her renal failure is due to extra-renal causes.

No. If you read **8.1** with care you would see that in extra-renal uraemia causing acute renal failure the urinary sodium is usually 60 mEq/1 or less; urinary osmolarity is often fairly well maintained and urinary urea concentration is more than

2 per cent. You should read **8.1** carefully and after that answer the question correctly.

8.6 Your answer – restrict the fluid intake because of oliguria.
You are wrong because if one makes the diagnosis of an extra-renal cause of renal failure it is necessary to correct the extra-renal factors e.g. by rehydration or blood transfusion. In cholera there is a massive loss of water and electrolytes causing a rapid fall in extracellular fluid volume and soon death from dehydration; the treatment is replacement of the lost fluid and not further fluid restriction. Now answer the question in **8.3** again.

8.7 Your answer – I don't know if she has renal or extra-renal causes for her renal failure. In **8.1** it was pointed out that there were the following findings in acute renal failure due to renal or extra-renal causes.

	Renal causes (more commonly acute tubular necrosis)	*Extra-renal*
Urinary sodium concentration	> 70 mEq/l	< 60 mEq/l
Urinary urea concentration	< 2 per cent	> 2 per cent

Now read **8.1** again and answer the question correctly.

8.8 Your answer – potassium ions are exchanged for potassium.
The purpose of using an ion-exchange resin is to exchange one ion for another. Resonium A is in the sodium cycle and will give up sodium in exchange for potassium. Read **8.14** again and give the correct answer to the question next time.

8.9 Your answer – urinary tract obstruction is present.
Good. Some indication that urinary tract obstruction is present may be obtained by ^{131}I hippuran renography but this should never be relied upon. It should be remembered that although absolute anuria is frequently caused by obstruction to the urinary pathways, the latter is not always associated with oliguria or even anuria. *Retrograde pyelography should be carried out in all cases suspected of obstructed urinary pathways*, but it may even rarely be normal in the presence of malignant infiltration of the ureters.

Renal disease, i.e. damage to the kidney parenchyma, is the commonest cause of renal failure. The types of renal disease commonly causing acute renal failure are:
  (1) Acute tubular necrosis.
  (2) Cortical necrosis.

(3) Acute glomerulonephritis.
(4) Collagen disease.
(5) Infarction of a solitary functioning kidney or of both kidneys.

First let us discuss *acute tubular necrosis* (ATN). In older textbooks of medicine and pathology this is referred to as lower nephron nephrosis, a term used by Lucké to describe the histology of the lesion which he thought was an ischaemic lesion of the distal tubule. J. J. Brown and his colleagues in Glasgow have produced evidence that renin is important in the pathogenesis of acute renal failure; they found high levels of renal vein renin at the onset of acute renal failure. Oken and his colleagues in Boston have demonstrated that it is possible to prevent acute renal failure due to glycerol poisoning in rats if they are saline loaded so as to suppress renin secretion and immunising rats with an antiserum containing antibodies to angiotensin II prevents acute tubular necrosis developing on subsequent challenge with glycerol, which causes severe tubular necrosis in non-immunised rats. These observations are particularly interesting because they shed light on a possible common pathway of acute renal failure independent of the aetiology i.e., acute renal failure may be due to vascular spasm of the cortex due to the release of renin, irrespective of aetiology. Oliver has described two histological lesions. (1) Necrosis of the tubular epithelium, leaving the basement membrane *intact*. This results from administration of nephrotoxic chemicals. (2) Necrosis of tubular epithelium *and* basement membrane, due to ischaemia. Oliver pointed out that the nephron was not only involved in its lower part, as the term lower nephron nephrosis indicated, but *all the nephron* could be involved, albeit often patchily. The glomeruli may be involved with hyalinisation of some glomeruli and occasionally periglomerular fibrosis. The tubular lesion usually heals completely and may be apparently normal histologically three to four weeks after an episode of acute tubular necrosis. Interstitial oedema present in the early stages disappears with healing. Sometimes there is tubular atrophy and interstitial fibrosis with occasional calcification. In *cortical necrosis* the entire nephron is infarcted. Sometimes the entire cortex is necrotic, but more often there is a patchy necrosis with areas of involved glomeruli. If cortical necrosis heals calcification of the affected areas occurs. This may be seen on plain X-ray of the abdomen as a 'monorail' or 'tramline' area outlining the cortex. Look at Fig. 8.9.

The causes of acute tubular necrosis are as follows:

(1) *Nephrotoxins:* carbon tetrachloride, ethylene glycol, and mercuric chloride are common causes. Mushroom poisoning will also cause acute tubular necrosis.

(2) *Haemoglobin and myoglobin:* mismatched blood transfusions, haemolytic anaemia, acute rhabdomyolysis.

(3) *Septic abortion:* how often this is due to the drugs used to induce the abortion or to the frequently observed accompanying infection, which may be haemolytic is not known.

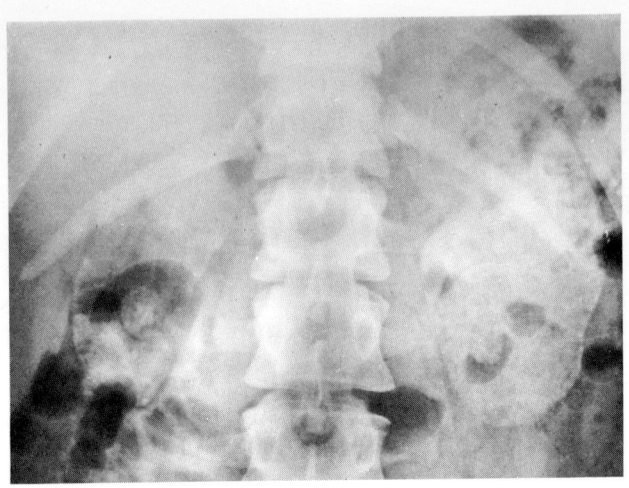

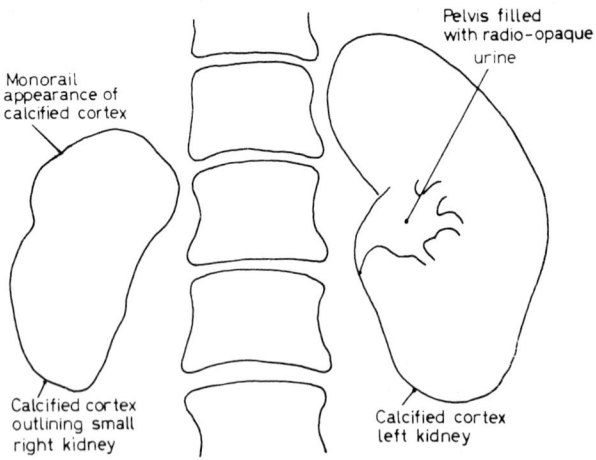

Fig. 8.9

(4) *Acute blood loss* e.g. gastro-intestinal haemorrhage, postpartum haemorrhage. Remember the clinical adage which states that anuria following abortion is usually due to acute tubular necrosis, whereas that following concealed accidental haemorrhage tends to be due to cortical necrosis. Like all adages it is partly true.

(5) *Post-operative:* particularly after infections on the biliary tract but also after virtually and abdominal operation, acute tubular necrosis (ATN) has been

recorded. The patient who is jaundiced is particularly liable to develop ATN: this combination is known as the hepato-renal syndrome, irrespective of the aetiology of the jaundice — obstructive or hepatogenous.

(6) *After radiography:* IVP or aortography. This is rare, but is commoner in myelomatosis after IVP.

(7) *Extensive burns:* these cause acute tubular necrosis most commonly.

(8) *Acute pancreatitis:* either by direct toxic action on the tubules causing ATN or by reducing the blood volume and by causing hypotension and acute tubular necrosis.

Now answer the question.

Question If tramline calcification is found in the kidneys on plain X-ray of the abdomen, what renal lesion has occurred?

Answer 1. Acute tubular necrosis. Go on to **8.10**.
2. Acute cortical necrosis. Go on to **8.13**.

8.10 Your answer — acute tubular necrosis has occurred if 'tramlines' are seen on X-ray.

You are wrong. 'Tramline' calcification is found when cortical necrosis has occurred. Read **8.9** again.

8.11 Your answer — renal infarction is present.

You are partly correct. To develop total anuria one requires massive bilateral renal infarction, or total infarction of the only functioning kidney. A more common cause of total anuria is obstruction of the urinary pathways giving rise to the necessity for cystoscopy and ureteric catheterisation in all cases of anuria where the aetiology is in doubt.

Go on to **8.9**.

8.12 Your answer — the patient is getting too little water.

You are wrong. The great danger in treating patients with acute anuria is to overhydrate them. It is advisable to give 300 to 400 ml of water a day plus the volume of fluid being passed as urine and in the gastro-intestinal tract: this is made more difficult by fever with its attendant increase in water loss. Consequently, the best check on adequacy of water intake is the daily weighing of the patient, aiming at a weight loss of 0.2 to 0.3 kg. Now read **8.17** again and answer the question correctly.

8.13 Your answer — acute cortical necrosis has occurred if 'tramline' calcification is present.

You are correct. If the possibility of the development of acute renal failure is recognised, e.g. during aortic surgery, it is worthwhile giving intravenous mannitol in 10—20 per cent solution to sustain an osmotic diuresis, before, during and after the operation for up to two days in order to prevent oliguria developing. The mechanism of the protective action of mannitol is unknown – one theory is that it keeps the tubular lumen wide open and sweeps out toxins (unspecified); another theory is that it directly protects the tubular cells. Nevertheless, there is now no doubt that during aortic surgery and genitourinary surgery mannitol will prevent renal failure in a considerable proportion of patients. Intravenous furosemide (Frusemide or Lasix) can be given in a dose of 100 mg hourly during operation to sustain urine flow and prevent acute tubular necrosis. Similarly, if mercuric chloride has been ingested, *before anuria develops* the patient should be given Dimercaprol.

Question How can you prevent oliguria developing after an aortic operation?

Answer 1. Dimercaprol. Go on to **8.15**.
2. Intravenous mannitol or lasix. Go on to **8.17**.

8.14 Your answer – the patient is receiving too much water.

You are correct. At one time the water was given as 5 per cent dextrose, either orally or through a stomach tube, or, if the patient were vomiting, as an intravenous infusion into the inferior or superior vena cava. This was at that time the sole source of calories for the patient. Nowadays it has been found that these patients can eat a 2000 calorie diet containing 16 g of protein but low in sodium and low in potassium (about 10 mEq of each) without an excessive rise in blood urea. The argument against feeding anuric patients with protein was that the patient would develop a high blood urea more rapidly, together with increasing acidosis caused by the ingestion of acid-producing sulphur compounds in the protein. This fear of feeding protein has been shown by Parsons to be largely unfounded; the ingested protein spares the patient's own protein, and a liberal diet provides adequate calories and thus prevents the patient from losing much weight during the illness. It is important to restrict sodium intake; increase in body sodium is associated with hypertension, peripheral and pulmonary oedema. Nevertheless, loss of sodium in diarrhoea or vomit should be replaced by equivalent volumes of normal saline. Hyperkalaemia is common in acute renal failure and was a frequent cause of death. Hyperkalaemia is predisposed to by acidosis, by tissue breakdown (as in the anuria of surgical or other trauma), or in the post-partum anuric patient. Hyperkalaemic intoxication is made worse by acidosis, hyponatraemia, hypocalcaemia. The clinical features of potassium poisoning include the following: cardiac arrhythmias leading to cardiac arrest; ECG changes of peaking of T waves; and muscular paralysis affecting the limbs first. Rapid increases in the level of serum potassium can be reversed quickly by intravenous insulin and glucose i.e. 20 units of soluble insulin and 100 ml of 50 per cent dextrose, but this affords only temporary relief. Intravenous molar sodium bicarbonate or lactate and calcium gluconate or chloride will reduce the lethal effects of hyperkalaemia. Cation exchange resins are useful in acute renal failure; sodium cycle polysterene sulphonate (Resonium A, or Kay-Exalate) is used widely for reducing the serum potassium level by exchanging sodium ion on the resin for potassium ion in the gut. Provided dialysis is carried out within a few hours, or resins are given for only a day or two, then sodium resins are fairly safe. Prolonged intake of sodium cycle resins without dialysis will result in sodium overload with oedema and heart failure. For more prolonged use, calcium cycle resins are safe, although they may cause hypercalcaemia.

In all patients with hyperkalaemia in acute renal failure, the above measures are not to be relied upon as anything more than **temporary**, and dialysis should be instituted (peritoneal or haemo-dialysis) to remove enough potassium from the body to prevent a fatal recurrence of hyperkalaemia – particularly in traumatic renal failure.

Question What ion is exchanged for potassium when Resonium A is given orally?

Answer 1. Sodium. Go on to **8.16**.
2. Potassium. Go on to **8.8**.
3. Don't know. Go on to **8.20**.

8.15 Your answer – Dimercaprol will prevent anuria in aortic surgery.
You are not correct. It is indicated in heavy metal poisoning. Read **8.13** again.

8.16 Your answer – sodium ions are exchanged for potassium ions.
You are correct. If the patient is vomiting and cannot be fed orally, he can be given intravenous carbohydrates such as 10–20 per cent dextrose, and Intralipid, a well tolerated fat emulsion giving the patient an adequate number of calories. Carbohydrate polymers such as caloreen and Hycal can be made into ice cream, popsicles (lollipops) and beverages to provide at least another 2000 calories per day if the patient is not vomiting. The disadvantages of the former method of giving the patient 50 per cent dextrose intravenously into the great veins were (1) infection introduced along the catheter, giving rise to thrombophlebitis; (2) clotting of the veins leading to inferior vena caval obstruction and sometimes pulmonary emboli. Intramuscular chlorpromazine or fentazine will often help to stop vomiting but sometimes vomiting will only respond to dialysis. A reduction in protein katabolism on administration of anabolic steroids can be demonstrated if the patient is on 40 g or more protein intake or has post-partum anuria. Decadurabolin (nandrolone decanoate) 25 mg i.m. twice a week is always indicated in the anurias of pregnancy accidents where there is a large post-partum uterus involuting. If the facilities for haemo-dialysis are freely available then there is no doubt that in hypercatabolic cases in particular, and in all other cases of acute renal failure, if possible, haemo-dialysis every alternate day with minimal fluid and food restriction is the method of choice for both patient and doctor. It enables the patient to be symptom free and eat as much as he is likely to want, and hyperkalaemia and uraemia are controlled very well.

Question If chlorpromazine does not control vomiting in acute renal failure, what should be done?

Answer 1. Dialyse. Go on to **8.18**.
2. Do nothing. Go on to **8.22**.

8.17 Your answer – intravenous mannitol or lasix will prevent anuria in aortic surgery.

Good. The clinical features of acute anuria depend on the cause of the anuria. Thus the patient with mercuric chloride poisoning will have a profound diarrhoea and abdominal pain and may not complain of anuria, which may go unnoticed until features of uraemia develop. In mismatched transfusion the patient has lumbar pain, rigors, and dark urine is passed in small amounts. After operations the oliguria may pass unnoticed in the midst of the other surgical complications. The features of uraemia are discussed in the next chapter on Chronic Renal Failure and are not described here. The management of anuria is dependent on the following principles:

(1) Do not overhydrate the patient.
(2) Do not give more sodium or potassium than is needed to replace losses from vomiting, diarrhoea, gastro-intestinal suction or fistulae.
(3) Keep the patient in the best possible state of nutrition.
(4) Choose antibiotics carefully if you need to treat an infection.
(5) Dialyse the patient early; don't wait until he is on the point of expiration.
(6) Treat surgical and post-traumatic cases vigorously from the beginning.

First let us deal with the problem of hydration. The water requirements of an adult weighing 70 kg *who is apyrexial* are 300–400 ml/day – plus the volume of water lost in urine and gastro-intestinal tract losses. The easiest way to check that the patient is being adequately hydrated is to weight him daily – this is of *the utmost* importance and cannot be overstressed – and see that the patient's weight *decreases* by 0.2–0.3 kg a day. If too much fluid is given and the patient gains weight he may be pushed into pulmonary oedema. It is overhydration which commonly gives rise to the X-ray picture of the so-called moemic lungs: this is really due to pulmonary oedema. Now answer the question.

Question A patient suffering from acute tubular necrosis weighs 67.4 kg one day. The next day he weighs 68.2 kg. Do you think his water intake is correct, assuming he was well hydrated the first day?

Answer 1. Too much water. Go on to **8.14**.
2. Too little water. Go on to **8.12**.
3. Being given the correct amount of water. Go on to **8.19**.

8.18 Your answer – dialyse the patient.

You are correct. The commonest cause of death in acute renal failure is infection. 30 per cent of anuric patients have positive blood cultures, and over $\frac{2}{3}$ of patients with acute anuria of any cause have positive urine cultures. First of all, one should not catheterise the patient without the strictest aseptic precautions. If possible, no indwelling catheters should be used. Antibiotics should be given according to the sensitivity of the organism isolated. Do not use the tetracyclines in renal failure for three reasons:

(1) They build up high blood levels.
(2) They tend to elevate the blood urea by their katabolic action on protein metabolism.
(3) They reduce GFR.

Antibiotics *not* to be used routinely in renal failure are streptomycin, kanamycin, gentamycin polymyxin and colistin. Antibiotics safe in normal or slightly modified dosage are penicillin, erythromycin, ampicillin, cloxacillin and chloramphenicol. See Appendix 5 for details of antibiotic dosage and other drugs in renal failure. Anaemia should be treated by transfusion of packed cells. Leucocytosis of 15,000 to 25,000 is common in renal failure and does not necessarily indicate that an infection is present. In acute tubular necrosis due, say to mismatched blood transfusion, the oliguric phase persists for two to three weeks; then gradually the urine volume increases until it reaches 1–2 litres/day. The so-called 'diuretic' phase where the patient passed several litres of urine a day is now rarely seen, presumably being a reflection of the overhydration of the early regimens for anuria.

Question Is tetracycline a safe antibiotic to use in acute renal failure?

Answer 1. Yes. Go on to **8.21**.
2. No. Go on to **8.25**.

8.19 Your answer – the patient is being given the correct amount of water.

No. The patient being given the correct amount of water should *lose* 0.2–0.3 kg per day. This patient is *gaining* weight. Read **8.17** again and answer the question correctly.

8.20 Your answer – I don't know what ion is exchanged for potassium when Resonium A is given.

Ion exchange resins in the sodium cycle are given to patients with potassium intoxication, so that potassium ions are exchanged for sodium ions. Now read **8.14** again very carefully. Do not day dream this time.

8.21 Your answer – tetracycline is a safe antibiotic in renal failure.

The tetracyclines cause a rise in blood urea due, it is thought, to their preventing incorporation of amino-acids into proteins: this is not desirable in renal failure. Moreover the tetracyclines build up high serum levels in uraemia. Now read **8.18** again because this chapter has several important facts about antibiotic therapy in renal disease and you *must know* these. Then answer the question again.

8.22 Your answer – do nothing to control the vomiting.

No. Vomiting makes both the nutrition and the fluid balance of the patient more difficult to control as well as being very unpleasant for the patient. Peritoneal or haemodialysis is usually successful in stopping the vomiting of acute renal failure. Now read **8.16** again and answer the question correctly.

8.23 Your answer – dialyse the patient.

You are correct. Peritoneal dialysis *cannot* be used if the patient has a recent abdominal wound or if the rise in blood urea is very rapid, as in renal failure following trauma. In non-traumatic and non-obstetric cases of anuria the blood urea increases 25–30 mg/100 ml a day; after trauma the blood urea rise may be up to 100–150 mg/100 ml/day with an accompanying rapid rise in serum potassium – hence the necessity for very frequent haemodialyses in these patients. The peritoneum has an area of about 2 m^2 in an average sized adult. The peritoneum itself is a membrane which permits the exchange of electrolytes between the plasma in the capillaries and the peritoneal cavity. Normally there are about 30 ml of fluid in the peritoneum but in acute renal failure an appreciable proportion of patients (about one in ten) has ascites. In peritoneal dialysis, fluid is introduced into the peritoneal cavity and allowed to come into equilibrium with the plasma for about 30–45 minutes after which it is evacuated. The peritoneal dialysis fluid initially contains sodium 140 mEq/l chloride 100 mEq/l, lactate 44 mEq/l, calcium 2.5 mEq/l, and magnesium 1 mEq/l. Potassium can be added up to a concentration of 4.0 mEq/l if hyperkalaemia is not present. The solution normally contains $1\frac{1}{2}$ per cent of glucose so that it has an osmolality of about 380 mEq/100 ml; this ensures that the solution is not absorbed from the peritoneal cavity so that the same volume can be removed 30–45 minutes after being instilled. Urea, potassium, phosphate, creatinine, methyl guanidine, methyl urea, guanidinosuccinic acid, other phenolic compounds and amines diffuse into the peritoneal fluid from the plasma. Water can be removed from the body by increasing the concentration of glucose to $4\frac{1}{2}$ per cent, or 7 per cent in exceptional circumstances. In peritoneal dialysis from 15 to 25 ml of plasma are cleared of urea each minute. This is $\frac{1}{5}$ to $\frac{1}{10}$ of the urea clearance of a Kolff twin coil artificial kidney with a blood flow of 200 ml/min. Now answer the question.

Question What is the osmolarity of peritoneal dialysis fluid containing $1\frac{1}{2}$ per cent glucose?

Answer 1. 380 mOsm/litre. Go on to **8.31**.
2. 600 mOsm/litre. Go on to **8.26**.
3. Don't know. Go on to **8.24**.

8.24 Your answer – I don't know the osmolarity of the peritoneal dialysis solution containing $1\frac{1}{2}$ per cent glucose.

Glucose has a molecular weight of about 180. Therefore 180 g/1 exerts a pressure of 1 osmol or 1000 milliosmols. Therefore $1\frac{1}{2}$ per cent glucose i.e. 15 g/1 exerts a pressure of $\frac{15}{180} \times 1000 = 83.3$ mOsm.

The solution itself contains about 297 mOsm/litre excluding glucose, so that with glucose its osmolarity is $297 + 83 = 380$ mOsm/litre. Now read **8.23** again and answer the question correctly.

8.25 Your answer – Tetracyclines are *not* safe in renal failure.

Good. The urine in acute tubular necrosis is brown and muddy; full of debris, granular casts, tubular and white cells; there are some red cells and many pigment casts with a brown appearance on conventional light microscopy.

The prognosis in acute tubular necrosis is good and, provided the associated precipitating disease is itself not fatal, recovery from the acute tubular necrosis can be expected with conservative management punctuated by dialysis at the appropriate times. Dialysis, either peritoneal dialysis or haemodialysis, is indicated for:

(1) Deterioration in the clinical condition, with nausea, vomiting, diarrhoea, pericarditis, fits, twitching, air hunger, left ventricular failure, overhydration presenting as oedema, clouding of consciousness or gastro-intestinal haemorrhage.

(2) Hyperkalaemia: a serum potassium of 7.5 mEq/1 or more where Resonium A or calcium resin cannot be used due to vomiting and diarrhoea.

(3) Severe acidosis: A plasma pH below 7.15, or total plasma CO_2 of 12 mM/1 or less.

(4) Blood urea of 300 mg/100 ml. Hess-Thayssen found that if a blood urea level of 300 mg/100 ml is used as the indication for dialysis, gastro-intestinal haemorrhage occurs much less frequently as a complication than when the blood urea is allowed to rise above 400 mg/100 ml before the patient is dialysed.

Dialyses will be required to be repeated at intervals of not more than 7 to 10 days during the severely oliguric phase, and when the urine volume rises the patient will probably require at least one further dialysis. Some patients have a very short oliguric phase of less than one week's duration; this group and those patients with a slightly longer oliguric phase (one to two weeks) often do not require a dialysis at all throughout the course of the illness. The patients with traumatic anuria often require daily or alternate daily dialyses during the first few days because of the rapid rise in serum potassium and blood urea. If you are in doubt, dialyse, rather than wait. Now answer the question.

Question If a patient with acute tubular necrosis has vomiting and diarrhoea, a serum potassium of 8 mEq/1, a pericarditis and a blood urea of 375 mg/100 ml, what would you do?

Answer 1. Dialyse. Go on to **8.23**.

2. Treat with Resonium. Go on to **8.27**.
3. Sedate. Go on to **8.29**.

8.26 Your answer – peritoneal dialysis fluid has an osmolarity of 600 mOsm/litre. You are partly correct in that the osmolarity of the stronger glucose solutions may sometimes be as high as 600 mOsm/litre, but the standard solution has a glucose content of $1\frac{1}{2}$ per cent: this solution has an osmolarity of 380 mOsm/litre. Read **8.23** again and then answer the question correctly.

8.27 Your answer – treat with Resonium A. How can you administer Resonium A, a drug given by mouth or rectum, to a patient with vomiting and diarrhoea? Think before you answer the question at the end of **8.25** again.

8.28 Your answer – no protein is lost during a peritoneal dialysis.
No. You have not concentrated adequately when reading **8.31**. Re-read **8.31** again.

8.29 Your answer – sedate the patient.
This is not enough therapy for a patient with a recoverable disease. For hyperkalaemia, dialysis would be needed; in any case the clinical conditions of pericarditis, nausea and vomiting are indications for dialysis: a blood urea of 375 mg/100 ml is itself a probable indication for dialysis. Now read **8.25** again and answer the question correctly.

8.30 Your answer – 10 g of protein are lost during the average peritoneal dialysis.
You are guessing. The average loss during a peritoneal dialysis is 40 g. If you did not recall this your learning is poor, presumably because you are not adequately concentrating. Go back and read **8.31**.

8.31 Your answer – peritoneal dialysis solution has an osmolality of 380 mOsm/kg.
You are correct. The peritoneal dialysis fluid is inserted through a plastic cannula (see Fig. 8.31) which is passed into the peritoneum through a trocar in the linea alba about 3 inches below the umbilicus, using local anaesthesia. One or two litres of fluid, warmed to 37°C, are allowed to run in after heparin has been added to prevent clotting in the cannula. The fluid takes 10 to 15 minutes to run in and is left in for 30–45 minutes before being quantitatively recovered. If less is recovered than is put in, the glucose concentration in the next 2 litres is increased to $4\frac{1}{2}$ per cent by addition of 50 per cent glucose. The peritoneum is not completely impermeable to protein, and many proteins, including albumin and IgG globulin are lost in amounts of about 40 g of total protein per dialysis. In addition at least 15 g of amino acids are lost/dialysis. Peritoneal dialysis is frequently painful, and patients often refuse to have a peritoneal dialysis repeated. Another disadvantage

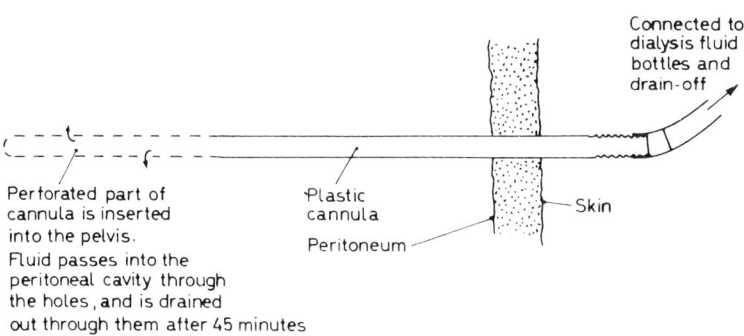

Fig. 8.31

is the occurrence of infection of the peritoneum, (peritonitis or abscess) although this can be treated by means of the appropriate antibiotics instilled into the peritoneal cavity and the dialysis continued. Pneumonia is a complication of peritoneal dialysis due to a combination of atelectasis and retention of bronchial secretions. It is reduced in frequency by using smaller volumes of peritoneal fluid for a shorter time. 2 litre volumes of dialysis fluid distend the peritoneal cavity and push up the diaphragms. The lung bases collapse and plate atelectasis results.

Question How much protein is lost, on the average, during a peritoneal dialysis?

Answer 1. None. Go on to **8.28**.
2. 10 g. Go on to **8.30**.
3. 40 g. Go on to **8.31**.

8.32 Your answer − cortical necrosis is usually fatal.

Quite right. Another cause of anuria is acute anuric glomerulonephritis. This has been mentioned in Chapter 5 on Acute Glomerulonephritis being a rare complication of acute glomerulonephritis. (Type I nephritis of Ellis). Very few cases of anuric glomerulonephritis with anuria for longer than seven days recover; hardly any recover if anuria has lasted for 50 days. Common features include hypertension, β haemolytic streptococci in throat cultures, and an elevated ASO titre. The scant urine is often very bloody, and total anuria may occur. In these patients, after the diagnosis is made by renal biopsy, the physician is again faced by the problem of whether the patient should be put on a programme of chronic haemodialysis with the possibility of leading a fairly normal life indefinitely, apart from twice weekly haemodialysis, or whether he should be allowed to die.

Infarction of the kidneys may be caused by embolisation or thrombosis of the renal arteries; the patient may develop severe loin pain, with hypertension and haematuria. If both kidneys are infarcted anuria results; if all the kidney tissue is infarcted the anuria may be total. Occlusion of both renal veins may result from thrombosis of the inferior vena cava or from amyloid disease, and may result in oliguria with haematuria or anuria. There is no curative therapy for bilateral renal vein occlusion causing venous infarction. Arterial infarction of both kidneys is equally without therapy other than that for acute renal failure, although recovery has been recorded from thromboembolectomy early after embolisation or thrombosis of the renal artery has occurred. Infarction of one of the kidneys *with* the development of severe hypertension is an indication for unilateral nephrectomy. Now answer the question.

Question What is the prognosis in a patient with acute nephritis who has been anuric for eight weeks?

Answer 1. Very bad. Go on to **8.46**.
2. Good. Go on to **8.37**.

8.33 Your answer – Pneumonia is a complication of peritoneal dialysis.
Good. There is no comparable loss of protein during haemodialysis which is indicated in the anuria of acute renal failure whenever dialysis is required but where peritoneal dialysis is contra-indicated by recent abdominal wounds (in which the peritoneum is no longer intact and water tight), peritonitis or in the hyperkatabolic state following trauma. Haemodialysis is discussed in detail in Chapter 9 – Chronic Renal Failure. In addition to trauma and the post-partum state, there is often a rapid rise in blood urea in patients with acute tubular necrosis and anuria due to burns and in patients who develop pneumonia during the course of the illness. In these conditions haemodialysis is to be preferred to peritoneal dialysis.

In cortical necrosis the patients have usually suffered a severe and rapid blood loss such as occurs in accidental haemorrhage of pregnancy or a fall in blood pressure due to myocardial infarction. The patient remains persistently oliguric and dies unless dialysis repeatedly. Very rarely will a patient with patchy cortical necrosis recover, with renal function improving so that the GFR reaches 15–20 ml/min i.e. quite adequate for an unrestricted life. There is no certain way of differentiating cortical necrosis from acute tubular necrosis in life other than by renal biopsy or, later on, by X-ray of the kidneys with the characteristic 'tramline' or 'monorail' calcification in the damaged cortex. Renal biopsy in cortical necrosis may go through a totally necrotic area, with glomeruli as well as tubules being necrotic; early calcification may be seen. Sometimes the biopsy reveals normal kidney tissue, if the necrosis is patchy. Look at the photomicrograph – Fig. 8.33:

If the diagnosis of cortical necrosis is made by renal biopsy a decision has to be made whether to place the patient on a chronic haemodialysis regimen or not. The possibility and difficulty of transplantation are considered in chapter 21.

Question What is the usual outcome of cortical necrosis?

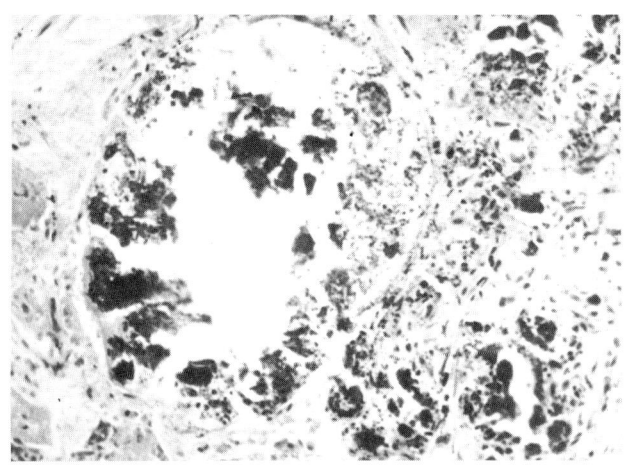

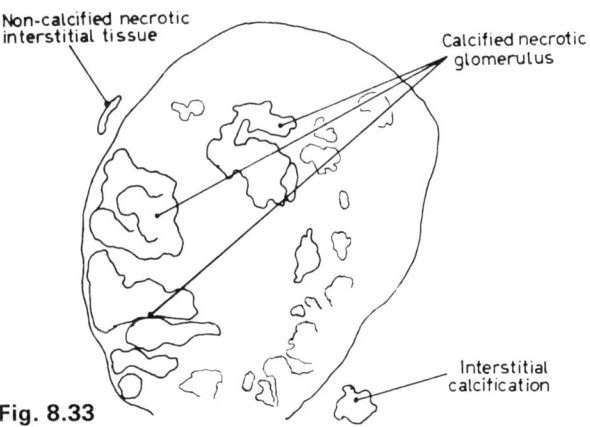

Fig. 8.33

Answer 1. Death. Go on to **8.32**.
2. Recovery. Go on to **8.35**.

8.34 Your answer — 40 g of protein is the average loss per dialysis.
Correct. Now answer the next question.
What serious pulmonary complications are found in peritoneal dialysis?

1. Pulmonary infarction. Go ontto **8.48**.
2. Pneumonia. Go on to **8.33**.
3. None. Go on to **8.49**.

8.35   Your answer – patients with cortical necrosis recover.
No. Very few recover. Read **8.33** again and then answer the question correctly.

8.36   Your answer – statements 1 and 2 are true, 3 is false.
You are wrong about statements 2 and 3. Go back to **8.17** and work through the chapter from there.

8.37   Your answer – the prognosis is good.
You are wrong; very few patients with anuric glomerulonephritis recover after five weeks of anuria. Read **8.32** again.

8.38   Your answer – statements 1 and 3 are true, 2 is false.
You are quite correct. Now you are ready to go on to the next chapter. If you want to read further work on acute renal failure the following can be recommended.
Merrill, J. Acute Renal Failure. The chapter by Merrill in Black's 'Renal Disease' is one of the best current reviews of acute renal failure available.
The chapter by Boen in the Symposium on 'Acute Renal Failure', edited by S. Shaldon (Blackwell Scientific Publications, Oxford 1964) contains up to date information of Peritoneal Dialysis.
Nephrotoxins: Hollenberg et al. New Eng. J. Med. 1970 **282**, 1329.
An earlier publication by Boen in Medicine (1961) **40**, 243 is the classical work on peritoneal dialysis. Papers by the author and his colleagues (Berlyne et al) in Lancet, 1964, **1** and in Transactions of European Dialysis and Transplant Association, 1964 deal with the protein loss problem in peritoneal dialysis. The pulmonary complications of peritoneal dialysis are dealt with in the author's paper in Lancet **2**, 75, 1966. Amino acid loss is dealt with in Lancet **1**, 1339, 1967. Hampers, C. and Schupak E., Long Term Haemodialysis – (Heinemann) is a good simple text on haemodialysis. A good German text is Hämodialyse und peritonealdialyse, edited by E. Wetzels Springer Verlag 1969.

8.39   Your answer – you would biopsy the patient who has been anuric for three days.
You are wrong. Biopsy itself is an added hazard in the uraemic patient – many recover spontaneously in the first fortnight of anuria so that little is to be gained by unnecessary biopsy. Read **8.37** again.

8.40   Your answer – only statement 1 is true.
You are partly correct but statement 3 is true. Go back to **8.25** and read on through the chapter from there.

8.41   Your answer – only statement 2 is true, 1 and 3 are false.
You are completely wrong. Start at the beginning of the chapter **8.1** and read through it again. You have not retained enough of the contents of this chapter to make it worth while proceeding further.

8.42 Your answer – statement 3 only is true.

You are partly correct but wrong about statement 1. Read **8.9** again and answer the question in **8.32** again.

8.43 Your answer – all the statements are true.

You are correct in so far as 1 and 3 are true, but statement 2 is obviously wrong. The usual requirement of fluid is stated in **8.17**. Go back and read it, then go on to answer **8.32** correctly.

8.44 Your answer – all the statements are false.

You are wrong about statements 1 and 3. Go back to **8.9** and read on through the chapter from there.

8.45 Your answer – do not biopsy the kidneys of a patient with three days' anuria.

Good. Now look at the following statements very carefully, and pick the appropriate answer – remember that a wrong choice may send you back to the beginning of the chapter again.

Statement 1 Cortical necrosis often follows accidental haemorrhage.

Statement 2 A fluid intake of 3 litres a day is essential for the anuric patient.

Statement 3 The prognosis in acute tubular necrosis is usually good. Now choose the answer which is correct.

Answer
1. All three statements are true. Go on to **8.43**.
2. All three statements are false. Go on to **8.44**.
3. Statement 1 is true, 2 and 3 are false. Go on to **8.40**.
4. Statement 2 is true, 1 and 3 are false. Go on to **8.41**.
5. Statement 3 is true, 1 and 2 are false. Go on to **8.42**.
6. Statement 1 and 2 are true, 3 is false. Go on to **8.36**.
7. Statement 1 and 3 are true, 2 is false. Go on to **8.38**.
8. Statement 3 and 2 are true, 1 is false. Go on to **8.34**.

8.46 Your answer – the prognosis is very bad.

You are correct. Acute renal failure develops very rapidly in some patients with systemic sclerosis; they develop very severe oliguria and hypertension and die within a few days. The diagnosis is usually obvious on physical examination with the shiny, tight, immobile skin of scleroderma over the hands and face; renal biopsy confirms the diagnosis. The renal failure of polyarteritis nodosa and systemic lypus erythematosus will be described in Chapter 10 on Collagen Diseases and the Kidney.

The importance of renal biopsy in the diagnosis of acute renal failure can hardly be over-emphasised. It is our practice to perform a percutaneous renal biopsy immediately after the second peritoneal dialysis has been carried out, or 1 to 2 days after the last haemodialysis, the latter delay being necessary to prevent bleeding due to the heparin remaining in circulation for some hours after a haemodialysis. It is not recommended that the biopsy be done earlier in view of the fact that many patients with presumed acute tubular necrosis recover after 10–14 days. Biopsy should never be done for its own sake. There is always a risk in biopsying the uraemic patient, primarily due to circulating inhibitors of plasma clotting factors and defects in platelet adhesiveness, but this risk is probably lower after dialysis. Biopsy gives diagnostic information not otherwise obtainable in majority of cases, and the management of the disease can be changed according to circumstances. Thus in the absence of facilities for chronic haemodialysis there is little point in further dialysing a patient with acute glomerulonephritis who has been anuric for 50 days or more. On the other hand, if acute tubular necrosis is found dialysis should be continued because of the very good chance of complete recovery. Most patients who have had acute tubular necrosis have renal lesions which heal completely leaving no impairment of renal functions subsequently. Now answer the question.

Question Would you carry out a renal biopsy on a patient who has been anuric for three days only?

Answer 1. Yes. Go on to **8.39**.
         2. No. Go on to **8.45**.

8.47 Your answer – only statement 1 is false.

You are wrong in that 1 is true and 2 is false. Go back to **8.9** and read through the chapter again.

8.48 **Your answer:** Pulmonary infarction is a complication.

No. There is no particular increase in the frequency of pulmonary infarction in patients subjected to peritoneal dialysis. Pneumonia is a complication of peritoneal dialysis because the elevation of the diaphragms (consequent upon distention of the peritoneal cavity) causes plate atelectasis in the lungs. The atelectatic areas become infected because there is a retention of bronchial secretions due to suppression of cough caused by the pain of peritoneal dialysis, and the uraemic patient has a lower resistance to bacterial infection than the healthy man. Now read **8.31** again.

8.49 Your answer: There are no pulmonary complications of peritoneal dialysis. You are wrong. The pulmonary complications are pneumonia and plate atelectasis. You have not read **8.31** carefully. Read it again.

Time for this chapter: 45 minutes

Chapter 9
Chronic renal failure

9.1 The understanding of some of the clinical features of chronic renal failure is conditional upon a knowledge of the disorded physiology in chronic renal failure. First of all let us consider what is going on in the kidney when the vast majority of functioning glomeruli have been destroyed, as in chronic glomerulonephritis. Platt and later Bricker have formulated the 'intact nephron hypothesis' which states that in chronic renal failure generally, any nephron that is damaged does not function, all the renal function being undertaken by the intact nephrons which are therefore working under an increased loan. There is an *osmotic diuresis* occurring in the few remaining functioning nephrons, which have to excrete an increased amount of solute nephron per nephron per minute compared to the solute load per nephron in the normal kidney. Bricker using animals with experimental unilateral renal disease, has demonstrated that solute load, ammonia excretion, free water excretion, T_mPAH, and T_mG were all reduced in proportion to the reduction in the GFR on the side of the diseased kidney. There are exceptions to this hypothesis; thus in distal tubular disease due to pyelonephritis or hydronephrosis, and in proximal tubular disease such as Fanconi syndrome or the heavy metal poisons, it is evident that the damaged nephrons still function.

Question What sort of diuresis is thought to occur in the few intact nephrons of chronic renal disease?

Answer 1. Water diuresis. Go on to **9.4**.
2. Osmotic diuresis. Go on to **9.6**.

9.2 Your answer — nocturia in a child of 4.
You are not correct, because children of this age usually present with problems of bed-wetting. Go back to **9.6** and read through it again.

9.3 Your answer — salt wasting is common in renal disease.
Good. The anaemia of renal failure is normochromic (MCHC 32—36 per cent) and is partly due to haemolysis with the red cells having a reduced half life, and partly due to inhibition of formation of red cells in the bone marrow. There is a reduction in renal erythropoietin, but this is not the sole cause of the anaemia. The haemoglobin may drop well below 5 g/100 ml. The only immediately effective therapy is transfusion with packed cells, but chronic haemodialysis and dietary measures can often keep the haemoglobin between 8 and 10 g/100 ml without repeated blood transfusion. In chronic renal failure there is often a defect in vitamin D metabolism in which there is a relative resistance to vitamin D. This gives rise to

renal rickets (osteomalacia secondary to renal failure). In some patients the hypocalcaemia of renal failure stimulates the parathyroid glands resulting in secondary hyperparathyroidism in which the serum calcium level is elevated to normal or supranormal figures in contrast to the low serum calcium concentrations usual in renal failure with osteomalacia. The osteomalacia and hyperparathyroidism of renal disease are collectively referred to as renal osteodystrophy. The patients suffer from bone pains in both types of disease, and frequently develop massive metastatic calcification in the soft tissues in renal hyperparathyroidism. Metastatic calcification occurs if the Ca P product in the serum is above 70. Metastatic calcification in the conjunctiva gives rise to reddening of the eyes, due to conjunctival irritation caused by hydroxyapatite crystals deposited in the superficial layers of the conjunctivae. In many patients the conjunctiva remain white yet there is massive deposition of crystals in the areas exposed when the eyes are open and also at the limbus — a limbal arc. Look at the Fig. 9.3.

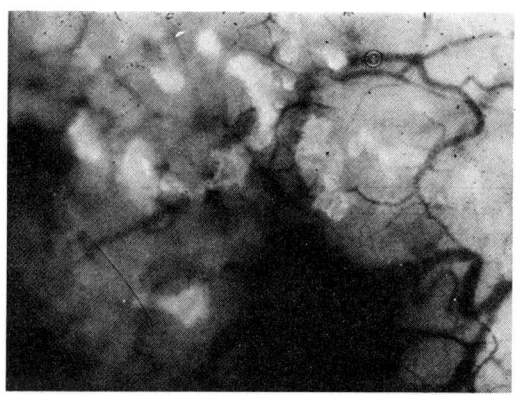

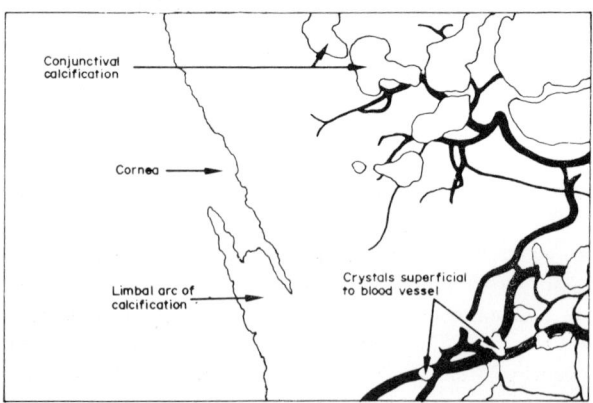

Fig. 9.3

Band Keratopathy, in which an opaque film of calcium salts extends across the front of the cornea, is extremely rare in chronic renal failure, and the term is usually used loosely to indicate an arc of calcification at the limbus – the corneo-conjunctival junction.

Question A patient with chronic renal failure with bone pains has the following biochemical findings.

Blood urea	250 mg/100 ml.
Serum calcium	11.0 mg/100 ml.
Serum inorganic phosphorus	12.0 mg/100 ml.
Serum alkaline phosphatase	36 KA units/100 ml.

What type of bone disease is present?

Answer 1. Osteomalacia. Go on to **9.11**.
2. Hyperparathyroidism. Go on to **9.13**.
3. Don't know. Go on to **9.15**.

9.4 Your answer – water diuresis occurs in the remaining intact nephrons.

No. There is a lot of solute to be excreted per minute by the remaining nephrons, so flow in each nephron is therefore high; the fluid is an ultrafiltrate of plasma and has a high content of urea as well as of the plasma cations and anions, particularly sodium and chloride. Hence an osmotic diuresis is occurring. Answer the question in **9.1** again, correctly.

9.5 Your answer – nocturnal enuresis in a child of 4.

Very good. The osmotic diuresis which occurs in the remaining functioning nephrons in chronic renal failure limits the ability to reabsorb sodium from the tubular lumen adequately, and this frequently leads to a loss of sodium in the urine which may be greater than the salt intake: this results in sodium depletion, postural hypotension, vomiting and pigmentation: this type of salt loss is known as 'salt wasting' or 'salt losing'. Chronic renal failure is the commonest cause of 'salt losing nephritis.' In these patients it is important to assess the sodium loss in the urine on a 20 mEq sodium dietary intake and then adjust the intake of salt to prevent sodium depletion. It is, however, easy to induce salt retention (with oedema and congestive heart failure) by giving sodium in excess of the kidneys' ability to excrete sodium. Thus patients in renal failure are poised on the razor's edge between salt depletion and salt excess. Severe salt loss may cause a reduction in the extracellular fluid volume and so depress renal function even further. Black has advocated the cautious use of 5 per cent saline intravenously in these circumstances. Potassium excretion is usually normal in chronic renal failure; this is achieved by a potassium clearance two to four times the glomerular filtration rate i.e. overall potassium secretion. This prevents hyperkalaemia from occurring until the last stages of renal failure or when sodium restriction reduces the amount of sodium in the distal tubule available for potassium exchange. Metabolic acidosis itself also causes hyperkalaemia. Potassium wasting occurs rarely in renal disease, but this is often due to thiazide diuretics and sometimes due to secondary aldosteronism. Metabolic acidosis is common in advanced renal failure, and is the rule if the GFR is below 3ml/min; this results from a reduction in the amount of NH_4^+ and titratable acid excreted in the urine: the acidosis is thought to cause a steady loss of calcium salts from the bone to buffer the excess acid production. It is often stated that capacity to lower urine pH is preserved in chronic renal failure: this is true only in part; many patients have a moderate impairment and a urinary pH of 5.5 to 6.0 is common in severe renal failure. Now answer the question.

Question Is salt wasting common in chronic renal failure?

Answer 1. Yes. Go on to **9.3**.
2. No. Go on to **9.7**.
3. Don't know. Go on to **9.9**.

9.6 Your answer – osmotic diuresis is present.

You are correct. The loss of concentrating ability caused by osmotic diuresis in the remaining nephrons in chronic renal disease results in an increased urine volume: the urine volume at night in health is low due to nocturnal urine concentration. This does not take place in renal failure, so that the amount of urine formed during the night is large and the older adult patient has to get out of bed at least once during the night to micturate. Young men do not often have this symptom, possibly because they have a larger bladder distensibility; in children there is a history of nocturnal enuresis rather than nocturia. Nocturia also occurs in prostatic hypertrophy, cardiac failure, and in people who drink much beer, tea or coffee before going to bed. Polyuria both day and night occurs in renal disease in congenital nephrogenic diabetes insipidus, pyelonephritis, hydronephrosis, amyloidosis, hypokalaemia, and hypercalcaemia. This will be discussed later in the chapter on Polyuria.

Question What nocturnal urinary symptom is to be expected in a child of four years of age with chronic renal disease?

Answer 1. Nocturia. Go on to **9.2**.
2. Nocturnal enuresis. Go on to **9.5**.
3. Diabetes insipidus. Go on to **9.8**.

9.7 Your answer – salt wasting is *not* common.

You are wrong. Salt wasting *is* common in chronic renal failure. Bear in mind that an osmotic diuresis is going on in the remaining tubules and that this saline diuresis causes an excess sodium loss in the urine. Read **9.5** again.

9.8 Your answer – diabetes insipidus.

You may be correct but diabetes insipidus is rare in chronic renal failure, more commonly being present in hydronephrosis, pyelonephritis and the rare inherited anomaly of congenital nephrogenic diabetes insipidus. In children renal failure is often associated with bed-wetting, not nocturia. In children with diabetes insipidus, bed-wetting is the rule. Now answer the question in **9.6** again.

9.9 Your answer — I don't know if salt wasting is common.

If you don't know you have not been reading **9.5** carefully. Go back and read it. Pay attention and avoid distractions: if you have no chance of this postpone your reading until you can read properly. Never waste time deceiving yourself that you are learning when you are looking at the words without thinking about the message.

9.10 Your answer — whole body heparinisation in uraemic pericarditis sometimes leads to haemopericardium and cardiac tamponade.

Good. Now let us go on to discuss the *treatment of chronic renal failure*. First of all hypertension, if present, should be controlled. The sodium intake of the patient should be reduced to 20 mEq/day for up to five days and the urine sodium loss per 24 hour period measured. After four or five days the extent of daily loss in the urine in excess of that taken in as dietary sodium will be known: this is known as the 'sodium leak.' The salt intake should be adjusted after this so that the patient remains in sodium balance. Thiazide diuretics occasionally cause natriuresis in severe uraemia, but as a rule they do not. On the other hand frusemide (lasix) in doses up to 2 grams per day by mouth will frequently cause an increase in urine volume and accompanying increase in sodium and urea excretion, even at G.F.R. levels of 2 to 3 ml per minute. There is an accompanying increase in urea and creatinine clearance even in very advanced chronic renal failure. Scribner has shown that hypertension can frequently be controlled by adjustment of the sodium intake, and the patient becomes sensitive to smaller doses of hypotensive drugs, α-methyldopa is a useful drug in controlling the hypertension if salt intake can be restricted to the desired quantity as outlined above. The dose of α-methyldopa (Aldomet) is 250 mg b.d. at the beginning rising to $1\frac{1}{2}$-2g per day if necessary. Guanethidine may also be required (starting dose 10 mg daily). In renal failure the dose increase should be gradual, 10 mg every four or five days, because of the cumulative effect of the drug being accentuated by renal failure. Propranalol (inderal) may be given in doses of 10 mg tds rising up to 80 mg tds if necessary, although heart failure may be precipitated. Oral diazoxide has been used in severe renal failure with good results.

Severe anaemia requires blood transfusion, either as packed red cells or as slow infusions of fresh cells. Older blood has a high *plasma* potassium content and is best avoided in renal failure. Digoxin may be required to control cardiac arrhythmias and larger doses may be required in hyperkalaemia: the excretion of digoxin is reduced in renal failure and high plasma levels build up. A method of giving digoxin is given on page 402. The treatment of hyperkalaemia itself is as follows:

(1) *Rapid fall in serum potassium*: this may be brought about by intravenous glucose 50 g (100 ml of 50 per cent) together with 20 units of soluble insulin, but the effect lasts only a few hours. The effects of hyperkalaemia may be alleviated by slow i.v. injection of calcium gluconate or lactate (20 ml of a 10 per cent solution) or equivalent $CaCl_2$, or slow, i.v. injection of 100 mEq of $NaHCO_3$.

(2) *Slower reduction in serum potassium* may be achieved by oral ion-exchange resins such as Resonium A, 15 g 6 hourly orally: it may be given more frequently in a dose of 15 g up to 2 or three hourly. Calcium zeokarb is safer than Resonium A, because it does not exchange sodium for potassium, but gives calcium ion in exchange instead. Sorbitol is best avoided. Its main use is in getting rid of sodium from the body by means of diarrhoea, rather than potassium loss.

Now answer the question.

Question What is the effect on the serum potassium of giving intravenous glucose and insulin?

Answer 1. Lowers serum potassium. Go on to **9.21**.
2. No effect. Go on to **9.23**.
3. Don't know. Go on to **9.25**.

9.11 Your answer – the patient has osteomalacia.

No. In renal osteomalacia S. W. Stanbury has shown that the tendency is for serum calcium figures to be depressed below normal – whereas in hyperparathyroidism secondary to renal disease the serum calcium tends to be normal or elevated and not depressed. Now answer the question in **9.3** correctly.

9.12 Your answer – whole body heparinisation may lead to 'bats wing' lungs.

No. The 'bats wing' lung is common in uraemia with pulmonary congestion. This has nothing to do with uraemic pericarditis in which anticoagulants may cause bleeding into the pericardial sac. Now read **9.16** again and answer the question correctly.

9.13 Your answer – patient has hyperparathyroidism secondary to renal disease.

You are correct. There are few effects from a high blood urea by itself, but there are various other substances (e.g., organic compounds such as methyl creatinine, methylguanidine, methyl urea, guanidinosuccinic acid which may be responsible for the symptoms of uraemia. The clinical features of uraemia can be divided into general symptoms – fatigue, dyspnoea on effort, malaise, pallor i.e. (1) *symptoms due to anaemia*. (2) *Pruritis* is a symptom which is of unknown cause and is intractable unless dialysis is undertaken. (3) A *bleeding tendency* appears later in the disease – skin purpura, vomiting of blood and bloody diarrhoea. This is frequently associated with thrombocytopenia and abnormalities in platelet adhesion and also inhibition of the circulating plasma coagulation factors, particularly Factor VII.

(4) *Gastro-intestinal symptoms* are very prominent in renal failure: nausea, vomiting, and anorexia are frequent; towards the end, bloody diarrhoea develops. The vomiting may be partly attributed to salt depletion and partly to the high ammonia

levels in the stomach. The mouth is dry, the tongue is coated, and the breath smells ammoniacal or like urine. The diarrhoea may cause severe salt depletion with profound hypokalaemia. The stomatitis itself is often ulcerative in type, with bloody sordes on the lips. (5) The cause of *the neuromuscular symptom* of twitching is unknown. Usually it is not attributable to hypocalcaemia: Trousseau's sign is usually negative. Likewise the occasional occurrence of a *severe peripheral neuropathy* is of unknown aetiology; our experience of this is limited, but it is common to find sensory disturbances such as 'burning feet' in severe chronic renal failure, particularly in those patients maintained alive on chronic haemodialysis. The neuropathy may be ultimately associated with profound muscular paralysis; the nerve conduction velocity in peripheral nerves is commonly decreased in uraemia. There is no reliable treatment of the neuropathy other than homo-transplantation of a kidney, although we have seen rapid improvement by more frequent haemodialyses. In chronic renal failure there is the occasional occurrence of gynaecomastia. This is enlargement of the male breast. Look at figures 9.13a and b. You will see that this actually was capable of milk secretion. Males with GFR's below 5 ml/min are commonly sterile and females – who usually have irregular periods or amenorrhoea, – are usually, but not always, sterile.

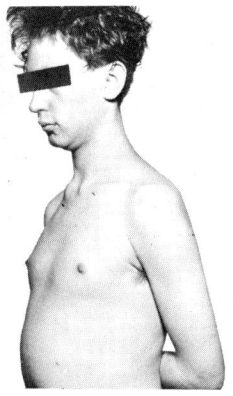

Fig. 9.13a

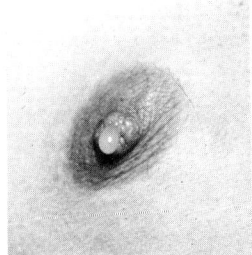

Fig. 9.13b

Question What is the mechanism of the bleeding tendency of uraemia?

Answer 1. Inhibition of some of the plasma coagulation factors. Go on to **9.14**.
2. Thrombocytopenia. Go on to **9.18**.
3. Thrombocytopenia, inhibition of platelet adhesion and inhibition of some of the circulating plasma coagulation factors. Go on to **9.16**.

9.14 Your answer – the bleeding tendency of uraemia is due to inhibition of some of the circulating plasma coagulant factors.

You are partly correct, but the uraemia is also associated with thrombocytopenia as well as deficiencies of several such coagulation factors as Factor VII. Now read **9.13** again and answer the question at the end correctly.

9.15 Your answer — I don't know what sort of bone disease is present.

In bone disease secondary to renal disease S. W. Stanbury has shown that in the group suffering from osteomalacia the serum calcium level is commonly depressed below normal; in renal hyperparathyroidism the serum calcium is normal or elevated in most cases. Now answer the question in **9.3** correctly.

9.16 Your answer — the bleeding tendency is partly due to thrombocytopenia and partly due to an inhibition of plasma coagulation factors.

Good. The cardiovascular changes of uraemia are: (1) *Congestive heart failure* due to anaemia with or without the superimposed effects of the hypertension so commonly associated with renal disease. Left ventricular failure is particularly common in uraemia and gives rise to the lung field changes on chest x-ray known as 'uraemic lung' in which congestion of the central lung fields due to pulmonary oedema causes a 'butterfly' or 'bats wing' appearance with *clear* peripheral lung zones (Fig. 9.16).

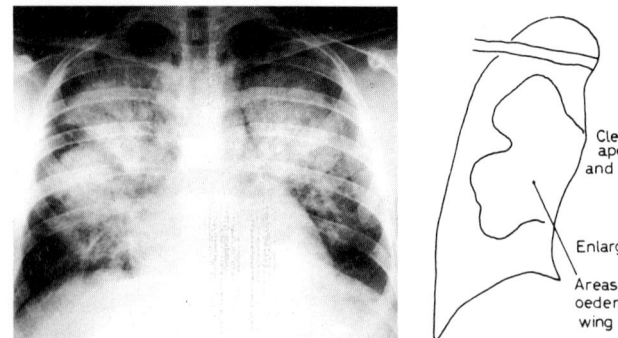

Fig. 9.16

(2) *Pericarditis and pericardial effusion*. Pericarditis occurs in at least half the patients with terminal uraemia, giving rise to a pericardial rub which is readily audible and which was formerly thought to indicate a fatal outcome within three weeks. With the advent of haemodialysis this is no longer true. Patients with a pericarditis who have a haemodialysis with whole body heparinisation may bleed into the pericardium, developing a haemopericardium. This may lead to cardiac tamponade with falling arterial blood pressure, rising venous pressure, tachycardia, and death in a few hours. Patients with uraemic pericarditis should therefore have 'regional heparinisation' during haemodialysis, in which the blood in the artificial

kidney is maintained in an anticoagulated state while the blood in the patient has a normal coagulation time due to the addition of protamine to the blood returning from the kidney.

Cardiac arrhythmias occur in about one patient in three with terminal uraemia. Now answer the question.

Question What is the danger of whole body heparinisation in a patient with uraemic pericarditis?

Answer 1. Cardiac tamponade due to haemopericardium. Go on to **9.10**.
2. 'Bats wing' lung. Go on to **9.12**.
3. Don't know. Go on to **9.17**.

9.17 Your answer – I don't know the dangers of whole body heparinisation in uraemic pericarditis.

The patient with an inflamed pericardium who is given anticoagulants runs an increased risk of bleeding into the pericardium with resultant haemopericardium and ultimately cardiac tamponade. Now read **9.16** again, paying more attention so that you do not miss any other facts of importance before you leave the paragraph. Then answer the question correctly: if you still cannot, then give up the attempt today or remove yourself to less distracting surroundings.

9.18 Your answer – the bleeding tendency in uraemia is due to thrombocytopenia.

You are correct in so far as this is one of the causes, but inhibition of Factor VII is present as well. Read **9.13** again and try the question again.

9.19 Your answer – the Giovannetti diet contains less than 20 g of protein.

You are correct. The dietary treatment of renal failure postpones death for some time but not forever. Furosemide has been used in the treatment of advanced chronic renal failure to increase the glomerular filtration rate and therefore to prolong life. It is given in large doses of up to 2.0 G/day orally; if the patient is vomiting it should be given intravenously at a rate of 100 mg per hour. If given at a faster rate there is a danger of reversible deafness developing. Renal function ultimately deteriorates so far that the patient's blood urea rises and he developes the terminal symptoms of anaemia, bleeding, agitation, pericarditis, etc. The pericarditis may be very painful, with pain in the precordium and epigastrium. Gastro-intestinal symptoms (hiccough, anorexia, vomiting or diarrhoea) are rare in patients on the Giordano-Giovannetti diet, but common in patients on standard low protein diets.

The two possible methods of keeping the patient alive at this stage are dialysis and renal transplantation. At present renal transplantation is still in its infancy, and will be considered in more detail in chapter 21. Dialysis, on the other hand, is of proven value and for a moderate financial outlay life can be preserved for years after the kidneys have ceased to function. There are two forms of dialysis, peritoneal and haemodialysis. Peritoneal dialysis is described in some detail in the previous chapter on Acute Renal Failure; it can be used to keep patients without renal function alive for up to 4 years. There is the ever present danger of infection being introduced even though peritonitis can be readily treated by infusing the appropriate antibiotic. If recurrent peritoneal dialysis is to be done, some physicians have an artificial 'belly button' made of plastic inserted permanently in the abdominal wall; through it a cannula can be inserted without making a fresh wound in the abdomen. In time all artificial 'belly buttons' become infected and may lead to generalised peritonitis. Boen prefers a multiple incision technique inserting the cannula for each dialysis through a new stab incision.

In chronic peritoneal dialysis, protein loss from the peritoneum into the dialysate can be considerable, an average loss being 20–40 G. per dialysis including albumin and IgG globulin. Amino acid loss is considerable, and combined with protein loss leads to protein malnutrition, with hypoalbuminaemia and reduced resistance to bacterial infection. Hypoalbuminaemia frequently occurs in patients on chronic peritoneal dialysis and protein replacement by intravenous plasma may be required to correct it. Pain is a prominent feature of peritoneal dialysis and requires alkaloids such as morphine for its relief: some patients refuse a second or third peritoneal dialysis because of the pain.

Question What are the major proteins lost in peritoneal dialysis?

Answer 1. IgG globulin. Go on to **9.35**.
2. Albumin. Go on to **9.33**.
3. Albumin and IgG globulin. Go on to **9.27**.
4. None. Go on to **9.29**.

9.20   Your answer – the bridge is made of Teflon.
Good. The second type of shunt is:
2. **Cimino-Brescia Subcutaneous A–V Fistula**. This is an advance on the Scribner shunt in that a side to side or end to side anastamosis is made between a limb artery (e.g. the radial artery) and a branch of major vein (e.g. cephalic vein). The vein gradually enlarges and becomes arterialised with a prominent thrill. Look at figure 9.20a. The enlarged vein is readily entered by a pair of 14 gauge needles passed through the skin at the time of dialysis. Each dialysis requires needling to gain access to the vessels and a blood pump must be used to drive the blood through the artificial kidney. Nevertheless these slight disadvantages are far outweighed by the advantage of fewer clotting episodes, and infections are rare. Shunt life is at least twice as long.

There are several types of artificial kidney, but the two in most common use will be described. First of all the Kolff twin coil kidney marketed by Baxter-Travenol uses disposable presterilised coils. These, together with connected tubes cost about $16–£19, dependent on the type and are designed for use once though some of them can be used 10–15 times using special precautions. They can be primed with saline. The structure of a standard Kolff twin coil kidney as shown in Fig. 9.20 (b).

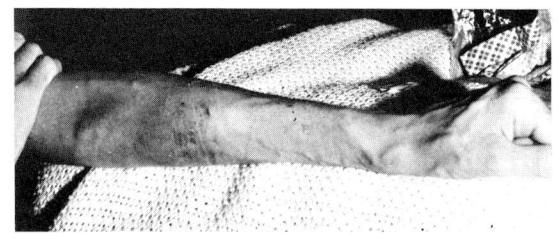

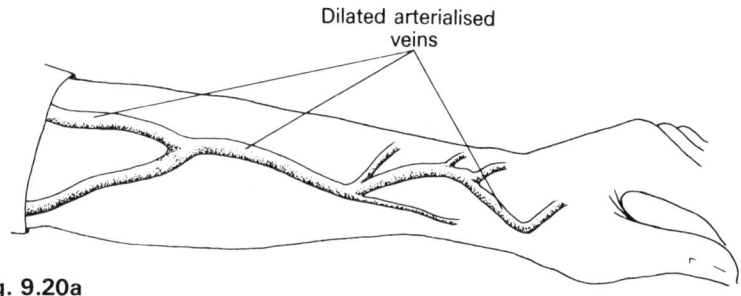

Fig. 9.20a

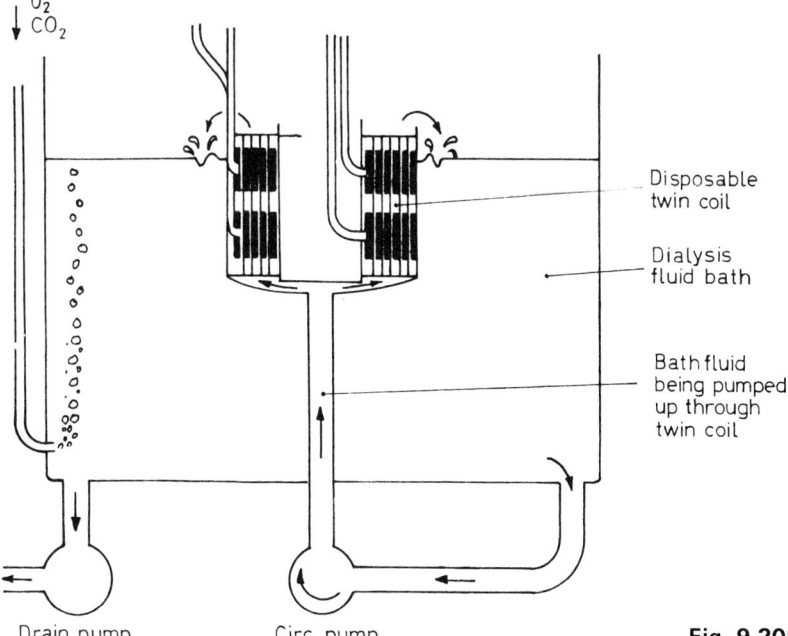

Dilated arterialised veins

Disposable twin coil

Dialysis fluid bath

Bath fluid being pumped up through twin coil

O_2
CO_2

Drain pump   Circ. pump

Fig. 9.20b

The stainless steel drum is filled with dialysis fluid (for composition see the appendix, p. 398) which is pumped round the coil. The coil itself consists of twin tubes of cellulose supported on fibreglass or plastic mesh and is disposable. A pump propels the blood through the coil. Increasing the pressure on the venous line enables one to remove fluid *from* the patient by ultrafiltration. The machine is efficient; dialyses take six to eight hours and its efficiency is greater than that of a two layer Kiil kidney. The requirement of blood for priming is a disadvantage. Look at the figure 9.20c – this is a photograph of a coil and its mounting.

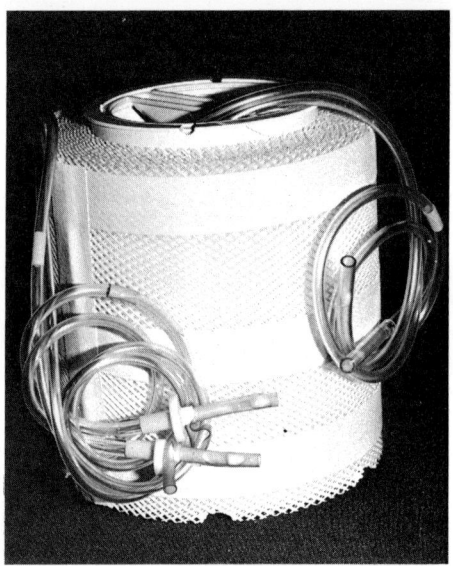

Fig. 9.20c

Question What is the advantage of a Cimino-Brescia fistula?

Answer 1. Less clotting and infections. Go on to **9.22**.
        2. More ease of access. Go on to **9.32**.

9.21 Your answer – insulin and glucose intravenously cause a fall in the serum potassium.

Good. The majority of patients suffering from chronic renal failure can have their lives prolonged with few symptoms of uraemia for some months by use of a low protein diet containing approximately 18 to 21 g of protein. The principles of this diet was designed in Italy by Giordano and Giovannetti and colleagues and it contains all the daily requirements of the essential amino acids in the form of the minimum amount of natural protein so that endogenous protein turnover is reduced to a minimum. The blood urea falls gradually and may reach normal levels despite advanced renal failure. The serum phosphate may also return to normal from the elevated levels common in uraemia. Serum urate levels in uraemia are usually very high and may be associated with a secondary gouty arthritis; the serum urate level falls to normal in patients with a GFR of 3 ml/min or more on a Giovannetti diet. The appetite returns and the patient may be able to return to work even when his GFR is 1.5 ml/min i.e., when he would have otherwise reached a vicious circle of uraemic vomiting and salt depletion, leading to death some weeks or months earlier. There is no indication for a diet with rigorous protein restriction such as the Giovannetti diet unless the patient has a blood urea of over 200 mg/100 ml. Dietary therapy of any disease requires enthusiasm and it is necessary to be sure that the enthusiasm is transmitted to the patient: otherwise patients gradually relax the diet and deteriorate. Now answer the question.

Question How much protein is in the modified Giovannetti diet described in this paragraph?

Answer 1. Less than 20 g. Go on to **9.19**.
2. 50 g. Go on to **9.24**.
3. No protein. Go on to **9.26**.

9.22 Your answer – less clotting and infections.

Good. The rapidity of dialysis with the Kolff twin coil kidney is such as to lead to the 'disequilibrium syndrome' described in detail by Kennedy in Glasgow. In this syndrome the patient during or after a rapid dialysis develops cerebral oedema with headache, twitchings, convulsions and loss of consciousness and sometimes death. EEG changes are found constantly in this syndrome. The cause of the disequilibrium syndrome has been found to be due to the slowness of diffusion of urea out of the brain into the extracellular fluid (ECF): the urea of the ECF is lowered more rapidly than that in the brain. During haemodialysis the brain therefore exerts a higher osmotic pressure than the perfusing plasma and so water passes into the brain with resultant cerebral oedema. The syndrome can be avoided by slower dialysis or by adding glucose, 1–1.5 g/100 ml to the dialysing bath. Now answer the question.

Question What is the pathological basis of the 'disequilibrium syndrome?

Answer 1. Cerebral haemorrhage. Go on to **9.36**.
2. Cerebral oedema. Go on to **9.37**.
3. Don't know. Go on to **9.39**.

9.23 Your answer – intravenous glucose and insulin have no effect on the serum potassium.

No. The serum potassium falls after insulin and glucose due to the potassium entering cells. Read **9.10** again and answer the question correctly.

9.24 Your answer – the modified Giovannetti diet contains 50 g of protein.

No. The diet contains less than 20 g of protein, just the bare minimum to provide the essential amino acids. Read **9.21** again before you answer the question.

9.25 Your answer – I don't know the effect of intravenous glucose and insulin on the serum potassium. You should have remembered that insulin and glucose cause a fall, albeit transient, in the serum potassium. Don't look at the text, read it; think about the words and concentrate on your reading. Now read **9.10** again.

9.26 Your answer – no protein is present in the Giovannetti diet.

No. You cannot use a 'no protein' diet because the patient will have an accelerated endogenous protein breakdown from his own muscles and other tissues which will lead to an elevation of the blood urea. The ideal diet causes the minimum amount of protein breakdown, and for this the patient should be in nitrogen balance or, if possible in positive balance – i.e. retaining nitrogen from the diet. Now read **9.21** again and answer the question again.

9.27 Your answer – albumin and IgG globulin are the major proteins lost in peritoneal dialysis.

Good. In chronic renal failure the indications for dialysis can be separated into two groups. (1) The indications for a single dialysis. (2) The indications for repeated dialysis, the so-called chronic dialysis programme, or RDT (regular dialysis treatment).

(1) *The indications for a single dialysis* (haemodialysis or peritoneal dialysis) are:

(a) *Every patient who has severe chronic renal failure (GER less than 2.5 ml/min) should be given the benefit of at least one dialysis*. This often has dramatic results, enabling the patients to be stabilised on a low protein diet and to live comfortably for several extra months. In these patients who have been precipitated into severe renal failure by a urinary tract infection or an infection elsewhere, a dialysis allows the patient extra time for treatment with antibiotics and improvements in renal function.

(b) Blood urea over 300 mg/100 ml or clinical features of drowsiness, severe oedema, fits, bleeding, twitching or confusion.

(c) Hyperkalaemia (serum potassium over 7.5 mEq/l), resistant to other treatment.

(d) Severe acidosis; plasma pH of 7.15 or less, total plasma CO_2 of 12 mM/l or less, in whom it is not advisable to give sodium bicarbonate, e.g. as in left ventricular failure.

If the patient has had no recent abdominal injuries or operations peritoneal dialysis should be carried out. Similarly, a bleeding tendency is an indication for peritoneal dialysis rather than haemodialysis. If the patient has had recent abdominal surgery, haemodialysis is indicated if peritoneal dialysis is impossible due to leakage and lack of an intact peritoneal surface.

(2) *Chronic haemodialysis*: RDT Patients with chronic renal failure in the absence of complicating disease of other organs can be maintained in reasonably good physical health for at least nine years by means of regular haemodialysis: this should be done 2 or 3 times weekly; the patients require a diet limiting their fluid, protein and salt intake. Haemodialysis can be carried out at home with automated, safe monitored apparatus as initially pioneered by Shaldon. There is no need for expensive nursing or technical staff and no risk of an outbreak of infective hepatitis. Now answer the question.

Question If a patient with chronic renal failure due to polycystic kidneys is admitted to hospital with a blood urea of 450 mg/100 ml vomiting and anaemia would you dialyse once, there being no facilities for chronic haemodialysis?

Answer 1. Yes. Go on to **9.28**.
         2. No. Go on to **9.31**.
         3. Don't know. Go on to **9.34**.

9.28 Your answer − dialyse the patient at least once.

Good. For chronic haemodialysis it is necessary to have access to arterial and venous blood. This is obtained through an arteriovenous shunt. There are two types of arterio-venous shunts.

1. Scribner shunt. This was the first chronic access to an artery and vein, and was achieved by putting a Teflon tube in a limb artery, and a similar one in an adjacent vein. The arterial teflon and venous teflon tube are connected by silastic (silicone-rubber) tubes which pass through the skin and are joined by a small Teflon bridge. Look at the figure 9.28a and b.

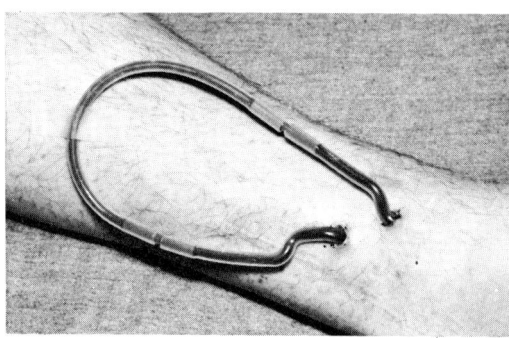

Fig. 9.28a

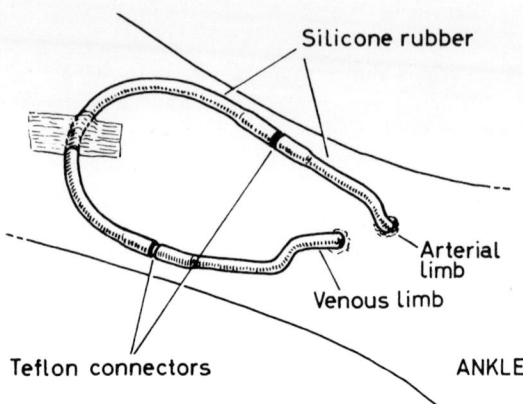

Fig. 9.28b

You can see the silastic tube which comes through the skin from the teflon tubes embedded beneath the skin in the artery and vein. At the time of a haemodialysis, the bridge is removed and the patient attached to the arterial and venous lines of the artificial kidney. Cannulas of this type often clot, and this is frequently associated with infections at the site of the entrance of the silastic through the skin. A Scribner shunt lasts about one year. Other types of shunts go into the femoral veins but are less satisfactory than the Scribner shunts described above. The blood flow through a teflon Scribner shunt should be about 150–250 ml/min.

Question What is the 'bridge' of a Scribner shunt made of?

Answer 1. Teflon. Go on to **9.20**.
2. Silicone rubber (or silastic). Go on to **9.30**.

9.29 Your answer – no proteins are lost in peritoneal dialysis.

No. In every peritoneal dialysis proteins are lost, the smaller proteins such as albumin and IgG globulin being lost in large amounts. You have not concentrated adequately when reading **9.19**. Go over it again and answer the question correctly.

9.30 Your answer – the bridge of a Scribner shunt is made of silicone rubber (or 'silastic').

You are not correct. The bridge is made of teflon and is removed at each dialysis. Teflon is cheaper than silicone rubber, and a leak proof joint is made easily. Now read **9.28** and answer the question again.

9.31 Your answer – I would not dialyse even once.

You are wrong not to dialyse the patient because the renal failure may have been precipitated by a renal tract infection which is common complication of polycystic kidney disease: the dialysis will give you time to treat the renal infection, and get the patient stabilised on a Giovannetti type diet. He may well be able to return to work even with marginal improvement in renal function. Now answer the question again after reading **9.27** carefully.

9.32 Your answer — easier access. You are wrong because needles have to be used to gain access through the skin to the circulation. Read **9.20** again and pay more attention this time.

9.33 Your answer — albumin is the major protein lost in peritoneal dialysis.
You are partly correct but IgG globulin is also lost in considerable amounts. Answer the question in 9.19 again.

9.34 Your answer — I don't know whether to dialyse or not.
If any patient comes in with chronic renal failure he should be given the benefit of at least one dialysis in order to gain time to treat intercurrent infections, and stabilise the patient on a Giovannetti diet. This may add months or years to the patient's life. Now read **9.27** again more carefully this time and answer the question.

9.35 Your answer — IgG globulin is the major protein lost in peritoneal dialysis.
You are partly correct. Albumin is also lost in large amounts in peritoneal dialysis. Read **9.19** again and answer the question correctly.

9.36 Your answer — the cause of the 'disequilibrium syndrome' is cerebral haemorrhage.
You are incorrect. You have not read **9.22** properly. Go back over it and then answer the question correctly.

9.37 Your answer — 'disequilibrium syndrome' is due to cerebral oedema.
Correct. The other common type of kidney is the Skeggs-Leonard and its simple modification, the Kiil kidney. The Kiil kidney will be considered in greater detail because it is the commonest type of kidney used in chronic haemodialysis. It is efficient, cheap to run, requires *no* priming with blood, and can be managed by nursing staff. Basically it consists of three polypropylene plates which are grooved so that dialysis fluid can run through them. Look at Fig. 9.37.

The blood runs between cellophane sheets which cost a few pennies only: the blood is separated from the dialysis fluid by the cellophane. The blood volume of

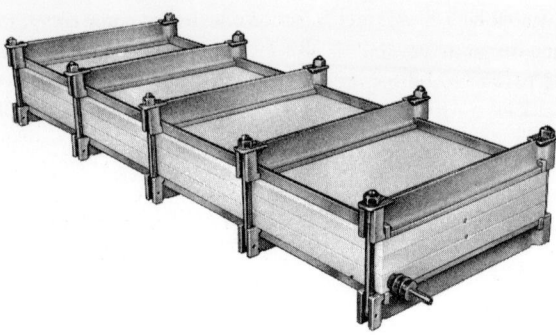

Fig. 9.37

the Kiil is less than 300 ml including all leads: the cellophane sheets require sterilisation before use. The resistance of the two layer Kiil kidney to blood flow is so low that a pump is not required to propel the blood from the artery to the vein: the arterial blood pressure is quite adequate. This applies only if a standard Scribner shunt is present. If Cimino-Brescia fistulae are used then a blood pump is needed whatever type of artificial kidney is used.

Question Does a Kiil kidney require priming with blood?

Answer 1. Yes. Go on to **9.40**.
2. No. Go on to **9.38**.

9.38 Your answer — the Kiil kidney does *not* need to be primed with blood.
Good. Patients must be dialysed for at least 14 to 18 hours twice a week on a two-layer Kiil kidney to remain alive and well without functioning kidneys. Blood transfusion is usually not needed, the haemoglobin reaching 8–9 g/100 ml spontaneously. Avoidance of blood transfusion prevents 2 complications — hepatitis of viral origin, and transfusion siderosis. The neuropathy which develops in chronic renal failure is not always relieved by haemodialysis. Metastatic calcification may develop. It disappears after lowering of the serum inorganic phosphorus level by oral aluminium hydroxide gel. Infections of the teflon shunt and clotting are constant hazards; the infections should be treated promptly with antibiotics. The use of antibiotics in renal disease depends on the following factors:

(1) The rate of degradation of the antibiotic in the body to nontoxic metabolites.
(2) The extent of excretion of the antibiotic or its metabolites in the urine in the normal person.

(3) The toxicity of high serum concentrations of the antibiotic. Firstly tetracycline should be avoided in renal disease because it has an adverse effect both on nitrogen metabolism, both elevating the blood urea and also exacerbating renal failure. Streptomycin, kanamycin and Colistin should be avoided in renal failure because of the toxicity of higher serum levels of these drugs. Polymyxin B and amphotericin B are nephrotoxic and should be avoided in renal disease. Penicillin, ampicillin, cloxacillin and methicillin are safe in reduced dosage in renal failure due to the lack of toxicity of high serum levels. 250,000 units a day of sodium penicillin G intramuscularly is a standard dose in renal failure. Erythromycin and chloramphenicol can be used in normal dosage in renal failure. Remember that the majority of deaths in acute renal failure nowadays are due to infections.

Question Would you give streptomycin intramuscularly 1 g b.d. to a patient with a blood urea of 400 mg/100 ml?

Answer 1. Yes. Go on to **9.42**.
2. No. Go on to **9.44**.
3. Don't know. Go on to **9.46**.

9.39 Your answer — I don't know what is the cause of disequilibrium syndrome.
If you don't know you have not read **9.22** with enough attention. Stop daydreaming and read **9.22** again.

9.40 Your answer — the two-layer Kiil kidney requires blood for priming.
No. The volume of all the blood circuit is less than 300 ml so that the machine can be primed with saline. Read **9.37** again.

9.41 Your answer — a rejection reaction is occurring.
You are correct. Rejection of a transplanted kidney can occur early, within a few hours or days of transplantation, or it may be delayed for several weeks or months. The kidney is swollen, and histological examination shows an infiltration with round cells in the early and reversible stages. The vessels in many patients show a specific rejection reaction which may progress and lead to vascular occlusion and infarction of the grafted kidney. There is no absolutely certain way of preventing rejection reactions, but prednisone and azathioprine (Imuran) can frequently suppress the rejection reaction at least temporarily. Lately promising results have come from the use of anti-lymphocyte serum with the other immuno suppressives — azathioprine and prednisone. Prior treatment of the recipient with deep X-rays was routinely practised in Hamburger's clinic in Paris in order to suppress the immune response. Like azathioprine this may suppress the marrow and lead to fatal bleeding or infections in spite of treating the patients in a 'sterile unit' with all precautions against the entry of micro-organisms. Some surgeons remove the thymus, spleen and appendix of the recipient and treat the graft with X-rays before or after grafting, to reduce the immune response. Drainage of the thoracic duct

lymph through a fistula in the neck causes a lymphopenia and an increase in the survival time of allografts, both skin and kidney.

The chance of permanent acceptance of a kidney graft from an unrelated donor is less than that from an identical twin or close relative; nevertheless, the problem at present is whether it is ethical to remove a kidney from a healthy person with a 50—95 per cent chance of the graft being successful for one year. This had led to the use of cadavers as kidney donors; the term 'cadaver' is somewhat misleading for the majority of the so-called cadavers undergo cardiac massage and artificial respiration from the actual moment of 'death' until the kidney is removed in the operating theatre. The kidney is usually damaged by anoxia and is frequently the site of acute tubular necrosis; The recipients may require haemodialysis until the transplanted kidney has recovered in a few weeks. It is at present too early to evaluate the usefulness of allografts and of hetero-transplantation, although it is known that a proportion of homografts develop the changes of membranous glomerulonephritis, probably as a type of rejection response. Transplantation and chronic haemodialysis complement reach other, and the view that transplantation with a cadaver donor is an invitation to play Russian Roulette is probably an exaggeration at the present state of the art. Transplantation is dealt with in chapter 21. Now answer the question.

Question What drugs are used to suppress the rejection reaction?

Answer 1. Prednisone. Go on to **9.50**.
2. Azathioprine. Go on to **9.48**.
3. Prednisone, azathioprine, and antilymphocyte serum. Go on to **9.57**.

9.42 Your answer — I would give systemic streptomycin to a patient in renal failure.

You should rarely give streptomycin in renal failure: it is excreted by glomerular filtration, and in renal failure a toxic plasma level of streptomycin is rapidly reached. Now read **9.38** again.

9.43 Your answer — proteinuria in a grafted kidney indicates urinary tract infection.

There may be a urinary tract infection, but the proteinuria from the grafted kidney is almost certainly due to a rejection reaction. Read **9.44** again

9.44 Your answer — streptomycin should not be given in this dosage to a patient with blood urea of 400 mg/100 ml.

Correct. Further details about antibiotics and other drug administration in renal failure is given in Chapter 20 and the Appendix. The only curative method of treatment in irreversible and progressive renal disease is renal transplantation. Organ transplantation is at an early stage both in our understanding of hostgraft response and in the practical experience of actual transplantation. First of all, let us have a look at the pertinent facts. Homotransplantation means transplantation of an organ from one member of the same species to another member of that species. This is an allograft. Heterotransplantation means transplantation of an organ from one species to a different species or xenografting. In man homotransplantation is usually practised, but heterotransplantation using baboon and chimpanzee kidneys, has been shown to be feasible. Homotransplantation usually succeeds if the donor of the kidney and the recipient are identical or very similar immunologically. In practice the only kidney transplants which are certain of success are those between identical twins because they have identical tissue antigens. After that, rather less successful but with a reasonable hope of success are transplantations of kidneys between dizygotic twins, between siblings and between parents and children. There are numerous recorded successful transplants between unrelated donors and even between persons with different ABO blood groups. The transplantation of organs usually fails *not* for technical reasons but because of immunological 'rejection' of the organ by the host. This rejection is an ill-understood subject but is thought to be due to the host producing humoral and cellular agents which attack the foreign transplanted organ. The rejection reactions are indicated by proteinuria, pyuria, fall in creatinine clearance, and in sodium excretion, oliguria, pyrexia and swelling of the kidney; anuria soon develops if the rejection reaction is not adequately controlled.

Question If proteinuria develops in the urine from a transplanted kidney what does this indicate is happening?

Answer 1. Rejection reaction occurring. Go on to **9.41**.
2. Urinary tract infection. Go on to **9.43**.
3. Don't know. Go on to **9.45**.

9.45 Your answer – I don't know what proteinuria in a grafted kidney indicates. It indicates a rejection reaction. Read **9.44** again.

9.46 Your answer – I don't know if streptomycin should be given to the patient in renal failure.
In **9.38** it is stated that streptomycin should not be given because of the toxicity of high plasma concentrations of streptomycin, which accumulates in the plasma in renal failure. Now read **9.38** again and answer the question correctly.

9.47 Your answer – 1 is true, 2 and 3 are false.
You are correct. If you want to read more about chronic renal failure read the Transactions of the American Society for Artificial Internal Organs, which are full of numerous articles dealing with the problems of chronic renal failure. Dietary treatment is discussed by Thomas Addis (1948) in his book on Glomerulonephritis. The Giovannetti diet is described in English by Giovannetti and Maggiore in the

Lancet, 1964, 1. and by Shaw et al., Quart, J. Med. **34**, 237, 1965. Peritoneal dialysis is discussed by Boen S. T. in Medicine, 1961, Xp. 40, 243, and a good review is by R. B. Miller and C. R. Tassiter (1969) New Eng. J. Med. **281**, 945. The chapters by Merrill and Relman and Levinsky in Diseases of the Kidney edited by Strauss and Welt, (Little Brown, 1971) are particularly good and stimulating. A useful book on haemodialysis is 'Haemodialyse' by K. W. Fritz, Georg Thieme 1966, but it is in German. Nephrology by Hamburger et al (translated by Walsh, Saunders 1968) has a very good chapter on transplantation. The symposium 'Uremia' edited by Kluthé R. Berlyne G. M. and Burton B. 1972 Thieme is useful. You can now go on to the next chapter.

9.48 Your answer – azathioprine is used to prevent the rejection reaction.

Yes, but prednisone and antilymphocyte serum are also used to suppress the host's immune response. Now go on to read **9.56**.

9.49 Your answer – statement 2 is true, the rest are false. You have learned nothing about nocturia, salt loss or dialysis as far as your answers go. Start again at **9.1** and work through the chapter.

9.50 Your answer – prednisone is used to suppress the rejection reaction.

You are correct but azathioprine and antilymphocyte serum are also used; now go on to **9.56**.

9.51 Your answer – statement 3 is true, the rest are false.

You are wrong about statements 1 and 3. Start reading the chapter again from **9.1**.

9.52 Your answer – statement 1 and 2 are true, 3 is false.

You are correct about 1 and 3 but 2 is false. Read **9.5** again, then answer the question in **9.56** again.

9.53 Your answer – statements 1 and 3 are true, 2 is false.

You are correct about statements 1 and 2 but wrong about 3. Read on from **9.27** again.

9.54 Your answer – statements 2 and 3 are true, 1 is false.

You are not correct on any point: 1 is true, 2 and 3 are false.
Start at the beginning of the chapter and read through it again.

9.55 Your answer – all the statements are false.

You are right about statements 2 and 3 but not about 1. Read from **9.1** to **9.5** then answer the question in **9.56** again.

9.56 Before answering this question read the following statements carefully. Then choose the answers after due thought: if you choose the wrong answers you may have to start reading the chapter again. The purpose of this paragraph is to determine how much you have learned in this chapter.

Statement 1 Nocturia is a common symptom in adults with chronic renal disease.

Statement 2 A salt leak is very rare in chronic renal failure.

Statement 3 Peritoneal dialysis is indicated in renal failure immediately after abdominal surgery.

Answer 1. All are true. Go on to **9.58**.
2. All are false. Go on to **9.55**.
3. Statement 1 is true, 2 and 3 are false. Go on to **9.47**.
4. Statement 2 is true, 1 and 3 are false. Go on to **9.49**.
5. Statement 3 is true, 1 and 2 are false. Go on to **9.51**.
6. Statements 1 and 2 are true, 3 is false. Go on to **9.52**.
7. Statements 1 and 3 are true, 2 is false. Go on to **9.53**.
8. Statements 2 and 3 are true, 1 is false. Go on to **9.54**.

9.57 Your answer – prednisone, azathioprine and antilymphocyte serum are commonly used at present to prevent the immune response.

Good. You are correct. There are several other drugs in use but prednisone and azathioprine are those used in most transplantation centres. Now go on to read **9.56**.

9.58 Your answer – all the statements are true.

You are partly correct in that statement 1 is true, but statements 2 and 3 are false. Go back to **9.5** and work on through the chapter.

Time for this chapter: 45 minutes

Chapter 10
Collagen diseases and the kidney

10.1 The collagen diseases are a heterogeneous group of unknown aetiology and include rheumatoid disease, systemic lupus erythematosus, polyarteritis nodosa, scleroderma and thrombotic thrombocytopenic purpura. Renal involvement is frequent in the collagen diseases. We shall first of all consider the renal involvement of systemic lupus erythematosus (SLE), which has been the most carefully documented. SLE has its maximum incidence in the 20 to 40 age group, but it should be remembered that it occurs at all ages. Thus the youngest patient with renal involvement in our own series was 9 and the oldest 79; the disease is commoner in females. In most series of cases of SLE, renal involvement is present in half to two thirds of the patients.

Question What sex is more commonly affected by SLE?

Answer 1. Males. Go on to **10.3**.
2. Females. Go on to **10.5**.

10.2 Your answer – of patients with SLE none get renal involvement.
No. Renal involvement occurs in half of two thirds of patients with SLE. Go back and read **10.6**, then answer **10.5** correctly.

10.3 Your answer – males are more commonly affected by SLE than females.
No. You have not read **10.1** carefully. Females are more commonly affected by SLE than males. Read **10.1** again and answer the question again.

10.4 Your answer – all patients with SLE have renal involvement.
No. You have not digested the content of **10.1** in which you were told that only half to two thirds of the patients have renal involvement. Answer the question in **10.5** correctly.

10.5 Your answer – females are more commonly affected than males.
Correct. Now go on to answer the next question.

Question What proportion of patients with SLE have renal involvement?

Answer 1. None. Go on to **10.2**.
2. All. Go on to **10.4**.
3. Half. Go on to **10.6**.

4. Two thirds. Go on to **10.7**.
   5. One third. Go on to **10.9**.

10.6 Your answer – one half of patients with SLE have renal involvement. Good. There are series which have an incidence as high as two thirds. Now go on to read **10.11**.

10.7 Your answer – two thirds of patients with SLE have renal involvement. You are correct in that some of the published series report an incidence as high as two thirds with renal involvement. Some series suggest that the incidence is as low as one half. Go on to **10.11**.

10.8 Your answer – IgG is present bound to the basement membrane.
You are correct. The clinical extra-renal manifestations of SLE have been mentioned in Chapter 6 (Nephrotic Syndrome), and will not be further described here. The earliest manifestation of renal involvement in systemic lupus is the presence of proteinuria, with white cells particularly prominent in the urinary sediment initially. As the disease progresses, the full blown picture of a 'telescoped' urinary sediment appears, with red cells, white cells, casts of all types, fat bodies, and tubular cells. By telescoped urine deposit is meant a telescoping of the time course of the nephritis as reflected in the urine deposit, i.e, there are at the same time the changes of acute, sub-acute, and chronic glomerulonephritis in the urine deposit. This 'telescoped' urine deposit is not specific for lupus nephritis but indicates the presence of a collagen disease. If the proteinuria becomes massive, the patient develops nephrotic syndrome. The proteinuria of patients with SLE contains a large proportion of IgG in addition to albumin, the serum IgG levels often being elevated.

Question Is a 'telescoped' urine deposit pathognomonic of SLE?

Answer 1. Yes. Go on to **10.17**.
   2. No. Go on to **10.19**.

10.9 Your answer – one third of patients with SLE develop renal involvement.
No. One half to two thirds of patients with SLE develop renal involvement. You have not absorbed this on your first reading of **10.1**. Be more careful with your subsequent reading. Now answer **10.5** correctly.

10.10 Your answer – pure membranous change is commoner.
No. In SLE the pure membranous type of change is rare. The wire loop type of change is many times more frequent. Now read **10.15** again.

10.11 The spectrum of renal disease in those patients with renal involvement is wide in SLE.

There are some patients who have the frank changes of nephrotic syndrome, with oedema, massive proteinuria, and hypoalbuminaemia; other patients have milder renal involvement with minimal proteinuria, while some are at the other end of the spectrum, with renal failure and hypertension. The variations in the clinical picture have been related to the histological changes by Kark's group in Chicago. Let us now examine these histological changes seen in the kidney. The first thing to learn is to forget the histology learned from textbooks of pathology which are based on post-mortem studies. The earlier changes of SLE are not so obvious in the patient with advanced renal disease, and this is the cause of the emphasis on the advanced renal lesions of SLE in the older textbooks. The earlier changes are as follows:

(1) There is a focal glomerulitis which consists of local areas of necrosis with cellular proliferation in *some* of the glomeruli only. This picture is not in itself diagnostic of lupus and is found in any focal glomerulitis, of any cause. It is called lupus glomerulitis. Look at Fig. 10.11a.

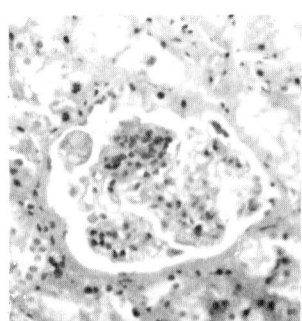 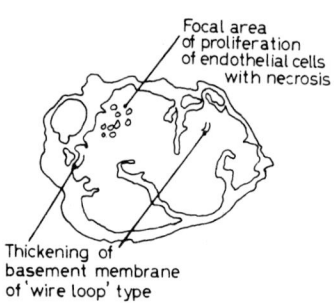

Fig. 10.11a

(2) The next stage of the pathology to be seen is a more advanced form of the disease with karyorrhexis of the tuft nuclei, fibrinoid necrosis, crescent formation, and interstitial infiltration with round cells. See Fig. 10.11b. This is known as lupus glomerulonephritis.

(3) The basement membrane is involved early in some patients but this is by no means constant, others having no obvious change until later. There is usually a patchy thickening of the basement membrane which gives rise to the 'wire-loop' appearance. Rarely there is a pure membranous form of SLE with uniform thickening of the basement membrane, indistinguishable histologically from non-lupoid membranous glomerulonephritis. This is, however, exceptional.

(4) The only certain way of identifying the renal lesion as that of SLE is by the presence of haematoxylin bodies or LE cells. These can certainly be found in

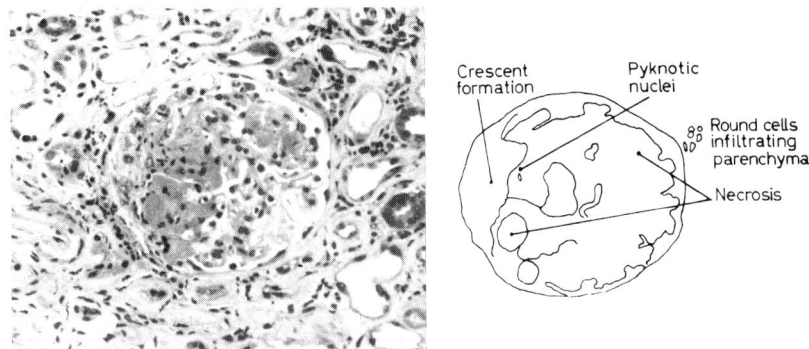

Fig. 10.11b

post-mortem material but are rarely found in biopsy specimens. It is difficult to understand how LE cells are ever present in biopsy material, for they are the phenomena associated with dying cells in SLE and are never found in situ in life otherwise. They may be formed in the anoxic biopsy core of tissue before penetration of fixative.

Immunofluorescent staining reveals a granular deposition of IgG and $C^1{}_3$ in SLE, typical of immune complex nephritis.

Now answer the question.

Question If you find histological evidence of a focal glomerulitis in a patient with proteinuria would you accept the statement that this patient has lupus on the basis of the renal findings only, there being no haemotoxylin bodies or LE cells seen?

Answer 1. Yes. Go on to **10.13**.
2. No. Go on to **10.15**.

10.12 Your answer — SLE causes a wire loop appearance most frequently.

Good. The end stages of lupus glomerulitis are variable in appearance. Some patients die with histological appearances which are identical to those of sub-acute or chronic glomerulonephritis. Others have no crescents at all, with a terminal picture of basement membrane thickening which obliterates the glomerular capillary lumen. Using fluorescein-conjugated antibodies, it has been shown that IgG and serum complement ($C^1{}_3$) are bound to the glomerular basement membrane in SLE: it is probable that this IgG globulin is *bound to* the basement membrane in an antigen-antibody reaction in which complement is consumed, although there is the less likely possibility that the IgG globulin is on its way *through* an abnormally permeable basement membrane. The antigen-antibody complex in SLE gives a granular appearance on fluorescent microscopy typical of immune complex nephritis. This fits in well with the electron microscope picture of electron dense deposits on the basement membrane. The antigen is probably an abnormal DNA and the antibodies are anti-DNA antibodies.

Question In what part of the glomerulus is IgG demonstrable using fluorescein-conjugated antibodies?

Answer 1. Basement membrane. Go on to **10.8**.
2. Bowman's space. Go on to **10.14**.

10.13 Your answer – I would accept a histological diagnosis of SLE on histology without any haemotyxlin bodies or LE cells being seen.

The histological diagnosis of SLE is not specific without the presence of LE cells or haematoxylin bodies. Focal glomerulitis occurs in many diseases and is in no way characteristic of SLE alone. Read **10.11** again, then answer the question correctly this time.

10.14 Your answer – IgG is bound to Bowman's space.

You are not correct. The IgG and complement are bound to the glomerular basement membrane, so that the question has arisen as to whether the proteins are passing through the basement membrane or whether they are bound to the basement membrane proper. Now answer **10.12** correctly.

10.15 Your answer – I would not be prepared to accept a diagnosis of SLE on these grounds only.

Correct. Now answer the next question.

Question Which is commoner in SLE – 1. a wire loop appearance; 2. pure membranous change with uniform thickening of basement membrane?

Answer 1. Wire loop is commoner. Go on to **10.12**.
2. Membranous change is commoner. Go on to **10.10**.

10.16 Your answer – IgG is present in the proteinuria of SLE.

Good. The nephrotic syndrome in SLE differs from that caused by other conditions in the frequent occurrence of a low or normal serum cholesterol level as opposed to the high serum cholesterol of the usual nephrotic syndrome. This low cholesterol group has been termed 'pseudo-nephrotic' syndrome, although a better term would be 'biochemical variant of the nephrotic syndrome'. In the original Chicago series of Muehrcke and his colleagues, this group of patients only survived a few months and had a worse prognosis than the group with SLE nephrotic syndrome and a high cholesterol. Soffer on the other hand, found that if anything the prognosis was no better in those with a high serum cholesterol than in the 'pseudonephrotic' group. The speed of deterioration of SLE nephritis is variable; sometimes there is rapid progression through a nephrotic phase to renal failure in a few months. Other patients have persistent proteinuria for years with no deterioration. Some patients lose all evidence of renal disease when given corticosteroids. It is impossible to determine the likely course of any given case on a single clinical examination early in the course of the disease, but renal biopsy may help: lupus glomerulonephritis with interstitial involvement, necrosis, crescents and widespread basement membrane changes is indicative of a bad prognosis although there is some evidence that large doses of prednisone and Imuran may prolong life and even prevent deterioration.

Now answer the question.

Question In Muehrcke's series, pseudo-nephrotic syndrome was associated with a bad prognosis. What is the serum cholesterol level which distinguishes this group from the other SLE nephrotic patients?

Answer 1. High. Go on to **10.18**.
        2. Low or normal. Go on to **10.20**.

10.17 Your answer – 'telescoped' urine sediment is pathognomonic of SLE.

You are incorrect. It indicates a glomerulitis and is not solely found in SLE. Read **10.8** again before answering the question again.

10.18 Your answer – serum cholesterol level in the pseudo-nephrotic group is high.

No. This group has a normal or low serum cholesterol in contrast to the usual finding in nephrotic syndrome of a high serum cholesterol. Read **10.16** before answering the question again.

10.19 Your answer – 'telescoped' urine deposit is *not* pathognomonic of SLE.

Good. Now answer the next question.

Question Is IgG as well as albumin present in considerable amounts in the urine of patients with renal involvement of SLE?

Answer 1. Yes. Go on to **10.16**.
        2. No. Go on to **10.21**.

10.20 Your answer – serum cholesterol level is low or normal in pseudo-nephrotic lupus nephrotic syndrome.

Correct. Now answer the next question.

Question Is the prognosis bad in lupus glomerulo*nephritis* with interstitial involvement?

Answer 1. Yes. Go on to **10.24**.
        2. No. Go on to **10.26**.

10.21 Your answer – IgG is *not* present in large amounts as well as albumin in the urine.

No. IgG is present in large amounts in the proteinuria of SLE. The glomeruli are not only permeable to the IgG molecule but there is often an elevated IgG serum level which will increase the γ globulinuria. Now answer the question in **10.19** again.

10.22 Your answer – prednisone therapy *is* indicated in lupus glomerulonephritis.

Good. The next type of collagen disease to be considered is polyarteritis nodosa. In this disease there is a panarteritis involving all the coats of the medium or small sized arteries: the disease affects many organs including the kidneys, which are involved in 3 out of 4 patients with polyarteritis nodosa. The first type of polyarteritis of the kidneys is a major vessel arteritis in which the arcuate vessels are frequently affected by a panarteritis, resulting in thrombosis and occlusion of the vessel lumen by thrombus, and infarction of the territory supplied by the occluded vessel; the infarcts in the cortex of the kidney ultimately atrophy leading to a series of irregular depressions on the surface of the kidneys.

Question How does panarteritis of the arcuate arteries lead to infarction of areas of the cortex?

Answer 1. Swelling of the intima occluding the vessel. Go on to **10.27**.
2. Thrombosis of the vessel lumen. Go on to **10.23**.

10.23 Your answer – thrombosis of the vessel lumen causes the infarction.

Good. The second type of renal polyarteritis is the so-called 'microscopic form,' in which there is a glomerulitis similar to that in acute glomerulonephritis (see Fig. 10.23a) with proliferation of the glomerular tuft, infarction of the glomeruli, panarteritis of the *small* vessels, and crescent formation (Fig. 10.23b).

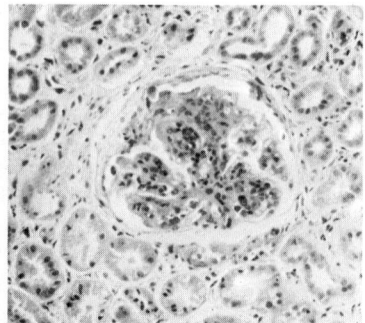
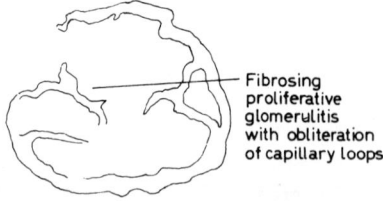

Fibrosing proliferative glomerulitis with obliteration of capillary loops

Fig. 10.23a

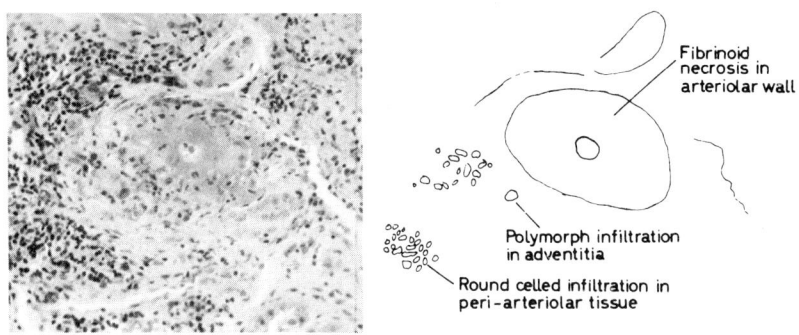

Fig. 10.23b

There are few lesions outside the kidneys although a careful search will reveal panarteritis in the small vessels of the spleen, adrenal, and pancreas. Unfortunately, the histological differentiation of this lesion from that of acute glomerulonephritis is difficult; panarteritis can occur in the small renal vessels in acute glomerulonephritis so that there is no absolute method of differentiation between acute glomerulonephritis and the 'microscopic form' of polyarteritis on renal biopsy examination.

Question What form of renal disease is histologically similar to the 'microscopic form' of polyarteritis nodosa?

Answer 1. Acute glomerulonephritis. Go on to **10.29**.
 2. Acute pyelonephritis. Go on to **10.31**.
 3. Don't know. Go on to **10.33**.

10.24 Your answer — lupus glomerulonephritis has a bad prognosis.

Correct. The treatment of lupus nephritis is far from agreed upon. The only useful therapy for lupus nephritis is corticosteroid therapy, usually prednisone, and immunosuppressive drugs such as azathioprine. Some authorities (e.g. the Kark group) advocate high prednisone dosage (40–60 mg/day) in *all* patients with lupus glomerulonephritis and lupus glomerulitis, suggesting from their experience initially that lupus glomerulitis could be prevented from progressing into lupus glomerulo*nephritis* and could increase the length of survival in lupus glomerulonephritis. Further work on this problem has not confirmed this initial suggestion. Some patients with lupus glomerulitis do not progress to lupus glomerulo*nephritis* in spite of the absence of prednisone therapy, but undeniably some do progress and it is probably wiser to maintain patients on high steroid dosage if there is glomerulonephritis. If there is only glomerulitis then smaller doses suffice.

Question Is prednisone therapy indicated in patients with lupus glomerulonephritis?

Answer 1. Yes. Go on to **10.22**.
2. No. Go on to **10.25**.

10.25 Your answer – prednisone therapy is *not* indicated in lupus glomerulonephritis.

No. There is some evidence that the only effective therapy for lupus nephritis of all types is the corticosteroid group of drugs possibly combined with Imuran or other immuno-suppresive drugs. Read **10.24** again.

10.26 Your answer – the prognosis is good in lupus glomerulo*nephritis*.

No. Lupus glomerulonephritis has a relatively bad prognosis, worse than focal lupus glomerulitis without interstitial involvement. Read **10.16** again before answering the question in **10.20** correctly.

10.27 Your answer – swelling of the intima causes the infarction.

No. You are correct in that all the coats of the arteries are involved in polyarteritis, but the lumen of a medium sized vessel is too large to be occluded by the intimal inflammatory swelling alone. Inflammation of the intima is associated with thrombosis in the vessel when the endothelial lining is involved. Now answer the question in **10.22** after reading the paragraph again.

10.28 Your answer – leucocytosis supports a diagnosis of polyarteritis nodosa.

Correct. The renal manifestations of polyarteritis nodosa are of several different types:

(1) An acute glomerulonephritic type with oliguria, haematuria, hypertension, raised blood urea, and 'telescoped' urine sediment. Sometimes the oliguria progresses to total anuria, from which there is little chance of survival.

(2) A chronic phase with proteinuria which may persist for years with or without hypertension; this proteinuria may become so great that it leads to:

(3) A nephrotic picture with massive proteinuria.

(4) Chronic renal failure may develop, not always associated with hypertension.

Question What is the prognosis in the anuria of renal polyarteritis?

Answer 1. Bad. Go on to **10.30**.
2. Good. Go on to **10.35**.

10.29 Your answer – acute glomerulonephritis is similar to the microscopic form of polyarteritis nodosa.

Good. The non-renal symptoms of polyarteritis nodosa include polyarthritis (often diagnosed as rheumatoid arthritis), an asymmetrical polyneuritis, pyrexia, hepatosplenomegaly, skin rashes with infarction of the skin, pulmonary lesions with cavitation, asthma, and eosinophilia. The sheep cell agglutination test (Rose-Waaler Test) is positive in 5 per cent of patients with polyarteritis. There is usually a leucocytosis and often an eosinophilia. The pulmonary form of polyarteritis is more frequently associated with an eosinophilia and the nasal, granulomas of Wegener's syndrome. A renal biopsy in a patient with Wegener's syndrome is shown in Fig. 10.29.

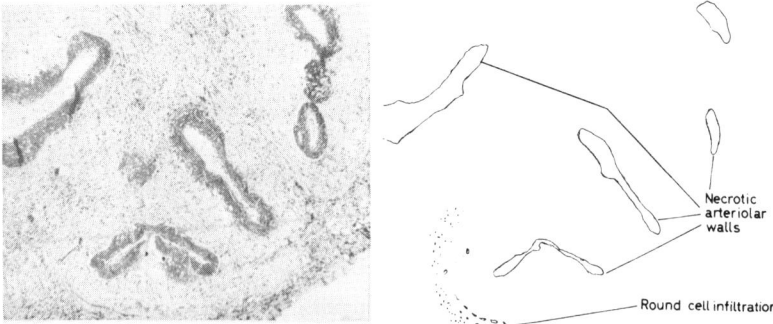

Fig. 10.29

Question In a patient with polyarthritis and a polyneuritis in whom there is hepatosplenomegaly, would a leucocytosis support or oppose a diagnosis of polyarteritis nodosa?

Answer 1. Support. Go on to **10.28**.
        2. Oppose. Go on to **10.32**.

10.30 Your answer – the prognosis is bad in anuric renal polyarteritis.
Correct. Now answer the next question.

Question If the proteinuria in the chronic phase of polyarteritis becomes massive, what clinical syndrome may result?

Answer 1. Nephrotic syndrome. Go on to **10.34**.
        2. Chronic renal failure. Go on to **10.36**.
        3. Don't know. Go on to **10.38**.

10.31 Your answer – acute pyelonephritis is histologically similar to the microscopic form of polyarteritis.

No. There is little similarity — in acute pyelonephritis there is a predominantly neutrophil polymorph infiltration with microabscess formation. The lesion in polyarteritis is quite different. Read **10.23** again and answer the question correctly.

10.32 Your answer — the presence of leucocytosis reduces the likelihood of a diagnosis of polyarteritis being correct.

No. Leucocytosis is the rule in polyarteritis. Read **10.29** again. It contains many facts about the non-renal aspects of polyarteritis nodosa. Then answer the question again.

10.33 Your answer — I don't know what renal disease is histologically similar to the microscopic form of polyarteritis nodosa.

Acute glomerulonephritis is remarkably similar histologically to this form of polyarteritis. Read **10.23** carefully then answer the question.

10.34 Your answer — massive proteinuria leads to the development of the nephrotic syndrome.

You are correct. Nephrotic syndrome is a rare manifestation of polyarteritis, but it does occur occasionally. The prognosis of polyarteritis nodosa is poor once renal involvement has occurred, and if glomerular involvement has progressed to anuria there is no chance of recovery. The treatment of the patient with non-anuric renal polyarteritis nodosa is with large doses of prednisone, 100 mg a day initially. This is particularly effective in medium vessel polyarteritis nodosa, with suppression of the arteritis the former presence of which can be detected histologically by the breaks in the elastic lamina of the arteries where the healed arteritic lesions were present. Immunosuppressive drugs such as azathioprine and cyclophosphamide should also be used.

Question What dose of Prednisone would you give in nephrotic syndrome caused by polyarteritis nodosa?

Answer 1. 100 mg a day. Go on to **10.37**.
          2. 300 mg a day. Go on to **10.40**.
          3. Don't know. Go on to **10.42**.

10.35 Your answer — the prognosis of anuria in renal polyarteritis is good.

No. The chance of survival from anuric renal polyarteritis is very small. Read **10.28** again and answer the question correctly.

10.36 Your answer – massive proteinuria leads to chronic renal failure.

You are correct in so far as renal failure ultimately develops, but the clinical syndrome produced by massive proteinuria is hypoproteinaemia, hypercholesterolaemia, and oedema. This is, as you know, nephrotic syndrome in itself: - now read **10.28** again and choose the correct answer to the question in **10.30** this time.

10.37 Your answer – the dose of prednisone initially is 100 mg a day.

Good. The next collagen disease to be discussed is systemic sclerosis. This usually is complicated by renal involvement as a terminal event in a patient with long-standing systemic sclerosis. The pathological features of renal involvement in systemic sclerosis are striking.

The salient histological features are multiple reduplications of the elastic tissue in the arteriolar wall, an appearance similar to that in malignant hypertension. The appearance of the arterioles on an haematoxylin and eosin stained section is one of a mucinous infiltration of the thickened arteriolar wall.

Now answer the question.

Question What is the appearance of the elastica in the renal arterioles in renal involvement in systemic sclerosis?

Answer 1. Reduplicated. Go on to **10.39**.
2. Necrotic. Go on to **10.41**.

10.38 Your answer – I don't know what massive proteinuria in PN causes clinically.

If the proteinuria is so large as to result in loss of massive quantities of protein, it may exceed the capacity of the liver; to synthesize albumin and to maintain a normal serum albumin concentration; the serum albumin level falls and hypoproteinaemic oedema results; serum cholesterol rising pari passu with the fall in serum albumin. This corresponds to the picture of the nephrotic syndrome, a rare manifestation of polyarteritis nodosa. Now read **10.28** again before choosing the correct answer to the question in **10.30**.

10.39 Your answer – the elastica of the renal arterioles is reduplicated in systemic sclerosis.

You are correct. The clinical picture is one of sudden onset of oliguria rapidly becoming total anuria in the course of a few days. Hypertension is not usually present until the last few days of life. There is no recorded case of spontaneous recovery from the anuria of systemic sclerosis, death occuring when dialysis is discontinued.

Question What is the prognosis if anuria develops in a patient suffering from systemic sclerosis?

Answer 1. Bad. Go on to **10.44**.
         2. Good. Go on to **10.46**.
         3. Don't know. Go on to **10.48**.

10.40 Your answer – the dose of prednisone is 30 mg/day in nephrotic syndrome due to polyarteritis nodosa.

You are not correct. The dose of prednisone used in polyarteritis nodosa should be very large so as to suppress the arteritis rapidly and reduce the chance of further renal damage occurring. Read **10.34** carefully once more and then answer the question correctly.

10.41 Your answer – the appearance of the elastica of renal arterioles in systemic sclerosis is necrotic.

No. The appearance of the elastica is quite striking in this disease and it is not necrotic. There is a reduplication of the elastica similar to that in severe hypertension. Pay more attention to the text of **10.37**, which you should read again before choosing the correct answer to the question.

10.42 Your answer – I don't know the dose of prednisone in nephrotic syndrome due to renal polyarteritis.

The purpose of giving prednisone in polyarteritis nodosa is to suppress the disease in the shortest possible time before the arteritis has damaged further vessels. This requires large doses of prednisone, even larger than are needed in nephrotic syndrome without 'light microscopical change' so that 100 mg of prednisone are given daily until all the signs of activity are suppressed and *then* the dose is gradually reduced. Now choose the correct answer to **10.34**.

10.43 Your answer – proteinuria is frequent in thrombotic thrombocytopenic purpura.

Good. The histological picture of thrombotic thrombocytopenic purpura is one of widespread occlusion of the small vessels by an amorphous eosinophilic material derived from fibrin or fibrinogen, not from platelets as was at first thought. This histological change is present in the glomerular arterioles as well as in the capillary loops.

Question What is the origin of the amorphous oesinophilic material which occludes arterioles and capillaries in thrombotic thrombocytopenic purpura?

Answer 1. Platelets. Go on to **10.47**.
         2. Fibrin or fibrinogen. Go on to **10.50**.

10.44 Your answer – the prognosis is bad.

Correct. In many patients with systemic sclerosis however, proteinuria is present for years and the severe anuric form may never develop. We shall now proceed to consider thrombotic thrombocytopenic purpura. This is a rare disease of unknown aetiology which is associated with a clinical picture of pyrexia, thrombocytopenia, jaundice, and central nervous system signs. In the majority of patients with this disease there is proteinuria, which may be occasionally massive and give rise to nephrotic syndrome. The blood urea is elevated in about three quarters of the patients.

Question Is proteinuria frequent or infrequent in thrombotic thrombocytopenic purpura?

Answer 1. Frequent. Go on to **10.43**.
2. Infrequent. Go on to **10.45**.

10.45 Your answer – proteinuria is infrequent in thrombotic thrombocytopenic purpura.

No. Proteinuria is found in the majority of patients with thrombotic thrombocytopenic purpura. You should read **10.44** again, more carefully this time, and then answer the question again.

10.46 Your answer – the prognosis is good.

You are wrong. The patient always dies within a few days and renal recovery does not take place. Read **10.39** more carefully before you answer the question again.

10.47 Your answer – the amorphous masses are derived from platelets.

No. They are immunologically identifiable as fibrinogen or fibrin, not platelets. Read **10.43** again before you answer the question again.

10.48 Your answer – I don't know the prognosis of the anuria of scleroderma.

The prognosis of this type of disease is uniformly fatal in a few days, unless the patient is dialysed. The disease is a contraindication to chronic haemodialysis. Now read **10.39** again and pay careful attention to the text before you answer the question.

10.49 Your answer – microscopic haematuria is common in this disease.

Correct. The clinical course is similar to acute, subacute, or chronic glomerulonephritis, the latter occasionally having a nephrotic phase. Histologically at biopsy there is usually a focal glomerulonephritis (look at Fig. 10.49a). At necropsy in the patients dying of renal failure all the glomeruli are uniformly affected by changes identical to those found in subacute and chronic glomerulonephritis (Fig. 10.49b). Immunofluorescent staining shows deposition of IgA, IgG, complement and fibrin in the glomeruli.

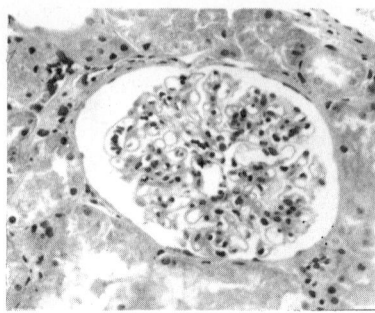
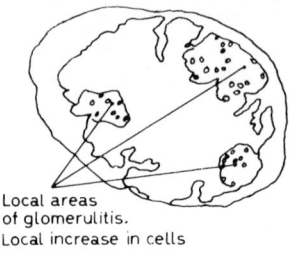

Fig. 10.49a

Question At necropsy is there any difference between the renal histological findings in a patient dying of chronic or subacute glomerulonephritis and those in a patient dying of Henoch-Schönlein syndrome with renal failure?

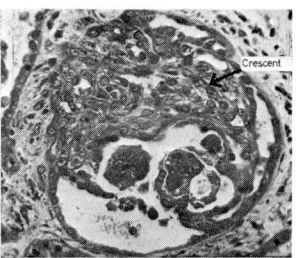

Fig. 10.49b

Answer 1. Yes. Go on to **10.53**.
2. No. Go on to **10.55**.

10.50 Your answer – the amorphous masses are derived from fibrinogen or fibrin.

Good. In the plasma there are fibrin degradation products. There is a low platelet count, the platelets having been consumed by the widespread (disseminated) intravascular clotting. The therapy for thrombotic thrombocytopenic purpura is corticosteroids such as prednisone, in high dosage. Not enough data are available to assess the effectiveness of this therapy in the renal failure of thrombotic thrombocytopenic purpura. Let us now discuss the syndrome of nephritis and anaphylactoid purpura, or Henoch-Schönlein syndrome. In this condition, commonest in children but also frequent in young adults, the clinical features are polyarthritis, abdominal pain, melaena and a purpuric rash. The aetiology is uncertain but may be related to a prior streptococcal infection in some. In almost all patients with this disease haematuria is present either macroscopical- or microscopically, and death may result within one or two years from renal failure. The prognosis in adults is generally worse than in children. There are many patients who recover completely from Henoch-Schönlein nephritis.

Question Is microscopic haematuria common in Henoch-Schönlein purpura?

Answer 1. Yes. Go on to **10.49**.
2. No. Go on to **10.51**.

10.51 Your answer – microscopic haematuria is *not* common in Henoch-Schönlein purpura.
No. Microscopic haematuria is very frequent in this syndrome. Read **10.50** again.

10.52 Your answer – anticoagulants *are* of benefit in haemolytic-uraemic syndrome.
Correct. You are now about to answer the paragraph testing your knowledge of Chapter 10. Choose your answers carefully.

Statement 1 In systemic lupus erythematosus, IgG is bound to the glomerular basement membrane.

Statement 2 The prognosis in the totally anuric patient with polyarteritis nodosa is good.

Statement 3 The prognosis of the anuria of systemic sclerosis is very bad.

Answer 1. Statement 1 is true, 2 and 3 false. Go on to **10.54**.
2. Statement 2 is true, 1 and 3 false. Go on to **10.56**.
3. Statement 3 is true, 1 and 2 false. Go on to **10.58**.
4. All the statements are false. Go on to **10.59**.
5. All the statements are true. Go on to **10.60**.
6. Statements 1 and 2 are true, 3 false. Go on to **10.61**.
7. Statements 1 and 3 are true, 2 false. Go on to **10.62**.
8. Statements 2 and 3 are true, 1 false. Go on to **10.63**.

10.53 Your answer – there is a difference between the histological changes in Henoch-Schönlein chronic or subacute nephritis and those in chronic or subacute glomerulonephritis.
No. There is no easy histological differentiation between them. Read **10.49** again and then answer the question correctly.

10.54 Your answer – 1 is true, 2 and 3 are false.
You are partially correct, but wrong in that 3 is true. Go back to **10.39** and read on from there.

10.55 Your answer — there is no histological differentiation between the two conditions at necropsy.

Correct. Treatment is purely symptomatic in patients with Henoch-Schönlein nephritis, and in our experience prednisone therapy has not materially altered the nephritis clinically or histologically. There is no certain way of differentiating between the patients who will develop a fatal subacute or chronic Henoch-Schönlein nephritis, and those who will develop a mild self-limiting focal glomerulitis.

Question Is the Henoch-Schönlein *nephritis* suppressed by prednisone therapy?

Answer 1. Yes. Go on to **10.57**.
2. No. Go on to **10.64**.

10.56 Your answer — 2 is true, 1 and 3 are false.

You are quite wrong. Start at **10.12** and work on through the chapter.

10.57 Your answer — Henoch-Schönlein nephritis is suppressed by steroid therapy.

You are not correct. In our experience steroid therapy makes little difference to the ultimate course of the nephritis in this disease. Read **10.55** again before answering the question.

10.58 Your answer — 3 is true, 1 and 2 are false.

You are partly correct, but 1 is also true; read from **10.12** to **10.27** inclusive, then answer the question in **10.52** again.

10.59 Your answer — all the statements are false.

No. Only 2 is false. Start at **10.12**, read from there up to **10.28** then from **10.39** onwards.

10.60 Your answer — all the statements are true.

You are partly correct, but 2 is not true. Read from **10.28** to **10.39**, then answer the question in **10.52** correctly.

10.61 Your answer — 1 and 2 are true, 3 is false.

You are correct about 1 only. Read on from **10.28** to the end of the chapter.

10.62 Your answer — 1 and 3 are true, 2 is false.

Correct. You can now start the next chapter.

For further reading the following references are suggested:

SLE
Muehreke R. C. et al. (1957) Medicine **36**, 1.
Pollak et al. (1961) Bull. rheumat. Dis. **11**, 249.

Pollak et al. (1964) J. lab. clin. Med. **63**, 537.
Simenoff M. L. & Merrill J. P. (1964) Nephron **1**, 348.
Gotoff S. P. et al. (1969). Annals Int. Med. **71**, 327.

Polyarteritis nodosa
Rose G. A. & Spencer H. (1957) Quart. J. Med. **26**, 43.
Davson et al. (1948) Quart. J. Med. **17**, 175.
Henoch-Schönlein syndrome; White et al. Quart. J. Med. 1972.

Systemic sclerosis
Moore H. C. & Sheehan H. O. (1952) Lancet **1**, 68.

Haemolytic-uraemic syndrome; leading article in New. Eng. J. Med. 1969 **281**, 1072.

Clarkson, A. R. et al. 1970. Quart J. Med. **39**, 227.

A general review of collagen diseases and the kidney is the chapter by Berlyne G. M. (chapter 20) in Renal Disease, edited by D. A. K. Black, published by Blackwell, Oxford, 1972, third edition.

10.63 Your answer – 2 and 3 are true, 1 is false.

You are wrong about 1 and 2. Read from the beginning of the chapter to **10.39**, then answer the question again.

10.64 Your answer – Henoch-Schönlein nephritis is not suppressed by corticosteroid therapy.

Correct. In rheumatoid arthritis (RA) proteinuria may be found. This is associated with several different causes:

1. A specific rheumatoid focal glomerulitis, the natural history of which is disputed and is predominantly unknown.
2. Amyloid disease. This is found often in rheumatoid arthritis at necropsy.
3. Gold induced nephritis due to the therapeutic administration of gold salts.
4. Pyelonephritis and papillary necrosis, partly due to the reduced resistance to bacterial infection in RA caused by an abnormal immune response to infection and, more frequently, also caused by the ingestion of large quantities of phenacetin in the form of analgesics. Phenacetin nephropathy is discussed in Chapter 20. (Drugs and the Kidney).
5. Lupus nephritis may be present coexistent with rheumatoid arthritis.

Question Is amyloid disease of the kidneys ever associated with rheumatoid arthritis?

Answer 1. No. Go on to **10.66**.
2. Yes. Go on to **10.68**.

10.65 Your answer – thrombocytopenia and bleeding are common.
Correct. The treatment of this disease depends on an understanding of the pathogenesis. It is suggested that the primary abnormality is a microangiopathy, in which the small blood vessels lose portions of their normally smooth endothelium. The red cells become damaged by contact with the roughened intimal surface, and are rapidly destroyed. The red cell damage is recognised by the abnormal irregularly-shaped red cells, termed 'burr cells.' In the areas of endothelial damage platelets adhere in such large quantities that thrombocytopenia develops. Due to the areas of local clotting in the arterioles fibrin emboli are formed which may occlude the glomerular capillaries and may be responsible for the anuria. The haemoglobin liberated from the red cells is another factor responsible for the development of anuria.

Question What is responsible for the damage to red cells in haemolytic-uraemia syndrome?

Answer 1. damaged intima. Go on to **10.69**.
2. uraemia. Go on to **10.70**.

10.66 Your answer – Amyloid disease is not caused by rheumatoid arthritis.
No. Amyloid disease is a renal complication of rheumatoid arthritis. You have not read **10.64** with sufficient care. Go back over it again more carefully before you answer the question.

10.67 Your answer – thrombocytopenia and bleeding are rare.
No. Bleeding complications are quite common, due to thrombocytopenia. Read **10.68** again.

10.68 Your answer – Amyloid disease is found often in rheumatoid arthritis. You are correct.
There is a syndrome known as the 'haemolytic-uraemic syndrome' which is rare, and mainly affects infants and children. It is of unknown aetiology in the majority of cases, but some are linked to preceding infections with haemolytic streptococci. Some evidence implicates a viral aetiology for the disease, including Cox-Sackie, Portillovirus and a rickettsial-like agent. The features of the disease are as follows: a severe haemolytic anaemia associated with a rapidly progressive acute renal failure, occuring after or during an infection with pyrexia, vomiting and diarrhoea. There is usually a severe thrombocytopenia with bleeding from the gastrointestinal tract and skin. There is a haemolytic jaundice with severe anaemia. The disease is fatal in the majority of cases. This disease is an example of a microangiopathy with excessive coagulation occurring in the circulation and obstructing the glomerular capillaries with fibrin and fibrin-degradation products. The consumption coagulopathy is responsible for the thrombocytopenia and bleeding.

Question In haemolytic-uraemic syndrome are thrombocytopenia and bleeding common or rare?

Answer 1. Common. Go on to **10.65**.
2. Rare. Go on to **10.67**.

10.69 Your answer – the damage to red cells is caused by a damaged intima.
Correct – treatment of the syndrome is divided into 2 parts
1. Dialysis and transfusion, to maintain life
2. Corticosteroid therapy and anticoagulation with heparin to prevent the damage to the endothelium; and reduce platelet adhesion in the afferent arterioles and plugging of the glomeruli with fibrin plugs. The use of anticoagulants in thrombocytopenic uraemic patients requires considerable courage, but is probably worth it, although the occasional patient has made a spontaneous recovery without the use of anticoagulants.

Question Are anticoagulants of any benefit in haemolytic-uraemic syndrome?

Answer 1. Yes. Go on to **10.52**.
2. No. Go on to **10.71**.

10.70 Your answer – the damage to red cells is caused by uraemia.

No. Uraemia is associated with a reduced life of the red cells, but this is not thought to be responsible for the massive haemolysis of 'haemolytic-uraemic syndrome.' It is more likely that a microangiopathy with discontinuity of the endothelium is responsible. Read **10.65** again, carefully this time.

10.71 Your answer – anticoagulants are of no benefit in haemolytic uraemic syndrome.

You are wrong. Anticoagulants prevent further loss of platelets in the clotting process on the damaged intima, and paradoxically reduce the bleeding tendency which is a prominent feature of the disease. Read **10.69** again so that you can answer the question correctly.

Time for this chapter: 20 minutes

Chapter 11
Diabetes mellitus and the kidney

11.1 Diabetes mellitus affects the kidney in many ways: such as glomerulosclerosis of specifically diabetic type, pyelonephritis and necrotising papillitis. Degenerative arterial disease of the kidneys is also very common in diabetes, but it will not be further considered here. First let us consider the pathology of renal diabetes mellitus. Glomerulosclerosis of diabetes is very common, being present in all patients who have had diabetes for ten or more years, as well as in many diabetics who have recently been diagnosed. In some who are in the 'prediabetic' stage there are changes of diabetic glomerulosclerosis. *All* the glomeruli are uniformly involved in diffuse diabetic glomerulosclerosis. Look at Fig. 11.1.

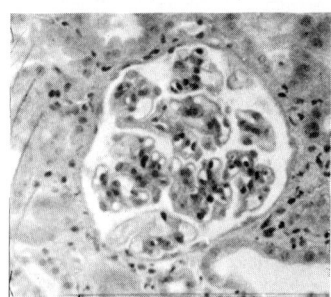
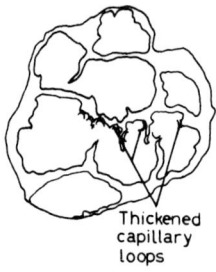

Fig. 11.1

The changes seen are a *diffuse* thickening of the glomerular capillary walls by a material staining with Periodic Acid Schiff stain, (PAS) i.e., a mucopolysaccharide is infiltrating the capillary walls. The aetiology and pathogenesis of diabetic glomerusclerosis are unknown. However, in giunea pigs sensitised to bovine insulin there is an increase in mesangial cells and mesangial proliferation. If the results can be extrapolated to man it suggests that insulin antibodies may play a part in the aetiology of the condition.

Question Does diabetic glomerulosclerosis uniformly affect all the glomeruli in the kidney or is a patchy change?

Answer 1. All the glomeruli are affected. Go on to **11.3**.
        2. The change is patchy. Go on to **11.5**.

11.2 Your answer – the nodule arises in the capillary wall.

Good. The clinical aspects of *diffuse* diabetic glomerulosclerosis and *nodular* glomerulosclerosis are difficult to differentiate from each other which is hardly surprising because all kidneys with the nodular lesion have the diffuse lesion throughout all the glomeruli as well, although not all kidneys with diffuse diabetic glomerulosclerosis have the nodular form as well. Read this last sentence again to make sure you have understood it. The majority of young diabetics have diffuse diabetic glomerulosclerosis, but few have any abnormality on clinical urine testing or renal function studies in the early stages. Very careful laboratory testing of diabetic urine has shown the earliest abnormality to be a slight increase in the quantity of proteinuria. At this stage light microscopy is normal but electron microscopy shows definite changes, with thickening of the basement membrane and deposition of electron-dense material close to or inside the endothelial cells. This ultimately encroaches on the lumen of the capillary and finally merges with other such capillary-occluding masses to form a nodule. Clinically detectable proteinuria occurs when the lesion has progressed; Gelman and his colleagues in Chicago showed a correlation between the extent of the proteinuria and the histological severity of the diffuse diabetic glomerulosclerosis. Now answer the question.

Question In a diabetic patient with mild and early diabetic glomerulosclerosis on renal biopsy, would you be surprised if little or no protein was present in the urine?

Answer 1. Yes. Go on to **11.7**.
2. No. Go on to **11.9**.
3. Don't know. Go on to **11.11**.

11.3 Your answer – the change is a uniform one affecting all the glomeruli.

Good. In some patients the Kimmelstiel-Wilson lesion is seen; this is known as nodular glomerulosclerosis, and appears to arise from one of the thickened walls of one of the capillary loops; the nodule stains positive with PAS and is probably mucopolysaccharide in nature. Gradually the nodule grows, encroaches on and crushes the other capillaries and finally makes the affected glomerulus into an ischaemic nodule in which the nuclei of the capillary loops can be seen, the nuclei embedded in the nodule wall.

The nodular lesion has two predominantly exudative types of lesion which are quite characteristic of diabetes. These are the *capsular drop* and the *fibrin cap*. The capsular drop is a droplet which is in the parietal layer of Bowman's capsule. It stains intensely eosinophilic with haematoxylin and eosin. 'Fibrin cap' is a lesion of intensely eosinophilic character on staining with haematoxylin and eosin which forms a 'cap' to the nodules of nodular glomerusclerosis. Both fibrin cap and capsular drop, can be shown by appropriate stains, to contain fibrin or other plasma proteins. Similarly the hyaline afferent arteriolar change so common in diabetes is associated with the staining reaction of fibrin or proteins infiltrating the arteriolar wall. Look at Fig. 11.3 a and b.

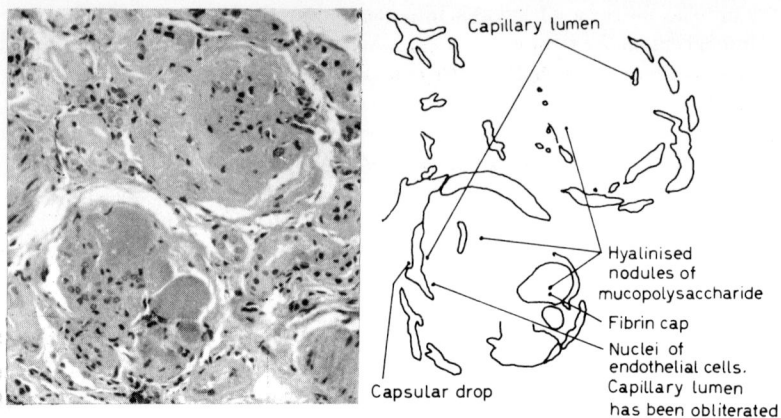

Fig. 11.3a

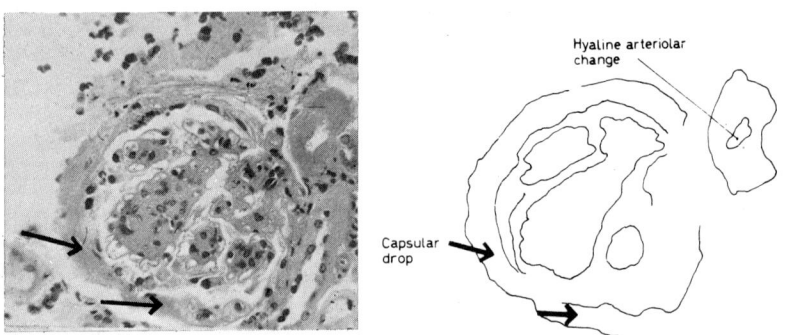

Fig. 11.3b

Now answer the question.

Question Where does the nodule of nodular glomerulosclerosis start?

Answer 1. In the capillary walls in the glomerulus. Go on to **11.2**.
2. In the glomerulus. Go on to **11.4**.

11.4 Your answer – the nodule arises in the glomerulus.

You are correct in so far as you give the answer, but it is not detailed enough. Read **11.3** again and then choose the correct answer.

11.5 Your answer – the change is patchy.

No. The change in diabetic glomerulosclerosis is diffuse and affects all the glomeruli uniformly. Read **11.1** again and look at Fig. 11.1 before answering the question again.

11.6 Your answer – both nodular and diffuse diabetic glomerulosclerosis are likely to be present.

Good. Early in diabetic glomerulosclerosis it is found that the glomerular capillaries appear dilated, and the GFR is increased due to increased filtration pressure. The patient with nephrotic syndrome due to diabetic nodular glomerulosclerosis will survive on the average for about three years, although some may survive for as long as ten years, and are often remarkably free from episodes of ketosis although this does not apply to *all* patients. Many patients never have proteinuria massive enough to cause hypoproteinaemic oedema i.e., nephrotic syndrome. They progress slowly and insidiously into chronic renal failure and hypertension, which is also the end stage of those who pass through the nephrotic stage. There is no known method of preventing of retarding the development of diabetic glomerulosclerosis, diffuse or nodular. The statement that adequate diabetic control will prevent or delay the onset of diabetic glomerulosclerosis is more partisan and optimistic than adequately proven.

Question Do all patients with diabetic glomerulosclerosis develop nephrotic syndrome?

Answer 1. Yes. Go on to **11.10**.
2. No. Go on to **11.12**.

11.7 Your answer – I would be surprised if little or no protein appeared in the urine in early diabetic glomerulosclerosis.

You are wrong, for the early cases often have no abnormality on clinical testing of renal function. Read **11.2** again and answer the question.

11.8 Your answer – you are not likely to find nodular and diffuse glomerulosclerosis in diabetic nephrotic syndrome.

No. Diabetics who have developed such a heavy proteinuria that nephrotic syndrome results, commonly have both nodular and diffuse diabetic glomerulosclerosis. Bear in mind that diffuse diabetic glomerulosclerosis is *always* present in the kidneys of patients with nodular glomerulosclerosis, but that nodular glomerulosclerosis is *not* constantly present in the kidneys of patients who have diffuse glomerulosclerosis. Now read **11.9** again and answer the question.

11.9 Your answer – I would not be surprised to see little or no proteinuria in early mild diffuse glomerulosclerosis.

Good. You are correct.

As the histological severity increases, the proteinuria becomes more and more severe, leading ultimately to hypoproteinaemia, hypercholesterolaemia and peripheral oedema, i.e., the nephrotic syndrome develops. The majority of diabetics who have nephrotic syndrome have diabetic nodular lesions as well as diffuse glomerulosclerosis. The nodular lesions were described in 1936 by Paul Kimmelstiel and Clifford Wilson hence the term Kimmelstiel-Wilson syndrome for the pathological picture of diabetic nodular glomerulosclerosis associated with nephrotic syndrome.

Question In a patient with diabetes who develops nephrotic syndrome, are you likely to find nodular glomerulosclerosis as well as diffuse glomerulosclerosis on biopsy of the kidney?

Answer 1. Yes. Go on to **11.6**.
2. No. Go on to **11.8**.

11.10 Your answer – all diabetics with glomerulosclerosis develop nephrotic syndrome.

No. Nearly all diabetics of long standing have diffuse diabetic glomerulosclerosis, but only a minority develop proteinuria severe enough to cause nephrotic syndrome. Read **11.6** again and answer the question correctly.

11.11 Your answer – I don't know if little or no protein is found in the urine in mild early diffuse glomerulosclerosis would surprise me.

There is a correlation between the histological severity of the glomerular lesion and the proteinuria in diabetic glomerulosclerosis. Early lesions are often associated with no proteinuria. Read **11.2** again in case you have missed other facts before going on to answer the question again.

11.12 Your answer – all patients with diabetic glomerulosclerosis do not develop nephrotic syndrome.

Correct. The treatment of diabetic glomerulosclerosis is purely symptomatic, that is: to keep the patient free of oedema, control hypertension and stabilise the diabetes. When chronic renal failure supervenes it is then well worth while to employ the symptomatic treatment described in the chapter on Chronic Renal Failure (Chapter 10).

Diabetics are more susceptible to infections of the genito-urinary tract than non-diabetics, and pyelonephritis is consequently a very common complication of diabetes mellitus, particularly in those patients who have been subjected to catheterisation and instrumentation. Catheterisation is often performed in diabetic ketosis to obtain a specimen of urine; it cannot be over-stated that diabetic patients should *not* be catheterised if it can be avoided; a blood sugar level is more useful than urinary sugar concentration in the diagnosis and control of diabetic ketotic coma, and acetone of the degree found in diabetic ketosis can be readily, accurately and rapidly detected in the patient's breath by the physician's nose. To leave an indwelling catheter in the bladder of a diabetic patient is courting disaster in the form of pyelonephritis and necrotising papillitis. Now answer the question.

Question Would you ever catheterise a diabetic if there were an alternative?

Answer 1. Yes. Go on to **11.13**.
   2. No. Go on to **11.15**.

11.13 Your Answer – I would catheterise a diabetic.

You are quite wrong. Catheterisation increases the chances of urinary tract infection, which diabetics readily develop. Read **11.12** again, answering the question correctly.

11.14 Your answer – urinary tract infection may be asymptomatic in the diabetic.

Your are correct. Diabetics are particularly liable to develop necrotising papillitis, in which there is a severe pyelonephritis with ischaemic necrosis of the papillae due to thrombotic occlusion of the medullary blood vessels involved by the infection. The symptoms are those of a rapidly progressing renal failure, often with evidence of urinary tract infection in the form of dysuria, frequency, and pyrexia; the hallmark of the disease and the absolutely diagnostic feature is the passage of the necrotic papillae in the urine, which should be strained through cheese-cloth to locate the papillary fragments. I.V.P. shows typical ring shadows of papillary necrosis. Retrograde pyelography demonstrates the loss of papillary tips. The occasional patient is asymptomatic until he becomes anuric, when one kidney is already functionless and a necrotic papilla blocks the ureter draining the sole functioning kidney. Vigorous antibiotic therapy should be undertaken in all patients with necrotising papillitis, but the results are often disappointing, the disease progressing slowly and relentlessly from one papilla to another until the kidney becomes functionless. Now answer the question.

Question If you suspected that a diabetic patient had necrotising papillitis, but had no facilities for X-ray, how could you confirm the diagnosis with absolute certainty?

Answer 1. Urine microscopy. Go on to **11.17**.
   2. Strain the urine through cheese-cloth to find necrotic papillary tissue. Go on to **11.19**.
   3. Don't know. Go on to **11.21**.

11.15 Your answer – *never* catheterise a diabetic unnecessarily.

Good. Diabetic renal tract infections are often difficult to control unless the diabetes is also well controlled; this may be partly because high tissue glucose concentrations are a better substrate for micro-organisms. The symptoms experienced by diabetics suffering from urinary infections are like those caused by pyelonephritis in non-diabetics — a spectrum ranging from the asymptomatic infection to the severely ill patient with a high pyrexia, frequency and strangury. Pyelonephritis may precipitate the patient into diabetic ketosis. Sometimes gas forming organisms grow in the high glucose concentrations of the bladder urine, giving rise to pneumaturia (the passage of gas in the urine). Commoner causes of pneumaturia are fistulae between the bladder and bowel caused by Crohn's disease or carcinoma of the colon. Now answer the question.

Question Can urinary tract infection be asymptomatic in the diabetic?

Answer 1. Yes. Go on to **11.14**.
2. No. Go on to **11.16**.

11.16 Your answer — urinary tract infection cannot be asymptomatic in the diabetic.
No. Infections may be quite asymptomatic in diabetics as well as in the non-diabetic, although it is true that diabetics tend to get frequently more severe infections which are harder to control. Read 11.15 again and answer the question correctly.

11.17 Your answer — Perform urine microscopy.
No. It is very difficult to find and be able to identify tiny papillary fragments in the urine sediment.
The correct answer is to find the pieces of papilla by sieving the urine through cheese-choth. Read **11.14** carefully and then choose the correct answer.

11.18 Your answer — statement 1 is true, 2 and 3 false.
You are correct only about statement 3. This is a very small chapter; read it through again from the beginning.

11.19 Your answer — strain the urine through a cheese-cloth.
You are correct. Bear in mind, however that you may have a long wait before another piece of papilla is sloughed into the urine. Monilial infections of fulminating type occasionally occur in the diabetic patient and rarely the entire renal pelvis may be blocked by the fungal growth, with fatal results: the diagnosis is somewhat difficult to make because yeasts are more frequently found in the lower urinary tracts of diabetics, but if they are present in large numbers a renal infection with Monilia should be suspected. Now answer the question.

Question Would the presence of a light growth of Monilia in a diabetic's urine imply the presence of a severe monilial renal infection?

Answer 1. Yes. Go on to **11.22**.
2. No. Go on to **11.24**.

11.20 Your answer – statement 2 is true, 1 and 3 are false.

Good. Before going on to the next chapter, the following references may be recommended for further reading:

Gellman D. D. et al. (1959). Medicine **38**, 321.
Kark R. M. & Gellman D. D. (1960) in Williams R. H. (ed.) Renal Diseases in Diabetes. Hoeber.
Lauler D. P. et al. (1961). Am. J. Med. **29**, 132.
Chapter on diabetes mellitus in the second edition of Strauss and Welt, 1971. Little Brown.
Mogensen C. E. Brit. Med. J. 1972 **4**, 257.

11.21 Your answer – I don't know how to diagnose papillary necrosis with certainty without radiological help.

The diagnosis is most certainly made in these circumstances by finding pieces of tissue in the urine which on histological section are shown to be necrotic papilla. This tissue is difficult to find unless the urine is filtered through a cheese-cloth or similar fine sieve. Now read **11.14** again and choose the correct answer.

11.22 Your answer – A light growth of Monilia in the urine suggests a severe monilial renal infection.

No. A few Monilia do not imply a severe monilial renal infection at all. They may well be contaminants from the lower urinary tract. Read **11.19** again and answer the question correctly.

11.23 Your answer – statement 3 is true, 1 and 2 false.

You are correct about statement 1, but not about 2 and 3. Start at the beginning of the chapter and read on from there.

11.24 Your answer – a light growth of Monilia would not imply a severe monilial renal infection.

Good. Now look at the statements below and pick the answer which you think is most suitable.

Statement 1 Nodular glomerulosclerosis is never found in Kimmelstiel-Wilson syndrome.

Statement 2 The average life duration in the nephrotic syndrome of diabetes (Kimmelstiel-Wilson syndrome) is three years.

Statement 3 Necrotising papillitis cannot cause renal failure.

Answer 1. Statement 1 is true, 2 and 3 false. Go on to **11.18**.
2. Statement 2 is true, 1 and 3 false. Go on to **11.20**.

3. Statement 3 is true, 1 and 2 false. Go on to **11.23**.
4. All are true. Go on to **11.25**.
5. All are false. Go on to **11.26**.
6. 1 and 2 are true, 3 false. Go on to **11.27**.
7. 1 and 3 are true, 2 false. Go on to **11.28**.
8. 2 and 3 are true, 1 false. Go on to **11.29**.

11.25 Your answer – all are true.

You are correct about statement 2 only, 1 and 3 being false. Start again and read through the chapter from **11.1**.

11.26 Your answer – all are false.

You are correct about statements 1 and 3 but not about 2. Go back and read from **11.9** onwards.

11.27 Your answer – statement 1 and 2 are true, 3 false.

You are correct about 2 and 3 but 1 is false. Read from **11.1** to **11.9**. Then answer the question in **11.24** again.

11.28 Your answer – statements 1 and 3 are true, 2 is false.

You are wrong about all the statements. Read the entire chapter through again.

11.29 Your answer – statements 2 and 3 are true, 1 is false.

Your are wrong about statement 3. Go back to **11.14** and read on from there.

Time for this Chapter: 20 minutes

Chapter 12
Polyuria

12.1 The total daily urine volume is dependent on several factors: the first of these is the osmotic load to be excreted: this is mainly composed of urea, sodium, chloride, potassium, ammonium and bicarbonate, although a number of other compounds are present in such small quantity as to be osmotically relatively unimportant. The quantity of urea excreted in the urine is dependent on exogenous protein ingested and also on endogenous protein metabolism: high protein diets produce large amounts of urinary urea; low protein diets produce small amounts of urinary urea. If you wish to get a rough idea of the amount of protein katabolism each day, multiply the daily urine urea excretion by 3. Diets containing large amounts of salt produce a urine containing more sodium chloride than low salt diets.

Question How much protein is being katabolised a day if 30 G of urea appear in the urine?

Answer 1. 90 G approximately. Go on to **12.3**.
          2. 10 G approximately. Go on to **12.5**.

12.2 Your answer – urine volume is related to the osmotic load.

Good. In renal disease the maximal concentration of urine which can be achieved is reduced. The same urine osmotic load will therefore require an increase in urine volume; in particular, the urine formed overnight which is concentrated in the healthy kidney will be more dilute and a greater nocturnal volume of urine will be formed. This leads to the early symptom of nocturia, a fairly constant concomittant of renal impairment, although young children often present with nocturnal enuresis rather than nocturia. Some patients with chronic renal disease never notice nocturia, having either a large bladder capacity or a low osmotic load due to low protein or low salt intake.

Now answer the question.

Question Is nocturia common in renal disease?

Answer 1. Yes. Go on to **12.7**.
          2. Go on to **12.9**.

12.3 Your answer – 90 G of protein are katabolised.

Good. By and large, for a given osmotic load in the urine, assuming a maximal ability to concentrate urine exists, then once this maximum concentration is attained the urine volume will be related to the osmotic load. This means that the greater the daily osmotic load in the urine (i.e., the urea and salt excreted each day), the larger the urine volume will be. Thus, the urine volume will be less on a low salt diet than on a normal salt intake, and a high salt diet will produce an increase in urine volume. This applies equally to the patient with renal disease, whose maximal concentrating ability is depressed; the urine volume on a low salt diet may be larger than in a normal person with a similar diet, and there will be some increase in urine volume on increasing oral sodium intake, until advanced renal failure has set in.

Now answer the question.

Question Is the urine volume related to the osmotic load to be excreted?

Answer 1. Yes. Go on to **12.2**.
2. No. Go on to **12.4**.

12.4 Your answer – the urine volume is not related to the osmotic load to be excreted.

You are wrong. The urine can only be concentrated up to a certain amount, say 1300–1400 mOsm/litre in health. If there are 3000 mOsm to be excreted per day even under conditions of maximum concentration there will be 3000/1300 litres of urine per day i.e. 2.3 litres. If only 1000 mOsm have to be excreted then 1000/1300 litres are obligated i.e. about 0.8 litres.

Now answer the question in **12.3** correctly.

12.5 Your answer – 10 grams of protein are katabolised. No. You have not read **12.1** with enough attention. 3 G of protein are broken down to 1 G of urea. Read **12.1** again to see if there is anything else you have missed, then answer the question correctly.

12.6 Your answer – $T_m^c H_2O$ remains constant as GFR falls.

No. $T_m^c H_2O$ is dependent on the GFR. When the GFR falls the $T_m^c H_2O$ is proportionately reduced in man. Some authorities use the term '$T_m^c H_2O$ per 100 ml of GFR' routinely to overcome errors introduced by the reduction in GFR. Read **12.7** again and answer the question.

12.7 Your answer – nocturia is common in renal disease.

Correct. The impairment of concentrating ability in renal disease can be measured conveniently by overnight fluid deprivation or by intramuscular injection of Pitressin tannate; these have been discussed in the chapter on renal function rests. As renal failure progresses, the urine concentration approaches that of plasma. This diminution in concentrating ability can be estimated with some difficulty during osmotic diuresis in the presence of excess exogenous vasopressin by measuring the maximal tubular reabsorption of free water, i.e., $T_m{}^cH_2O$, which is *reduced* in generalised renal disease *in proportion to the reduction in GFR*. The term $T_m{}^cH_2O$ is a sophisticated way of deriving a relationship based on the urine: plasma osmolality ratio. If $T_m{}^cH_2O$ decreases, there comes a time when it is zero, i.e., when urine and plasma are of equal osmolality; on a normal diet the patient at this stage will pass 2 to 3 litres of urine a day, usually drinking more than necessary and so keeping the urine below its maximal concentration.

Question Does $T_m{}^cH_2O$ remain constant as the GFR falls?

Answer 1. Yes. Go on to **12.6**.
2. No. Go on to **12.8**.
3. Don't know. Go on to **12.10**.

12.8 Your answer – $T_m{}^cH_2O$ does not remain constant as GFR falls.

Correct. A patient whose urine is permanently hypotonic to plasma (i.e., in whom the urine osmolality is lower than plasma osmolality) irrespective of the quantity of fluid taken in, has the condition known as diabetes insipidus. There are two types of diabetes insipidus.

(1) Vasopressin sensitive, due to an absolute reduction in the production of antidiuretic hormone (ADH) from the posterior lobe of the pituitary gland. It is caused by posterior pituitary-hypothalamic disease, such as pituitary tumor, trauma, operations, and encephalitis. This will not be further considered here.

(2) Vasopressin insensitive or pitressin resistant diabetes insipidus in which antidiuretic hormone is liberated by the posterior pituitary gland but the renal tubules are refractory to its action. $T_m{}^cH_2O$ is negative in this condition. Alternative names for this condition are renal diabetes insipidus and nephrogenic diabetes insipidus.

The distinction between these two conditions is readily made by the response to injected vasopressin. In vasopressin sensitive or pituitary diabetes insipidus, the urine becomes hypertonic to plasma on injection of intramuscular or intravenous vasopressin; whereas in renal or vasopressin resistant diabetes insipidus, the urine remains hypotonic to plasma after vasopressin injection, i. e., the urine osmolarity remains lower than that of plasma. Radio-immunoassay of vasopressin shows levels of ADH in circulating plasma in nephrogenic diabetes insipidus, but not in pituitary diabetes insipidus.

Question A man with a polyuria of 4 litres a day has a urine osmolarity of 150 mOsm/1. He is given an injection of 5 units of vasopressin tannate and his urine osmolarity rises to 700 mOsm/1. What is the diagnosis?

Answer 1. Vasopressin-resistant diabetes insipidus, i.e. renal diabetes insipidus. Go on to **12.11**.
2. Vasopressin-sensitive diabetes insipidus. Go on to **12.13**.

12.9 Your answer – nocturia is not common in renal disease.

No. It is quite common but there are occasional exceptions due either to a large bladder capacity or a small osmotic load to be excreted. Read **12.2** again.

12.10 Your answer – I don't know if $T_m^cH_2O$ is GFR dependent.

$T_m^cH_2O$ is related to the amount of functioning distal tubular tissue present, and this is usually related *in generalised renal disease affecting the glomeruli and the proximal and distal tubules equally* to the mass of functioning glomeruli, expressed as GFR. As the GFR falls, $T_m^cH_2O$ falls. The exception of this rule is disease predominantly affecting the distal convoluted and collecting tubules, as found, for example, in pyelonephritis and hydronephrosis. In these conditions $T_m^cH_2O$ is reduced more than would be expected from the reduction in the GFR; in some patients this reduction in $T_m^cH_2O$ reaches levels when urine osmolality remains lower than plasma osmolality i. e. $T_m^cH_2O$ is negative. This is known as diabetes insipidus. Now answer the question in **12.7** again.

12.11 Your answer – vasopressin resistant diabetes insipidus is present.

No. This patient has a good response to pitressin injection with an increased osmolality well above that of plasma, therefore his diabetes insipidus is pitressin sensitive. Now read **12.8** again.

12.12 Your answer – the carriers are male.

No. This is a sex-linked disease and the affected children are males inheriting the disease from mildly affected carrier mothers. Now read **12.13** again and answer the question.

12.13 Your answer – vasopressin sensitive diabetes insipidus.

You are correct. There are many causes of renal diabetes insipidus. The first to be considered, although it is rare, is inherited congenital diabetes insipidus. This is inherited in a sex-linked dominant manner, the affected children commonly being male and inheriting the disease from their mothers who carry the trait. Although the female carriers do not have diabetes insipidus, they have an impaired urine concentrating ability on stressing them by overnight fluid deprivation.

Question Are the carriers of congenital nephrogenic diabetes insipidus male or female?
Answer 1. Male. Go on to **12.12**.
2. Female. Go on to **12.14**.

12.14 Your answer – the carriers are female.

You are correct. Congenital nephrogenic diabetes insipidus usually goes unrecognised in the first few months of life, although the parents may notice the great thirst; more often the child becomes severely dehydrated and is admitted to hospital where hypernatraemia is found and the disease is recognised. Severe dehydration may lead to brain damage. The majority of patients with this disease are mentally retarded, which is particularly tragic when it is realised that adequate hydration would have prevented brain damage. The random urine osmolality is usually about 150 mOsm/kg.

Question Are the majority of patients with congenital nephrogenic diabetes insipidus of average or of less than average intelligence?

Answer 1. The majority are of average intelligence. Go on to **12.16**.
2. Less than average intelligence. Go on to **12.18**.

12.15 Your answer – I don't know the cause of the polyuria.

12.18 is devoted to hypercalcaemia as a cause of reversible renal diabetes insipidus. In vitamin D resistant rickets treated by large doses of vitamin D, hypercalcaemia may develop due to vitamin D intoxication; polyuria and polydipsia are therefore early indications that hypercalcaemia due to vitamin D intoxication is present and is causing renal diabetes insipidus. Now read **12.18** again and learn the common causes of hypercalcaemia, which may cause this condition; then answer the question.

12.16 Your answer – the majority of patients with congenital nephrogenic diabetes insipidus are of average intelligence.

No. They often have mental retardation due to brain damage caused by severe dehydration before the disease is diagnosed. Read **12.14** before answering the question again.

12.17 Your answer – renal diabetes insipidus caused by hypercalcaemia due to vitamin D intoxication.

You are correct. Hypokalaemia is another reversible and common cause of nephrogenic diabetes insipidus. Like hypercalcaemia, it first causes impairment of renal concentrating ability before the development of the diabetes insipidus. Among the causes of hypokalaemia are the administration of diuretics, steatorrhoea, Cushing's syndrome (particularly those cases associated with bronchial neoplasm, primary and secondary aldosteronism, renal tubular acidosis, and Fanconi syndrome. Hypokalaemic nephropathy is often complicated by pyelonephritis; correction of the hypokalaemia does not necessarily lead to amelioration of the pyelonephritis. Although the urine concentrating defect is associated with distal convoluted and collecting tubular dysfunction, the more obvious light miscoscopic changes are in the proximal tubules in hypokalaemia. Now answer the question.

Question What renal disease commonly complicates hypokalaemic nephropathy of any aetiology?

Answer 1. Pyelonephritis. Go on to **12.21**.
2. Renal tubular acidosis. Go on to **12.23**.

12.18 Your answer – the majority have less than average intelligence.

You are correct. The next cause of vasopressin resistant diabetes insipidus to be considered is hypercalcaemia. The cause of the hypercalcaemia may be vitamin D overdosage, hyperparathyroidism, sarcoidosis, immobilisation, carcinoma (e.g., of bronchus) with parathyroid like hormone being secreted by the tumour cells, non-endocrine metastatic bony deposits, Paget's disease, and thyrotoxicosis. In all these diseases hypercalcaemia causes damage to the distal convoluted and collecting tubules, resulting first of all in impairment of concentrating ability and later in nephrogenic diabetes insipidus. The diabetes insipidus may be reversible if the hypercalcaemia is treated early and normal serum calcium levels restored before renal failure has developed.

Question If a patient with vitamin D resistant rickets receiving vitamin D therapy develops polyuria and polydipsia *without* glycosuria, what is the likely cause?

Answer 1. Don't know. Go on to **12.15**.
2. Renal diabetes insipidus due to hypercalcaemia caused by vitamin D intoxication. Go on to **12.17**.
3. Diabetes mellitus. Go on to **12.19**.

12.19 Your answer – diabetes mellitus is present.

You are incorrect because glycosuria is specifically excluded in this patient. Read **12.18** again.

12.20 Your answer – renal diabetes insipidus due to hydronephrosis.

You are correct. There are several other and rare causes of renal diabetes insipidus including chronic glomerulonephritis, malignant hypertension, Sjögren's syndrome, polyarteritis nodosa, and renal amyloid disease. Some patients with malignant hypertension develop renal diabetes insipidus at night only. This has been called nocturnal nephrogenic diabetes insipidus and is apparently due to a massive nocturnal excretion of sodium chloride and water; in the daytime these patients can concentrate the urine above the osmolality of plasma but have a pitressin resistant hypotonic polyuria at night. The cause of the natriuresis is unknown.

Question If a patient with malignant hypertension has a massive nocturnal polyuria what cation is found in large quantities in the nocturnally produced urine?

Answer 1. Potassium. Go on to **12.25**.
2. Chloride. Go on to **12.27**.
3. Sodium. Go on to **12.29**.

12.21 Your answer – pyelonephritis commonly accompanies hypokalaemic nephropathy.

Correct. Renal diabetes insipidus may be caused by hydronephrosis due to obstruction of the urinary pathways or by pyelonephritis; the young patient with renal diabetes insipidus of *any* aetiology may have mildly dilated urinary pathways on pyelography, so that one should be hesitant in attributing renal diabetes insipidus to hydronephrosis in the absence of gross hydrocalycosis (i.e. dilated calyces). Dilatation of the renal pelves and ureters may be the consequence and not the cause of the polyuria.

In hypokalaemia, hypercalcaemia, pyelonephritis and hydronephrosis there may be disturbance of distal tubular function in addition to the defect in urine concentration. There may be inappropriate urinary sodium loss, inability to acidify the urine and reduction in ammonium and total hydrion excretion. Now answer the question.

Question A patient with a benign prostatic hypertrophy develops a sterile vasopressin-resistant hypotonic polyuria. What diagnosis is more likely?

Answer 1. Renal diabetes insipidus due to hydronephrosis. Go on to **12.20**.
2. Renal diabetes insipidus due to pyelonephritis. Go on to **12.22**.

12.22 Your answer – renal diabetes insipidus due to pyelonephritis.

The urine in this patient was specifically stated to be sterile, but it is possible that pyelonephritis was present. It is more likely that hydronephrosis was the cause of the renal diabetes insipidus, because benign prostatic hypertrophy is a common cause of obstruction of the urinary pathways. Now read **12.21** again and choose the correct answer.

12.23 Your answer – the renal disease most commonly complicating hypokalaemic nephropathy is renal tubular acidosis.

While you are correct in that renal tubular acidosis is often accompanied by hypokalaemia and the nephropathy of hypokalaemia, it should be realised that renal tubular acidosis is a rare disease whereas hypokalaemia is common. Renal tract infection is a common concomitant of hypokalaemia. Read **12.17** again and answer the question correctly.

12.24 Your answer – they all respond with a hypertonic urine.

You are incorrect. Many compulsive water drinkers have developed a refractory state of the distal convoluted and collecting tubules to the action of vasopressin and these patients do not therefore respond to vasopressin injection by the production of hypertonic urine. Now read **12.29** more carefully and then choose the correct answer.

12.25 Your answer – the principal cation is potassium.

No. The principal cation is sodium. You have not absorbed the message in **12.20** adequately. Read it again and then choose the correct answer.

12.26 Your answer – some compulsive water drinkers do not produce a hypertonic urine after an injection of pitressin.

Good. The treatment of nephrogenic diabetes insipidus is first of all to allow the patients free access to fluids to prevent their becoming dehydrated; reduction in urine volume can be accomplished by administration of thiazide or mercurial diuretics or chlorpropamide. These act partly by causing sodium depletion and so producing a fall in GFR although this is by no means the sole story. Chlorpropamide is not a diuretic yet it works quite well as an anti-diabetes insipidus agent. It is thought to have a vasopressin-like affect on cyclic AMP. Diuretic induced sodium loss may be associated with orthostatic hypotension and in our experience is a cause of the patients' abandoning the treatment. In any case the urine does not become hypertonic to plasma, although it may reach 270–280 mOsm/kg and the urine volume may drop to 2 litres a day.

Question Do diuretics used in the treatment of nephrogenic diabetes insipidus cause the urine to become hypertonic to plasma?

Answer 1. No. Go on to **12.28**.
2. Yes. Go on to **12.31**.

12.27 Your answer – the principal cation is chloride.

No. Chloride ions are *anions* not cations. Think before you answer the question after reading **12.20** again.

12.28 Your answer – diuretics used in the treatment of nephrogenic diabetes insipidus do *not* cause the urine to become hypertonic to plasma.

Correct. Let us now consider the prognosis in nephrogenic diabetes insipidus. Congenital nephrogenic diabetes insipidus is a life-long disability with mental retardation as a complicating factor; hypercalcaemia and hypokalaemia cause a readily reversible diabetes insipidus on correction of the electrolyte abnormality, although hypercalcaemia will itself cause renal failure which may ultimately be irreversible. The diabetes insipidus of hydronephrosis, if relieved early, is often reversible, as is the concentrating defect of pyelonephritis. There is no adequate published datum about the prognosis of nephrogenic diabetes insipidus in chronic glomerulonephritis, renal polyarteritis, sickle cell anaemia, Sjögren's syndrome, and renal amyloid.

Question What is the prognosis in nephrogenic diabetes insipidus due to hydronephrosis if the obstruction to the urinary pathways is relieved?

Answer 1. Some chance of recovery. Go on to **12.30**.
2. No chance of recovery. Go on to **12.34**.

12.29 Your answer – the major cation is sodium.

You are correct. The diagnosis of renal diabetes insipidus is made by demonstrating that the urine remains hypotonic after adequate dosage of vasopressin i.e., 5 units of vasopressin tannate in oil, well shaken and warmed in the hand, given by the intramuscular route. Unfortunately, as de Wardener has shown, people who suffer from the psychological state of compulsive water drinking (potomania) may develop a temporary state of refractoriness to pitressin after days or weeks of drinking many litres of water daily. Barlow and de Wardener found that some of these patients respond to fluid deprivation by an increase in the urinary osmolality to levels greater than after exogenous pitressin stimulation. This suggests that either the fluid deprivation causes a greater production of anti-diuretic hormone than is administered in the vasopressin test, or that the fluid deprivation test causes a fall in glomerular filtration rate responsible for urine concentration. Remember that the fluid deprivation test in diabetes insipidus is potentially dangerous; it should only be carried out inside hospital with hourly weighing of the patient. The test should be terminated when the weight has fallen by 5 per cent or when the patient has been deprived of fluid for 24 hours, whichever is the *sooner*.

Question Do patients with compulsive water drinking all respond to vasopressin injection by producing urine which is hypertonic to plasma?

Answer 1. Yes. Go on to **12.24**.
2. No. Go on to **12.26**.

12.30 Your answer – some chance of recovery.

Good. Now you are about to choose the answer to statements testing your knowledge of the contents of the chapter. Think carefully before you answer.

Statement 1 $T_m^c H_2O$ has a positive value in diabetes insipidus of renal origin.

Statement 2 Sex linked congenital nephrogenic diabetes insipidus is carried by females.

Statement 3 Hypokalaemic diabetes insipidus is reversible on correction of the potassium deficit.

Answer 1. All the statements are true. Go on to **12.35**.
2. All the statements are false. Go on to **12.36**.
3. Statement 1 is true, 2 and 3 false. Go on to **12.37**.
4. Statement 2 is true, 1 and 3 false. Go on to **12.38**.
5. Statement 3 is true, 1 and 2 false. Go on to **12.39**.
6. Statements 1 and 2 are true, 3 false. Go on to **12.40**.
7. Statements 2 and 3 are true, 1 false. Go on to **12.33**.
8. Statements 1 and 3 are true, 2 false. Go on to **12.32**.

12.31 Your answer – diuretics used in the treatment of nephrogenic diabetes insipidus cause the urine to become hypertonic to plasma.

No. The urine may approach the osmolality of plasma but does not usually exceed it. Read **12.26** again and answer the question correctly.

12.32 Your answer – statements 1 and 3 are true, 2 false.

You are correct about 3 only. Read from **12.1** to **12.17** then answer the question in **12.30** correctly.

12.33 Your answer – 2 and 3 are true, 1 is false.

You are correct. You may want to read the subject in more detail before starting the next chapter. The following references are recommended:

de Wardener H. E. (1962) in Black D. A. K. (ed.) Renal Disease, p. 566. Blackwell, Scientific Publications, Oxford (general review of polyuria).

Carter C. & Simpkiss M. (1956) Lancet **2**, 1069 (carrier state in 'nephrogenic diabetes insipidus').

Crawford J. D. & Kennedy G. C. (1959) Nature, Lond. **183**, 89 (treatment of D. I. with thiazide diuretics).

Barlow E. D. & de Wardener H. E. (1959) Quart. J. Med. **28**, 235 (compulsive water drinking).

Milne M. D., Muehrcke R. C. & Heard B. E. (1957) Brit. med. Bull. **13**, 15 (potassium deficiency and the kidney).

Cohen S. I., Fitzgerald M. G., Fourman P., Griffiths W. J. & de Wardener, H. E. (1957) Quart. J. Med. **26**, 1923 (hypercalcaemia and polyuria).

Berlyne G. M. (1961) Quart. J. Med. **30**, 339 (hydronephrosis).

12.34 Your answer – no chance of recovery.

No. There is sometimes a complete recovery in concentrating ability in patients with urinary tract obstruction causing renal diabetes insipidus. Read **12.28** again before answering the question.

12.35 Your answer – all the statements are true.

You are correct about 2 and 3 only; 1 is false. Read **12.7** and **12.8** again, then choose the correct answer to **12.30**.

12.36 Your answer – all the statements are false.

You are correct about 1 only; read on from **12.8**, working through the chapter.

12.37 Your answer – statement 1 is true, 2 and 3 false.

You are quite wrong. Start at **12.1** again and work right through this short chapter.

12.38 Your answer – statement 2 is true, 1 and 3 false.

You are correct about 1 and 2 but 3 is true. Read on from **12.17** to the end of the chapter, then answer **12.30** again.

12.39 Your answer – statement 3 is true, 1 and 2 are false.

You are wrong about statement 2. Read on from **12.8** to **12.17** then answer the question in **12.30** again.

12.40 Your answer – 1 and 2 are true, 3 is false.

You are wrong about 1 and 3. Read through the chapter again from the beginning.

the endocrine secretions of pregnancy rather than to the mechanical effects of a large uterus. The dilated ureters and pelvis have decreased to normal size in over 90 per cent of patients within six weeks of delivery, although in an occasional patient hydronephrosis may persist for up to six months. The dilated ureters and pelvis of pregnancy have a large, slowly-moving pool of urine in them – ideal surroundings for micro-organisms to multiply and cause pyelitis of pregnancy. Pyelitis of pregnancy is a urinary tract infection which occurs in over a third of patients with persistent and significant bacilluria in pregnancy. (Significant bacilluria, you will remember, is 100,000 colonies or more per ml of urine.) An additional factor is probably the sugar in the urine – glycosuria is commoner in pregnant women than in non-pregnant women, and towards the end of pregnancy lactosuria becomes more frequent.

Question A woman is found to have hydronephrosis on IVP carried out two weeks after delivery. Would you view this with alarm or complacency?

Answer 1. Alarm. Go on to **13.9**.
2. Complacency. Go on to **13.11**.

13.5 Your answer – renal function is increased.

No. In the normal pregnant woman the GFR increases to a peak of 40 per cent above the normal non-pregnant values. This patient's GFR is depressed below normal. Read **13.1** again before answering the question.

13.6 Your answer – the exchangeable sodium is increased by 2000 mEq in pregnancy.

No. The total exchangeable sodium is not increased by anything like this vast amount. Remember that the increase in exchangeable sodium in pregnancy can be accounted for by the sodium content of the increased extracellular fluid volume of pregnancy plus the sodium content of the foetus, placenta, uterus and amniotic fluid. Now read **13.7** again; then choose the correct answer.

13.7 Your answer – renal function is depressed.

Correct. Exchangeable sodium is increased in pregnancy by up to 400 to 500 mEq, which is accounted for by the sodium in the uterus, placenta, amniotic fluid, and foetus, plus the increase in extracellular fluid volume in pregnancy. The mechanism of how this sodium is retained is uncertain. There is some evidence (which is disputed) that aldosterone secretion is increased in pregnancy. This would cause sodium retention. At the same time there is an increase in secretion of progesterone which antagonises the sodium retaining properties of aldosterone. In addition, the filtered load of sodium is increased in pregnancy because of the increase in GFR but tubular sodium reabsorption is also increased.

Question By how much is exchangeable sodium increased in pregnancy?

Time for this chapter: 20 minutes

Chapter 13
The kidney and pregnancy

13.1 Renal function is abnormal in pregnancy, and the pregnant woman is subject to renal diseases peculiar to pregnancy as well responding in a different manner to diseases not peculiar to pregnancy. The changes of renal function will be first considered.

The GFR is to 40–50 per cent *higher* than normal non-pregnant levels, and the renal plasma flow is also elevated; there is an increase in plasma volume, red cell volume, and cardiac output which reaches a peak in the ninth month of pregnancy. The blood urea is lowered in normal pregnancy to 15–20 mg/100 ml, on a normal protein intake.

In the normal pregnant woman urea clearance and uric acid clearance are increased. Glucose is commonly found in the urine in up to 40 per cent of pregnant women and TmG per 100 ml of GFR is reduced. Histidine excretion in the urine is so increased that it was at one time proposed as a test of the presence of pregnancy.

Question If a pregnant woman has a GFR measured by inulin clearance of 90 ml/min per 1.73 m^2, is renal function normal, increased or decreased?

Answer 1. Normal. Go on to **13.3**.
2. Increased. Go on to **13.5**.
3. Decreased. Go on to **13.7**.

13.2 Your answer – I don't know how much the exchangeable sodium is increased in pregnancy.

The exchangeable sodium is increased by the amount calculated from the sodium content of the uterus and its contents, and the increased extracellular fluid volume of pregnancy. This amounts to 400–500 mEq on the average. Read **13.7** again so as to make sure you have not missed any other facts.

13.3 Your answer – renal function is normal.

No. Renal function as measured by GFR is elevated in pregnancy up to a peak of 40 per cent above control values in the last trimester. This woman has a GFR depressed below control values. Read **13.1** again and answer the question.

13.4 Your answer – the exchangeable sodium is increased by 400–500 mEq.

You are correct. The structural changes in the urinary tract in pregnancy consist of hydrocalycosis, hydropelvis, and hydroureter; these changes are due to

Answer 1. Don't know. Go on to **13.2**.
2. 400–500 mEq. Go on to **13.4**.
3. 2000 mEq. Go on to **13.6**.

13.8 Your answer – all patients develop pyelonephritis.
No. Just over 1 in 3 develops pyelonephritis, but less than 1 in 40 of patients without significant bacilluria later develops a renal tract infection. Read **13.4** again, then answer the question in **13.11** again.

13.9 Your answer – I would view the presence of a hydronephrosis two weeks after delivery with alarm.
You are wrong. A large number of patients have hydronephrosis two weeks after pregnancy has terminated. Read **13.4** again.

13.10 Your answer – more than one third develop pyelonephritis.
You are correct. The patient with significant bacilluria in pregnancy should be treated with the appropriate antibiotic, after checking that the particular antibiotic chosen has no teratogenic action i.e., will not harm the foetus.

Now we can consider toxaemia of pregnancy. This is an ill-understood disease in which there is no certain knowledge of the aetiology or pathogenesis of the condition. There are two types of toxaemia:

(1) Pre-eclamptic toxaemia (PET), in which there is albuminuria, hypertension and oedema.

(2) Eclampsia in which there are convulsions in addition to the manifestations of PET. Eclampsia is now fortunately rare due to better obstetric care.

The major renal lesion of PET is a swelling of the glomerular tuft due to hypertrophy and hyperplasia of the *endothelial* cells: this change is reversible, as renal biopsy studies have shown. In addition there may be thickening of the basement membrane and the vascular changes of hypertension. These changes may persist for at least 4 years.

Question Are the endothelial cells of the glomeruli hypertrophied or atrophied in PET?

Answer 1. Hypertrophied. Go on to **13.14**.
2. Atrophied. Go on to **13.16**.

13.11 Your answer – I would be complacent.
Good. Now answer the next question.

Question In what proportion of pregnant patients with *untreated* significant bacilluria will pyelonephritis develop?

Answer 1. All. Go on to **13.8**.

2. More than one third. Go on to **13.10**.
3. Don't know. Go on to **13.12**.

13.12 Your answer – I don't know what proportion of patients develop pyelonephritis.

In **13.4** you have read that over 1 in 3 patients with significant bacilluria develops pyelitis of pregnancy. If you have forgotten this, you need to read **13.4** again, then answer the question in **13.11**.

13.13 Your answer – plasma urate levels are increased in PET.

Good. The GFR is reduced in PET and the filtered load of sodium is therefore decreased; in addition, aldosterone secretion is increased and sodium retention occurs, causing oedema formation and contributing to arterial hypertension. The albuminuria of PET is caused by the glomerular lesion which has been described above, in which there is an endothelial cell proliferation and hypertrophy and basement membrane thickening.

Question What is the mechanism of sodium retention in PET?

Answer 1. Reduced filtered load of sodium. Go on to **13.18**.
2. Increased aldosterone secretion. Go on to **13.20**.
3. Both increased aldosterone secretion and reduced filtered load of sodium. Go on to **13.22**.

13.14 Your answer – the glomerular endothelial cells are hypertrophied.

You are correct. Renal function in PET is impaired: the GFR is reduced when compared to the normal values for pregnant women and some reduction in renal plasma flow is also present. The filtration fraction is lower than in normal pregnant women. There is hyperuricaemia which is caused by a reduced urate clearance. This reduced urate clearance is associated with the elevation of plasma lactate levels in the patient with PET. This has been demonstrated by showing that infusion of lactate in normal pregnancy as well as in PET will depress urate clearance.

Question Is the plasma urate level in PET higher or lower than that in normal pregnancy?

Answer 1. Higher. Go on to **13.13**.
2. Lower. Go on to **13.15**.

13.15 Your answer – plasma urate levels are lower in PET than in normal pregnancy.

No. Plasma urate levels are elevated in PET: this is due to a reduction in urate clearance associated with elevated plasma levels of lactate in the patient with PET. Now read **13.14** again and answer the question correctly.

13.16 Your answer – the glomerular endothelial cells are atrophied.

No. The glomeruli are swollen in PET and this is largely due to the endothelial cells being hyperplastic and hypertrophied. Answer the question in **13.10** correctly after re-reading that paragraph.

13.17 Your answer – the evidence is conclusive.

No. If you think it is conclusive you have not read **13.22** carefully. Go back and read it again.

13.18 Your answer – the sodium retention of PET is due to a reduced filtered load of sodium.

You are partly correct in that GFR is depressed and so the filtered load of sodium is reduced. Aldosterone is also secreted in a greater amount than is found in uncomplicated pregnancy and this causes further reabsorption of sodium. Now answer the question in **13.13** again.

13.19 Your answer – the evidence is inconclusive:

You are correct. Arterial hypertension is a common condition and it is not surprising that pregnancy and hypertension frequently are present in the same patient. The physician can readily distinguish between PET and essential benign hypertension because oedema is absent in the latter group in the absence of heart failure, but only a knowledge of the patient's blood pressure *before* pregnancy can differentiate between PET and the combination of PET with pre-existing hypertension. It has been suggested that a blood pressure of 150/100 in the first trimester of pregnancy is indicative of hypertension antedating pregnancy.

Question In an untreated pregnant woman with severe hypertension there is no oedema or albuminuria. What diagnosis would you make?

Answer 1. PET. Go on to **13.23**.
2. Hypertension not due to PET. Go on to **13.25**.

13.20 Your answer – aldosterone secretion is increased.

You are partly correct, but the filtered sodium load is also reduced due to a reduction in the GFR, and this also contributes to the sodium retention. Now answer the question at the end of **13.13** again.

13.21 Your answer – I don't know if the evidence is conclusive or not.

The evidence in the literature is bedevilled by conflicting reports using different racial and ethnic groups. The subject of the long term effects of PET is as controversial as that of the inheritance of essential hypertension. Now read **13.22** again to savour the controversy surrounding the subject, then choose the correct answer to the question.

13.22 Your answer − both aldosterone secretion increase and a reduction in the filtered load cause the sodium retention of PET.

You are correct. The long term effects of PET on the patient after the affected pregnancy are the subject of conflicting reports. Thus Gibson and Platt adduced evidence of mild or moderate hypertension on follow up four years after the episode of PET, whereas in a follow up averaging 20 years after PET by Cosgrove and coworkers, it was concluded that eclampsia did not cause hypertension. Tillman found that a four year follow up of normals and PET patients revealed no difference in the mean blood pressure levels.

Question Is the evidence conclusive about the occurrence of hypertension in the long term follow up of PET?

Answer 1. Conclusive. Go on to **13.17**.
2. Inconclusive. Go on to **13.19**.
3. Don't know. Go on to **13.21**.

13.23 Your answer − the diagnosis is PET.

No. Pre-eclamptic toxaemia is a symptom complex consisting of oedema, proteinuria and hypertension. If there is no oedema or proteinuria the diagnosis remains that of hypertension. Read **13.18** again before answering the question.

13.24 Your answer − essential hypertension is *not* associated with an increased incidence of PET.

No. There is a definite correlation between pre-existent essential hypertension and pre-eclamptic toxaemia of pregnancy. Read **13.25** again and then answer the question correctly.

13.25 Your answer − the diagnosis is hypertension.

You are correct. In the non-pregnant woman suffering from benign essential hypertension, the occurrence of pregnancy is associated with an increased incidence of PET. The evidence about whether pregnancy causes a *permanent* increase in the severity of pre-existing hypertension after the end of pregnancy is suggestive but not conclusive. 30 per cent of patients with pre-existing hypertension have an exacerbation of their hypertension due to the pregnancy, and there is a 50 per cent foetal mortality. The aetiology of the hypertension has some bearing on the effects it produces in pregnancy. In one type of hypertension − that associated with coarctation of the aorta − there is no increase in the frequency of PET. In all other types of hypertension, PET is more frequent than in the woman who is normotensive before pregnancy. The reason for the lack of PET in coarctation of the aorta is that the arterial blood pressure distal to the site of coarctation of the aorta is not elevated, and therefore the kidneys and uterus do not suffer from the effects of high arterial pressure, and so the pregnancy carries on as if the patient were normotensive.

Question What cause of arterial hypertension is *not* associated with an increased incidence of PET?

Answer 1. Essential hypertension. Go on to **13.24**.
2. Coarctation of the aorta. Go on to **13.26**.

13.26 Your answer — coarctation of the aorta is *not* associated with an increased incidence of PET.

You are correct. Let us now consider pregnancy and acute, subacute and chronic glomerulonephritis. These affect both the morbidity and mortality rate of the mother and also the foetal mortality rate and will now be considered not from the point of hypertension, which may or may not be present, but mainly from the point of view of the renal disease.

First of all, acute glomerulonephritis — Type 1 nephritis. If this disease occurs in pregnancy there is usually foetal death and abortion or premature labour. Very *few* pregnant patients who develop acute glomerulonephritis have a normal pregnancy and are delivered of a live baby at term. Now answer the question.

Question If acute glomerulonephritis develops in a pregnant woman are the chances that she will continue on with a normal pregnancy and delivery of a live baby at term good or bad?

Answer 1. Good. Go on to **13.27**.
2. Bad. Go on to **13.29**.

13.27 Your answer — the prognosis is good for foetal survival and the normal continuation of pregnancy in acute glomerulonephritis.

No. Very few pregnant women who develop acute glomerulonephritis continue in pregnancy. Usually the pregnancy terminates with abortion and foetal death in utero. Read **13.26** again before answering the question correctly.

13.28 Your answer — two out of three die.

Correct. The effect of pregnancy on membranous glomerulonephritis is undefined, much of the data on the effect of renal disease on pregnancy having been gathered before percutaneous renal biopsy became widespread. Nevertheless, in nephrotic syndrome caused by membranous glomerulonephritis, there is little evidence of deterioration in maternal or foetal prognosis *in the absence of hypertension or renal failure*. Some women develop a recurrent nephrotic syndrome in each pregnancy which remits between pregnancies. The aetiology in some of them is PET in which the albuminuria has become massive, and in others the aetiology is unknown: they are normotensive and may be exhibiting some immune response to the foetus. This group is referred to as cyclical nephrotic syndrome of pregnancy.

Question Is nephrotic syndrome ever caused by pre-eclamptic toxaemia?

Answer 1. Yes. Go on to **13.31**.
2. No. Go on to **13.33**.

13.29 Your answer – the outlook for foetal survival and normal continuation of pregnancy is bad.

You are correct. In chronic proliferative glomerulonephritis (slowly progressive Type I nephritis of Ellis) the prognosis in pregnancy for maternal and foetal survival is dependent on the degree of reduction in renal function and hypertension; if there is little reduction in renal function and no hypertension, there is a good chance that pregnancy will be normal and little direct evidence of any acceleration in the progress of the chronic nephritis. In patients with chronic glomerulonephritis, the RPF and GFR increase in pregnancy, and toxaemia is very frequent. The patient with renal disease and hypertension before pregnancy or in whom the blood pressure rises before the 30th week of pregnancy tends to develop toxaemia and the chance of foetal survival is less. If there is severe renal damage (i.e., GFR of 5–10 ml/min) and the patient is not sterile, there is foetal death with abortion or premature labour in *2 out of 3*, and frequently evidence of some maternal deterioration in renal function after pregnancy. The occasional patient may undergo rapid deterioration in renal function, particularly if a renal tract infection is superimposed.

Question If a patient with severe renal impairment due to chronic glomerulonephritis becomes pregnant, what is the likelihood of foetal death?

Answer 1. 2 out of 3 die. Go on to **13.28**.
2. All survive. Go on to **13.30**.

13.30 Your answer – all survive.

No. Many patients with chronic and severe renal disease are sterile but if they become pregnant a minority of the patients are delivered of live infants. Read **13.29** carefully before you choose the correct answer.

13.31 Your answer – PET sometimes causes the nephrotic syndrome of pregnancy.

Correct. Lupus erythematosus is a common cause of nephrotic syndrome in pregnancy. Pollak and Kark found that although the renal disease is not accelerated by pregnancy, SLE in pregnancy may deteriorate in the middle trimester and in the first two months after delivery. Advanced lupus nephritis, as in any other form of chronic renal disease, is associated with a high incidence of foetal death and abortion.

In all cases of renal failure caused by chronic renal disease in which pregnancy occurs, the question arises whether pregnancy should be terminated or not. There is little to guide one in the fragmented experience and small series of which much of the literature is composed. Each case must be dealt with on its merits, the major consideration has to be the possibility of further deterioration in the mother's condition with the probability that the foetus will not survive, although the ultimate decision must be left to the mother. Patients who come for advice before embarking on pregnancy can be advised that advanced renal disease and hypertension are relative contra-indications to pregnancy; the absence of an adequate statistical survey of all forms of renal disease in pregnancy makes counselling difficult.

Question In what trimester of pregnancy is renal SLE most likely to deteriorate?

Answer 1. First, Go on to **13.32**.
2. Second. Go on to **13.34**.
3. Third. Go on to **13.36**.

13.32 Your answer – SLE tends to deteriorate in the first trimester of pregnancy.
No. It deteriorates most commonly in the middle trimester of pregnancy and in the early post-partum period. Read **13.31** again more carefully and choose the correct answer to the question.

13.33 Your answer – nephrotic syndrome is never caused by PET.
No. PET sometimes causes a massive proteinuria which is sufficient to cause hypoproteinaemia and oedema i.e. nephrotic syndrome. Read **13.28** again before choosing the correct answer.

13.34 Your answer – SLE deteriorates more commonly in the second trimester. Irreversible post partum renal failure was first described by Robson and colleagues in Edinburgh. It occurs within the first 6 weeks of the puerperium, usually beginning at least 2 weeks post-partum. The patient develops acute oliguric renal failure, with focal glomerular necrosis and thrombus in the interlobular arteries and arterioles. Recovery has been claimed after heparin therapy to prevent arterial thrombus formation.

Good. Now choose the correct answer after careful consideration of the statements below.

Statement 1 Hydronephrosis is common in pregnancy.

Statement 2 Serum urate levels are elevated in pre-eclamptic toxaemia.

Statement 3 The prognosis for survival of the foetus in a pregnant woman who develops acute glomerulonephritis is bad.
Which of the answers is correct?

Answer 1. All the statements are true. Go on to **13.39**.
2. All the statements are false. Go on to **13.40**.
3. Statement 1 only is true, 2 and 3 false. Go on to **13.35**.

4. Statement 2 only is true, 1 and 3 false. Go on to **13.37**.
   5. Statement 3 only is true, 1 and 2 false. Go on to **13.38**.
   6. Statements 1 and 2 are true, 3 false. Go on to **13.41**.
   7. Statements 1 and 3 are true, 2 false. Go on to **13.42**.
   8. Statements 2 and 3 are true, 1 false. Go on to **13.43**.

13.35 Your answer – only statement 1 is true.

You are correct about statement 1 but wrong about 2 and 3. Read on from **13.14** through the remainder of the chapter.

13.36 Your answer – SLE deteriorates in the third trimester of pregnancy.

No. You have forgotten the correct answer. Go back and read **13.31** again, then choose the correct answer.

13.37 Your answer – statement 2 only is true.

You are wrong about 1 and 3. Read from the beginning of the chapter to **13.14** and then from **13.26** to the end of the chapter.

13.38 Your answer – only statement 3 is true.

You are correct about 3, but not about 1 and 2. Start from **13.1** and read on to **13.26**, then answer the question in **13.34** again.

13.39 Your answer – all the statements are true.

You are correct.

The following references may be of help in further reading of the subject:
Dill et al. (1942) Am. J. Obst. and Gynae. **43**, 32.
Gibson G. B. & Platt R. (1959) Brit. Med. J. **2**, 159.
Kass E. H. (1960) Arch. Int. Med. **105**, 194; (1962) Ann. Int. Med. **56**, 46.
Handler J. S. (1960) J. Clin. Invest. **39**, 1526.
Pollak V. E. & Nettles, J. B. (1960) Medicine **39**, 469.
Kincaid-Smith P. et al. (1964) Lancet **2**, 61.
Brumfitt W. et al. (1961) Lancet **2**, 1059.
Hamburger et al. (1968) Nephrology.
Robson J. S. et al. (1968) Quart J. Med. 37,423.

Now you can begin the next chapter.

13.40 Your answer – all the statements are false.

No. You are wrong about all three statements. Start at the beginning of the chapter and work through it again.

13.41 Your answer – statements 1 and 2 are true.

You are partially correct but statement 3 is also correct. Read on from **13.26**.

13.42 Your answer – statements 1 and 3 are true.

You are wrong about statement 2. Read from **13.14** to **13.26** and then answer the question in **13.34** again.

13.43 Your answer – statement 1 is false, 2 and 3 are true.

You are partly correct, but wrong about 1. Read from **13.1** to **13.14**, then answer the question in **13.34** again.

Time for this chapter: 30 minutes

Chapter 14
The kidney and Hypertension

14.1 The problem of the kidney and hypertension can be likened to a jigsaw puzzle with a few pieces in place and the remainder either unrelated at present or not yet discovered. There are two ways in which one can approach the kidney-hypertension problem: the first one is by the consideration of the pathophysiology of renal hypertension; the other method is to consider the various types of renal hypertension, benign and malignant, in an unconnected manner. For a book of this type it is more appropriate to use the pathophysiological approach in so far as current knowledge permits. In the early 19th century it was known that left ventricular hypertrophy was commonly found in patients suffering from nephritis of any type. The invention of the sphygmomanometer by Riva-Rocci in the latter half of the 19th century enabled the blood pressure to be measured accurately, and so the left ventricular hypertrophy found in nephritic patients was shown to be due to high blood pressure. Shortly after this, in 1898, Tigerstadt and Bergman discovered a substance capable of elevating the blood pressure in saline extracts of the kidney: this pressor substance was called 'renin'.

Question Does 'renin' increase or decrease the blood pressure?

Answer 1. Increase. Go on to **14.3**.
2. Decrease. Go on to **14.5**.

14.2 Your answer – the changes of severe hypertension are visible in the kidney with the clipped renal artery.

No. The renal artery occlusion is such that there is a pressure gradient across the clamped renal artery, the artery distal to the clamped portion being at a much lower pressure than the general systemic arterial pressure. Now read **14.3** again and answer the question correctly.

14.3 Your answer – renin causes an increase in blood pressure.

Correct. The next piece of work which added another piece to the jigsaw was Goldblatt's finding, in 1934, that constriction of the renal artery in the dog caused a rise in blood pressure if the other kidney were first removed. The histological changes of severe hypertension were absent in the kidney which was 'protected' by the clip on the renal artery, but they were present elsewhere in the body where the full systemic blood pressure was felt. The implications of this in man were rapidly realised, and unilateral diseased kidneys in man were soon being removed for the cure of hypertension.

Question Are the changes of severe hypertension visible in the kidney with the clipped renal artery in the Goldblatt experiment?

Answer 1. Yes. Go on to **14.2**.
2. No. Go on to **14.6**.

14.4 Your answer – renal artery stenosis does not always cause hypertension.

Good. Renal artery stenosis may be unilateral or bilateral: its diagnosis by means of arteriography has been discussed in the chapter on morphological renal function tests. Intravenous pyelography in unilateral renal artery stenosis shows a smaller kidney on the affected side, at least 1.5 cm smaller than its fellow. The shadow of the renal pelvis may be denser than normal on the affected side in a minority of patients because water reabsorption from the affected side makes the radio-opaque medium more concentrated than in the normal kidneys. The Stamey test has been considered in the chapter on biochemical renal function tests. The radio-active renogram is that of a screening test only: it is of some use in the precise diagnosis of renal artery stenosis, but errors of up to 20 per cent in apparent renal function may be caused by slight malposition of the scintillation counters. Improvements in percutaneous angiographic techniques now enable direct measurements of the pressure gradient across the stenotic segment *through the lumen* of the artery. If the pressure drop is less than 25 mm Hg, the stenosis is unlikely to be the cause of hypertension and operation on the renal artery is contra-indicated.

Question In a hypertensive man with renal artery stenosis the renal artery is cannulated and the pressure drop across the stenotic segment is found to be 5 mm Hg. Would you advise operation on the renal artery to cure the hypertension?

Answer 1. Yes. Go on to **14.9**.
2. No. Go on to **14.11**.
3. Don't know. Go on to **14.13**.

14.5 Your answer – renin causes a decrease in blood pressure.

No. The saline extract of kidney described by Tigerstadt and Bergman in 1898 was noteworthy because it had a pressor action, i.e. it caused an elevation of the blood pressure.

Read **14.1** again and choose the correct answer.

14.6 Your answer – the changes of severe hypertension are *not* visible in the kidney with the clipped renal artery.

Correct. The clipped or ischaemic kidney is smaller than the normal kidney, and has atrophic tubules and normal looking glomeruli. This appearance is common in renal artery stenosis which occurs in man as a result of atheroma, fibromuscular hyperplasia, trauma, and thrombosis, and can cause severe hypertension. Recent work has shown that hypertension in man is frequently *absent* in spite of renal artery stenosis or occlusion, and this implies that in man hypertension and renal artery stenosis are not necessarily always directly related; this accounts for the frequent failure of arterioplastic operations or nephrectomy in renal artery stenosis to relieve the hypertension.

Now answer the question.

Question Does renal artery stenosis always cause hypertension?

Answer 1. No. Go on to **14.4**.
2. Yes. Go on to **14.7**.

14.7 Your answer – renal artery stenosis always causes hypertension.

No. Necropsy and arteriographic series have shown that renal artery stenosis is often found in the normotensive patient. Read **14.6**. again.

14.8 Your answer – the juxta-glomerular apparatus is the site of renin secretion. Correct.

It has been shown experimentally that most of the renin content of the kidney is situated in the part of the glomerulus where the afferent and efferent vessels join the tuft. The action of renin is on plasma angiotensinogen, which is converted to angiotensin I, a decapeptide. A converter enzyme then converts angiotensin I to angiotensin II, the active octapeptide, whose structure was discovered by Peart.

Question What is produced by the action of renin on angiotensinogen?

Answer 1. A polypeptide. Go on to **14.14**.
2. Angiotensin 1. Go on to **14.16**.
3. Don't know. Go on to **14.18**.

14.9 Your answer – I would advise operation if the gradient were 5 mm Hg.

You would be given the patient bad advice, for a gradient of that size is unlikely to cause hypertension itself. Read **14.4** again.

14.10 Your answer – renin secretion is from the juxtamedullary glomeruli.

Your are confusing juxtaglomerular apparatus with juxtamedullary glomeruli. Read **14.11** before going on to answer the question again.

14.11 Your answer – I would advise against operation.

Good. Your would be correct. How does renal artery stenosis cause hypertension? The answer seems to lie in the renin-angiotensin-aldosterone system. Let us summarise what is known of the physiology of this system.

Renin is an enzyme produced by the juxta-glomerular apparatus; the stimulus to the secretion of renin by the juxta-glomerular apparatus is unknown with certainty but it is either the blood pressure in the afferent arteriole or, more likely, the sodium concentration and content of the distal tubule at the level of the macula densa, or the gradient between plasma sodium and macula densa concentration of sodium.

Question What is the site of renin secretion?

Answer
1. Juxta-glomerular apparatus. Go on to **14.8**.
2. Juxta-medullary glomerulus. Go on to **14.10**.
3. Distal tubule. Go on to **14.12**.

14.12 Your answer – the distal tubule is the site of renin secretion.

No. You are confusing the macula densa with the juxta glomerular apparatus: the macula densa is closely related to the latter but is itself not the site of renin secretion, which is thought to come from the juxta-glomerular apparatus itself. The macula densa may well have specialised cells to detect flow rates and salt concentration in the distal tubule. Now read **14.11** again.

14.13 Your answer – I don't know what to advise.

If the patient has renal artery stenosis it is important to realise that the renal arterial constriction is commonly *not* the cause of the patients hypertension, and this is particularly liable to be true if his stenosis is inadequate to cause a gross pressure gradient across the stenosis. A fall of 5 mm Hg indicates that the stenosis is itself not likely to be significant cause of the hypertension. Now answer the question in **14.4** correctly.

14.14 Your answer – a polypeptide is formed by the action of renin on angiotensinogen.

You are correct but you have forgotten the name of the polypeptide. Choose the correct answer to **14.8** after re-reading the paragraph.

14.15 Your answer – angiotensin II causes the adrenal cortex to secrete aldosterone.

Good. The aldosterone secretion may be so marked as to lead to the clinical features of 'secondary' aldosteronism with hypokalaemia, nocturnal polyuria, alkalosis, hypertension etc. This commonly occurs in renal artery stenosis together with proteinuria which may be due to the direct effect of the renin on the kidney. It may give rise to nephrotic syndrome. In the male rat renin regularly produces a heavy proteinuria.

Question What is the syndrome produced by excessive angiotensin production?

Answer
1. Don't know. Go on to **14.20**.
2. Proteinuria. Go on to **14.21**.
3. Aldosteronism. Go on to **14.24**.

14.16 Your answer — angiotensin I is formed by the action of renin upon angiotensinogen.

You are correct. The actions of angiotensin II appear to be dual: (1) Upon the arterioles causing a rise in blood pressure. (2) Upon the adrenal cortex, stimulating the secretion of aldosterone.

Question What does the action of angiotensin II on the adrenal cortex cause the secretion of?

Answer 1. Aldosterone. Go on to **14.15**.
2. Renin. Go on to **14.17**.
3. Aldactone. Go on to **14.19**.

14.17 Your answer — angiotensin II causes the adrenal cortex to secrete renin.

No. Angiotensin II causes the adrenal cortex to secrete aldosterone. Read **14.16** again and then answer the question again.

14.18 Your answer — I don't know what is formed by the action of renin on angiotensinogen.

Renin is an enzyme which has the action of converting a plasma, protein, angiotensinogen, to angiotensin, a pressor polypeptide. Now answer the question correctly, after reading **14.8** once more.

14.19 Your answer — angiotensin II causes the secretion of aldactone.

No. Aldactone is not secreted by the adrenal cortex. It is a synthetic compound which antagonises the renal tubular action of aldosterone. Go back to **14.16** and answer the question after reading the paragraph.

14.20 Your answer — I don't know what syndrome may be produced by excessive angiotensin production.

The production of angiotensin is likely to lead to stimulation of the adrenal cortex with the production of secondary aldosteronism. Read **14.15** again to make sure you have not missed anything else in this paragraph. Then go on to answer the question correctly.

14.21 Your answer — proteinuria is caused by excessive angiotensin production.

You are correct and this is important in animals, particularly the rat, although it may very rarely give rise to nephrotic syndrome in man with renal artery stenosis. More commonly and more strikingly there is the profound hypokalaemic polyuria due to secondary aldosteronism. Go on to **14.24**.

14.22 Your answer — plasma renin is low in primary aldosteronism.

You are correct. You have now seen a possible mechanism for hypertension caused by renal artery stenosis. Renal artery stenosis is a cause of hypertension at any age; the majority of patients in the age groups 35 to 55 have 'essential' hypertension, whereas in hypertension in those below 35 or above 55 it is necessary to exclude with certainty other diseases such as renal artery stenosis, chronic pyelonephritis, and chronic glomerulonephritis because this age group contains the majority of secondary (non-essential) hypertension. Renal vein renin levels have been found to be high in the blood which has circulated through the kidney supplied by a stenosed renal artery and is useful in predicting a successful result from a plastic repair of a unilateral renal artery stenosis. Renal venous renin assays are at least as reliable as split renal function studies. In a patient with renal artery stenosis shown to have a significant pressure drop across the stenosis or, where it is not technically possible for this to be measured, with a positive Stamey test, the affected renal artery should be reconstructed or the kidney removed if reconstructive surgery is not possible. The results of such surgery are disappointing, about 50 per cent of the patients having a persistent hypertension after operation. This is presumably due to the contralateral kidney being irreversibly affected by hypertension. The hypertension may be due to a disease other than renal artery stenosis.

Question Does nephrectomy for renal artery stenosis invariably cure the hypertension?

Answer 1. Yes. Go on to **14.25**.
2. No. Go on to **14.27**.

14.23 Your answer – Plasma renin is high in primary aldosteronism.

Wrong. You have not read **14.24** with enough care; go back and read it carefully, then choose the correct answer to the question.

14.24 Your answer – aldosteronism.

Your are correct. In patients with malignant hypertension bioassay often reveals low or normal peripheral plasma concentrations of renin, and it is difficult to obtain hypertensive effects with physiological doses of renin in short term experiments, although Dickinson has shown by ingenious long term experiments in rabbits that a minute dose of angiotensin given intravenously will over many days produce a definite hypertensive effect, whereas the same dose in acute experiments will produce no rise in blood pressure. It is therefore possible that renin produced in the stenosed kidney stimulated by a fall in distal tubular sodium content or blood pressure reduction in the afferent arteriole may be responsible for the hypertension. The renal vein renin level is usually elevated in samples of blood taken from the renal vein on the same side as the stenosed renal artery. Some authorities use this test to decide if it is worthwhile to operate on the stenosed side to cure renal hypertension. It is thought that if the renal vein renin on the stenosed side is 1.5 or more times greater than the level on the contralateral side, then operation to relieve the renal artery stenosis is likely to be followed by a fall in blood pressure to normal levels.

If the plasma aldosterone level is high and the renin level is low it is likely that severe hypertension present is due to an aldosterone producing adenenoma (Conn's syndrome). This is known as primary aldosteronism. In secondary aldosteronism the aldosterone plasma levels are low and the renin levels are high.

Conn has suggested that as many as 1 in 7 cases of essential hypertension may be caused by adrenal cortical adenomata which secrete aldosterone. So far little or no evidence has been provided in careful autopsy series to confirm this suggestion.

Question In primary aldosteronism is plasma renin low or high?

Answer 1. low renin level. Go on to **14.22**.
2. high renin level. Go on to **14.23**.

14.25 Your answer – nephrectomy invariably cures the hypertension of renal artery stenosis.

You are not correct. It is one of the unfortunate facts of modern surgery that nephrectomy for unilateral renal disease associated with hypertension is frequently unsuccessful in curing hypertension: the success rate in those patients where the indications for surgery are restricted to those with a positive Stamey test or with an adequate pressure gradient across the renal artery is better, approaching 1 in 2. Now read **14.22** again.

14.26 Your answer – there are ischaemic areas in the chronic pyelonephritic kidney.

Correct. The problem of essential hypertension and the kidney will be considered next. First of all it should be remembered that essential hypertension, a disease of unknown aetiology, is the commonest cause of hypertension. Benign essential hypertension differs from malignant essential hypertension both clinically and pathologically. The diastolic blood pressure in malignant hypertension is 130 mm Hg or more; in benign hypertension it is lower than this. Malignant hypertension is always associated with papilloedema and renal damage. In benign hypertension papilloedema is not present, nor is renal damage necessarily present.

Question A man of 52 has a diastolic blood pressure of 110 mm Hg, no albuminuria or other evidence of kidney damage, and normal optic fundi. From what type of hypertension is he suffering?

Answer 1. Benign. Go on to **14.30**.
2. Malignant. Go on to **14.32**.

14.27   Your answer – nephrectomy does *not* invariably cure hypertension due to renal artery stenosis.

You are correct. Unilateral renal disease due to the chronic pyelonephritis causes hypertension, and at one time nephrectomy was advocated to cure the hypertension, but the results were disappointing. The position at present in patients with unilateral renal disease and hypertension is that the hypertension should be controlled by drug therapy first and that surgical intervention should be the last resort in view of the uncertain results of surgery.

Question   Would you first employ drug therapy in the treatment of hypertension due to renal artery stenosis?

Answer   1.   Yes. Go on to **14.29**.
2.   No. Go on to **14.31**.

14.28   Your answer – there are no ischaemic areas in the chronic pyelonephritic kidney.

You are incorrect. The depressions seen on the surface of the pyelonephritic kidney are largely attributable to infarcted areas of kidney, the end result of ischaemia being infarction. Read **14.30** again.

14.29   Your answer – I would use drug therapy first.

You are correct. Many renal diseases are associated with hypertension, although in the majority the reason for this is unknown; in unilateral chronic pyelonephritis there are many infarcted areas: these are caused by a reduction in the arterial blood supply following inflammation of the arteries with arterial narrowing or total arterial occlusion. The cause of the hypertension in glomerulonephritis is uncertain. In rapidly progressive glomerulonephritis there is an elevation of plasma renin levels however. In polyarteritis nodosa the presence of vascular infarcts due to the panarteritis suggests that there may be ischaemic areas similar to those in chronic pyelonephritis. These ischaemic areas may produce renin in a similar manner to the ischaemic kidney of renal artery stenosis.

Question   Are there ischaemic areas in the kidney in chronic pyelonephritis?

Answer   1.   Yes. Go on to **14.26**.
2.   No. Go on to **14.28**.

14.30   Your answer – he has benign hypertension.

You are correct. Essential hypertension is a common condition which appears to be inherited as an autosomal dominant character, although the evidence is at present conflicting. The vast majority of hypertensive patients develop benign hypertension, only 1 per cent to 5 per cent developing malignant hypertension. Benign hypertension is misleading in its name – it is far less benign in men than in women, as Bechgaard has shown. The age of onset of benign hypertension is ill-defined, the majority of the patients being below 50 years old when hypertension appears; if female they may survive for 20 years. Male patients tend to survive for considerably less than this.

Question Has benign hypertension a better prognosis in men or women?

Answer 1. In men. Go on to **14.34**.
2. In women. Go on to **14.36**.

14.31 Your answer – I would not employ drug therapy in the treatment of hypertension due to renal artery stenosis.

You are incorrect. Drug therapy should always be tried first, for if it is successful there is no need to embark upon operation. The operations for renal artery stenosis are often disappointing in that the hypertension persists after the operation. Read **14.27** again and select the correct answer.

14.32 Your answer – he has malignant hypertension.

To have malignant hypertension a patient has to have a diastolic blood pressure higher than this patient's, together with papilloedema and renal damage. You have not read **14.26** with sufficient concentration. Read it again and answer the question correctly.

14.33 Your answer – hyaline thickening of the afferent arterioles.

Correct. The majority of patients with benign hypertension have no symptoms until a complication develops, although a minority have headaches, dyspnoea on exertion, dizziness, nosebleeds and a host of minor symptoms. The complications of benign essential hypertension are as follows: *one third to one half the patients die of heart disease* – left ventricular failure or myocardial infarction: *one sixth die of cerebral vascular disease* – cerebral haemorrhage or thrombosis, and *only one tenth die of uraemia*. The remainder die of causes unrelated to hypertension.

Question Do the majority of patients with *benign* essential hypertension die of uraemia?

Answer 1. Yes. Go on to **14.37**.
2. No. Go on to **14.39**.

14.34 Your answer – benign hypertension has a better prognosis in men.

No. In **14.30** you have read that the prognosis in benign hypertension is worse in men than in women. Go back and read this again.

14.35 Your answer – The major histological change in benign essential hypertension is fibrinoid necrosis. Wrong. The major histological change in benign hypertension is hyaline thickening of the afferent arterioles. You should read

14.36 with more care to ensure that you have not missed any more facts in the paragraph.

14.36 Your answer – benign hypertension has a better prognosis in women than in men.

Your are correct. The pathological changes in benign nephrosclerosis will be considered next. The kidney is finely granular and normal in size in the majority, although occasionally it is contracted in those patients with the rare type of long standing benign hypertension leading to renal failure. The major histological change in the kidney is a hyaline thickening of the affferent arterioles which begins subintimally and spreads into the media. Renal function tests show that the GFR remains normal for a long time with an increase in the filtration fraction and there is a very gradual reduction in GFR, RPF and in Tm_{PAH}. Ultimately a small proportion of the patients develop renal failure.

Question What is the major histological change in the arterioles of kidneys in benign hypertension?

Answer 1. Hyaline thickening of the afferent arterioles. Go on to **14.33**.
2. Fibrinoid necrosis. Go on to **14.35**.

14.37 Your answer – the majority of patients die of uraemia.

No. In benign essential hypertension only one patient in ten develops uraemia, in contrast to the stituation in malignant hypertension where uraemia is much the most important complication. Read **14.33** again and then answer the question.

14.38 Your answer – the major histological change in malignant hypertension is hyaline thickening of the arterioles.

No. The arteriolar hyaline change is characteristic of benign, not malignant hypertension. In malignant hypertension necrosis of the arteriolar wall occurs due to the high diastolic blood pressure; the 'fibrinoid' appearance is probably due to fibrin which enters from the arteriolar lumen. Read **14.39** again and answer the question correctly.

14.39 Your answer – the majority of patients do not die of uraemia.

Your are correct. The deterioration of renal function which has been shown to take place in untreated benign hypertension is reduced by treatment with hypotensive agents, but no twenty years-follow-up has as yet been made of patients with benign essential hypertension who have been adequately treated by drugs. In malignant hypertension the entire clinical and pathological picture is dramatically different. The prognosis is much worse, the majority of untreated patients being dead within 18 months of the onset of the malignant phase. The precise relationship between benign and malignant essential hypertension is ill-defined, only a small proportion of known benign hypertensives developing malignant hypertension, but the majority of malignant hypertensive patients develop the disease *out of the blue* with no certain evidence of prior hypertensive disease. The kidneys in malignant essential hypertension are large and have petechial haemorrhages on the surface. On histological examination the key features are endothelial proliferation of the arterioles, fibrinoid necrosis of the arteriolar walls and fibrinoid necrosis of the glomerular tufts. It is the glomerular necrosis which is responsible for the rapidly progressing renal failure in malignant essential hypertension. It is because of the relentless and unremitting destruction of glomeruli caused by the persistently high diastolic blood pressure that it is essential to lower the blood pressure *as soon as possible* to limit the glomerular destruction.

Question What is the major histological change in malignant essential hypertension?

Answer 1. Hyaline thickening of the arterioles. Go on to **14.38**.
2. Fibrinoid necrosis of the arterioles, glomeruli and endothelial arterial proliferation. Go on to **14.40**.

14.40 Your answer – the major change is fibrinoid necrosis of the glomeruli and afferent arterioles.

You are correct. There are also changes of fibrosis of glomeruli and even epithelial crescents which may make differentiation from acute or subacute glomerulonephritis difficult on histological grounds. It is possible that some of these patients are actually suffering not from malignant *essential* hypertension but from malignant hypertension secondary to acute or subacute glomerulonephritis. Other patients suffering from secondary malignant hypertension have many other diseases such as pyelonephritis, glomerulonephritis, renal artery stenosis, renal hypoplasia, Cushing's syndrome, Conn's syndrome, polyarteritis, polycystic kidneys, phaechromocytoma, hydronephrosis, and toxaemia of pregnancy.

Question If a patient with polycystic kidneys develops hypertension with a blood pressure of 250/160 mm Hg, would you make a diagnosis of malignant *essential* hypertension or malignant hypertension *secondary* to polycystic kidneys?

Answer 1. Malignant hypertension secondary to polycystic kidneys. Go on to **14.42**.
2. Malignant *essential* hypertension. Go on to **14.44**.

14.41 Your answer – the prognosis is better in patients with renal impairment at the beginning of treatment.

No. If there is renal impairment at the beginning of therapy, as shown, say, by a raised blood urea, this is presumptive evidence of severe glomerular damage due to the severity of the hypertension, and this usually progresses irrespective of subsequent control of the hypertension, leading to death from renal failure. The absence of evidence of renal impairment indicates much less glomerular damage and thus the prognosis is better. Now answer the question in **14.45** again.

14.42 Your answer – the patient is suffering from malignant hypertension secondary to polycystic kidneys.

Correct. This is certainly the most likely diagnosis if you wish to avoid making two diagnoses – polycystic kidneys and malignant essential hypertension.

The majority of patients with malignant essential hypertension are males, in a ratio of male to female of 2 to 1. The average age of patients with this disease is 40 years.

Question Is malignant essential hypertension commoner in females or males?

Answer 1. In females. Go on to **14.47**.
2. In males. Go on to **14.45**.

14.43 Your answer – the prognosis is worse if renal impairment is present at the beginning of treatment.

You are correct. What is meant by the term 'renal impairment' in malignant hypertension? Albuminuria is very common in malignant hypertension and may be so massive that it causes nephrotic syndrome. *Microscopic* haematuria is usually present in malignant hypertension and sometimes reaches such massive proportions that *macroscopic* haematuria appears. An elevated blood urea is presumptive evidence of severe renal damage, which affects the prognosis adversely.

Question Is albuminuria rare in patients with malignant hypertension?

Answer 1. Yes. Go on to **14.46**.
2. No. Go on to **14.48**.

14.44 Your answer – the patient is suffering from malignant essential hypertension.

You may of course be perfectly correct, in that anybody can suffer from two diseases simultaneously, but it is axiomatic in medicine to attempt to make a single diagnosis to fit all the known facts. In this case malignant hypertension secondary to polycystic disease is a single diagnosis which is to be preferred; read **14.40** again and check over some of the other causes of malignant hypertension secondary to renal disease. Then answer the question again.

14.45 Your answer – it is commoner in males.

Correct. The main symptoms of malignant essential hypertension are defective vision (due to papilloedema, exudates and haemorrhages), headaches, dyspnoea on effort, and paroxysmal nocturnal dyspnoea, nocturia and haematuria. *About half the patients develop renal failure*, and with the advent of effective hypotensive drug therapy the major cause of death is renal failure, with cerebral haemorrhage, left ventricular failure, and myocardial infarction as common complications. In benign hypertension, renal failure is found much less frequently than in malignant hypertension. Untreated malignant hypertension causes death in 80 to 90 per cent of patients within 15 months, but with adequate hypotensive treatment in the patients without renal failure 25 per cent will survive 7 years. Patients with a blood urea level above 60 mg/100 ml at the beginning of treatment do badly, and the majority are dead in 5 years.

Question Does renal impairment at the beginning of treatment make the prognosis in malignant hypertension better or worse than in patients without initial renal impairment?

Answer 1. Better. Go on to **14.41**.
2. Worse. Go on to **14.43**.

14.46 Your answer – albuminuria is rare in malignant hypertension.
No. It is very common in malignant hypertension, in contrast to the rarity of albuminuria in benign hypertension. Read **14.43** again, the answer the question correctly.

14.47 Your answer – it is commoner in females.
No. Before picking the alternative answer to this question read **14.42** again to pick up any other facts you have missed.

14.48 Your answer – albuminuria is not rare in malignant hypertension.
You are correct. If a group of patients with untreated malignant hypertension is investigated, a significant proportion are found to have *hypokalaemia with an associated alkalosis*. This is probably due to secondary aldosteronism caused by hypersecretion of aldosterone, which has been demonstrated in malignant hypertension by Laragh and his co-workers, although in the treated case thiazide diuretics are frequently responsible. Buchborn has found that in malignant hypertension a defect in urine concentrating power is frequent, causing diabetes insipidus with negative values of $T_m{}^cH_2O$; sometimes the diabetes insipidus is nocturnal, but this is rare.

Question If a patient with *untreated* essential malignant hypertension has a serum potassium level of 2.7 mEq/l and a plasma pH of 7.52, what is likely to be the cause of this?

Answer 1. Aldosteronism. Go on to **14.49**.
2. Thiazide diuretics. Go on to **14.51**.

14.49 Your answer – the hypokalaemia is caused by aldosteronism.
You are correct. *The treatment of malignant hypertension should be considered an emergency*, because of the danger of widespread irreversible glomerular damage if the hypertension is allowed to persist. This means that the diastolic blood pressure should be brought down rapidly to about 100 mm Hg, using hypo-

tensive drugs such as guanethidine and thiazide diuretics with dietary salt restriction. Care should be taken to increase the dosage of guanethidine gradually if renal failure is already present, because of the tendency for a *sudden* fall in blood pressure to occur due to accumulation of the drug in the body. α Methyldopa has sometimes little hypotensive action in patients with malignant hypertension, and should not be selected as the sole drug in malignant hypertension, although it may be useful as a supporting drug in guanethidine therapy. Propranalol is useful but may cause heart failure.

Question Is it important to commence hypotensive treatment of malignant hypertension with minimal delay?

Answer 1. Yes. Go on to **14.52**.
2. No. Go on to **14.54**.

14.50 Your answer – statements 2 and 3 are true, 1 is false.

You are correct. You can now proceed to the next chapter. If you wish to read further about hypertension and the kidney the following references are well worth reading:

Books
Fishberg A. M. (1954) Hypertension and Nephritis. Lea & Febiger, Philadelphia.
Pickering G. W. (1955) High Blood Pressure. Churchill, London.
Smirk F. H. (1957) High Arterial Pressure. Charles C. Thomas, Springfield.
Articles
Shapiro A. P. et al. (1969), Am. J. Med. **47**, 175.
Breckenridge et al (1967) Quart. J. Med. **36**, 549.
Kincaid-Smith P., McMichael J. & Murphy E. A. (1958) Quart. J. Med. **27**, 117.
Bechgaard P. (1946) Acta Med. Scand. Suppl. **172**, 3.
Tobian L. (1960) Physiol. Rev. **40**, 280.
Schottstaedt M. F. & Sokolow M. (1953) Am. Heart J. **45**, 331.
Amsterdam et al. (1969) Am. J. Med. **47**, 860.
Dustan, H. P. (1969). New Eng. J. Med. **281**, 1348.
Brunner H. R. et al. New Engl. J. Med. (1972) **286**, 441.
Laragh, J. H. et al. Amer. J. Med. (1972) **53**, 649.
Guedon M. et al. Europ. J. Clin and biol. research 1972 **17**, 757.
Kaufman J. J. et al. J. Urol (1970) **103**, 702.

14.51 Your answer – the hypokalaemia is caused by thiazide diuretics.

In the question it was emphasized that no treatment has been given to the patient. Read **14.48** again before going on to answer the question correctly.

14.52 Your answer – it is important to commence hypotensive treatment with minimal delay.

Correct — You should read the following statements carefully and then choose the appropriate answer: this paragraph is an overall test of some important points in the chapter, and failure to choose the correct answer is indicative of poor learning and may oblige you to re-read some paragraphs.

Statement 1 Renal artery stenosis invariably causes hypertension.

Statement 2 1 in 10 patients with benign hypertension die of renal failure.

Statement 3 Proteinuria is common in malignant hypertension.

Answer   1. All the statements are true. Go on to **14.53**.
          2. All the statements are false. Go on to **14.55**.
          3. Only statement 1 is true. Go on to **14.56**.
          4. Only statement 2 is true. Go on to **14.57**.
          5. Only statement 3 is true. Go on to **14.58**.
          6. Statements 1 and 2 are true, 3 is false. Go on to **14.59**.
          7. Statements 1 and 3 are true, 2 is false. Go on to 14.60.
          8. Statements 2 and 3 are true, 1 is false. Go on to **14.50**.

14.53   Your answer — all the statements are true.

You are correct about 2 and 3, but incorrect about statement 1. Go back to **14.6** and read on from there to **14.33** and then answer the question in **14.52** again.

14.54   Your answer — it is not important if the treatment of malignant hypertension is delayed.

You are wrong. The treatment of malignant hypertension is as much an emergency as is the treatment of subacute bacterial endocarditis. Failure to reduce the diastolic blood pressure may lead to necrosis of glomeruli and irreversible renal failure. Read **14.49** again carefully before you answer the question.

14.55   Your answer — all the statements are false.

You are correct about the first statement only, having forgotten some very important facts about benign and malignant hypertension. Read from **14.33** on to the end of the chapter.

14.56   Your answer — only statement 1 is true.

You are entirely incorrect. Start at the beginning of this chapter and work through it.

14.57   Your answer — only statement 2 is true.

You are correct about statements 1 and 2 but incorrect about statement 3. Read **14.43** and continue through to the end of the chapter.

14.58 Your answer — only statement 3 is true.

You are correct about 1 and 3 but are wrong about statement 2. Read from **14.33** to **14.43** and then answer **14.52** correctly.

14.59 Your answer — only statement 3 is false.

You are correct about statement 2 only. Read from **14.6** to **14.33** and from **14.43** to the end of the chapter.

14.60 Your answer — only statement 2 is false.

You are correct about statement 3 but wrong about 1 and 2. Start at the beginning of the chapter and work back through it to **14.43**. Then answer the question in **14.52** correctly.

Time for this chapter: 50 minutes

Chapter 15
Renal tubular disorders

15.1 In this chapter various syndromes associated with renal tubular dysfunction will be discussed.

The arrangement of the chapter will be to consider proximal tubular abnormalities first, followed by distal tubular and then mixed proximal and distal tubular abnormalities. The functions of the proximal renal tubule were described in Chapter 2, and included reabsorption of filtered water, sodium and potassium, chloride, bicarbonate, reabsorption of amino acids, glucose, phosphate and urate, some acidification of tubular fluid and some ammonia production.

Let us first consider the commoner disturbances of amino acid metabolism.

Cystinuria is a condition in which cystine stones are formed, although urinary lysine excretion is twice that of cystine. Cystine is, however, much less soluble than lysine in urine with a pH less than 7, so that cystine stones form in the urinary pathways, the lysine remaining inconspicuously in solution. Cystine stones in the urinary tract cause pain, haematuria and urinary tract infection.

Question In cystinuria, why is it that lysine stones are not prominent if more lysine is excreted than cystine?

Answer 1. Lysine stones *are* common. Go on to **15.3**.
2. Cystine is less soluble than is lysine in acid urine. Go on to **15.5**.

15.2 Your answer — cystine stones are more soluble in acid solution.

No. The solubility of cystine is less in acid urine than in alkaline solution. You should read **15.5** again then answer the question correctly.

15.3 Your answer — lysine stones are common.

No. Lysine is much more soluble in water than is cystine; cystine is remarkably insoluble in acid urine, but is more soluble in alkaline urine. Hence cystine stones are common in cystinuria, but their frequency may be reduced by alkalinisation and dilution of the urine. Read **15.1** again and answer the question correctly.

15.4 Your answer — cystine stones are more soluble in alkaline solution.

You are correct. An alternative and effective form of treatment in cystinuria is to reduce the solubility of cystine in the urine by administration of penicillamine, which in cystinurics is excreted as the mixed penicillin — cystine disulphide. This mixed disulphide is soluble. Penicillamine however has nephrotoxic side effects, nephrotic syndrome being the most serious. Nevertheless, Kincaid-Smith has found that penicillamine is more likely to succeed in causing cystine stones to disappear than is an alkaline-diuretic regimen. This is probably because it is easier to take a few tablets each day than 3 litres of water. The chance of nephrotoxicity from penicillamine is probably worth taking. The inheritance of cystinuria will now be considered. There are two main groups of cystinuric patients. In group 1, the disease is inherited as a recessive, and the homozygote excretes large amounts of crystine, lysine, arginine and ornithine — you will recall that these four amino acids have a common transport mechanism — whereas the normal and the heterozygote excrete a normal urinary amino acid pattern. In group 2, the homozygotes are similar to those in group 1, but the heterozygotes have an increased urinary excretion of cystine and lysine only. In group 1 the inheritance is recessive in type; in group 2 the inheritance is 'incompletely' recessive: the homozygotes form cystine stones; the heterozygotes in group 2 are found on familial investigation but have no stone formation or other symptoms.

Question Is the inheritance of cystinuria by a dominant or recessive gene?

Answer 1. Dominant. Go on to **15.7**.
2. Recessive. Go on to **15.9**.

15.5 Your answer — cystine is less soluble than is lysine.

You are correct. Because of the solubility of cystine being greater in alkaline urine, Dent and his co-workers suggested that cystine stones could be dissolved or their formation discouraged by increasing the urine volume to 3 litres over the 24 hours (*including the night period*), together with the administration of alkalies to keep the urine pH persistently over 7. This treatment is remarkably effective, and cystine stones can be shown to disappear.

Question Is cystine more soluble in acid or alkaline urine?

Answer 1. More soluble in acid. Go on to **15.2**.
2. More soluble in alkaline. Go on to **15.4**.

15.6 Your answer — cystine stones are radio-opaque.

You are correct. Lignac-Fanconi syndrome is found in two different forms, that seen in infants, and that seen in adults. It should be understood at the outset that *the infantile form is a quite different disease from the adult form*. The infantile disease is inherited as a recessive trait and is probably due to an abnormality in the enzyme *cystine reductase*. The absence of this enzyme increases the cystine concentration in body fluids and thus causes the deposition of cystine crystals throughout the body, cystine crystals being visible in the cornea and conjunctiva, bone marrow, leucocytes and throughout the reticulo-endothelial system. The main renal change is a 'swan neck' deformity of the proximal tubule. This change is also found in adult Fanconi syndrome.

Question What crystalline substance is found to be visible in the leucocytes in infantile Lignac-Fanconi syndrome?
Answer 1. Cystine. Go on to **15.11**.
2. Lysine. Go on to **15.13**.

15.7 Your answer – cystinuria is inherited by a dominant mode of inheritance.

No. There are two types of inheritance in cystinuria, the 'recessive' and the 'incompletely recessive' form. In both these forms the homozygote suffers from cystine stones. In group 1 (purely recessive) the heterozygote form is not recognisable biochemically or clinically. In group 2 (incompletely recessive) the urinary excretion of the amino acids cystine and lysine is found to be abnormally high in the heterozygote form although it is not extensive enough to be associated with cystine stone formation. Now answer the question in **15.4** correctly.

15.8 Your answer – cystine stones are not radio-opaque.

You are incorrect. In **15.9** it is stated that cystine stones are radio-opaque because the cystine molecule contains sulphur atoms. Now read **15.9** again, paying more attention, then answer the question.

15.9 Your answer – cystinuria is inherited as a recessive.

You are correct. One thing which you must bear in mind about cystinuria is that cystine stones are radio-opaque although they are not as radio-opaque as oxalate stones. They can be detected on a plain X-ray of the abdomen. The radio-opacity is due to the sulphur atoms present in the cystine molecule. Cystine stones are often found in the bladder as large solitary stones, and then they may be coated with calcium phosphate, being made even more radio-opaque by this coating.

Question Are cystine stones radio-opaque?
Answer 1. Yes. Go on to **15.6**.
2. No. Go on to **15.8**.

15.10 Your answer – in infantile Lignac-Fanconi syndrome there is a pure proximal tubular lesion.

No. You should look at **15.11** again more carefully. You will read that there are distal tubular abnormalities as well as proximal tubular defects. Now answer the question again.

15.11 Your answer – cystine crystals are visible in the leucocytes in Lignac-Fanconi syndrome.

Correct. In this disease there are both proximal and distal tubular abnormalities giving rise to the following clinical picture:

The infant of six months to one year old develops vomiting, refusal to eat and failure to thrive; weight gain stops; there is polyuria and thirst due to inability to concentrate the urine, and rickets may be present due to hypophosphataemia. There is glycosuria and amino-aciduria. The child may be weak or suffer muscular paralysis from hypokalaemia; he may be acidotic and ketotic from starvation and may suffer from photophobia due to the ocular deposits of cystine.

Question Are the abnormalities in infantile Lignac-Fanconi syndrome characteristic of a pure proximal tubular lesion or are they due to both proximal and distal tubular lesions?

Answer 1. Pure proximal tubular lesion. Go on to **15.10**.
2. Mixed proximal and distal tubular lesions. Go on to **15.14**.

15.12 Your answer — the child has Lignac-Fanconi syndrome.

No. You would expect more evidence of proximal tubular abnormalities if the diagnosis were Lignac-Fanconi syndrome. As it stands the diagnosis in this patient would be renal glycosuria. Read **15.14** more carefully and answer the question again.

15.13 Your answer — Lysine is the crystalline substance found in the leucocytes in Lignac-Fanconi syndrome.

No. The answer to this question is given in **15.6**. One of the major histological findings in this disease is the deposition of cystine crystals in various tissues throughout the body, including the leucocytes. Go back and read **15.6** more carefully, then answer the question correctly.

15.14 Your answer — mixed proximal and distal tubular lesions are present.

Correct. The amino-aciduria is a widespread non-specific type involving a moderate increase in the excretion of alanine, valine, cystine, serine, glycine, ornithine, glutamine and asparagine. The amino-aciduria is due to an abnormality in the proximal tubular reabsorption of amino acids and is not associated with elevated plasma amino acid levels. There is also a defect in phosphate reabsorption leading to a *lower* tubular reabsorption of phosphate and consequently a low plasma phosphate. This leads to the development of rickets. Renal glycosuria is present due to a reduction in TmG. Plasma urate levels are abnormally low because of the reduction in tubular urate reabsorption. In practice, therefore, one can diagnose Lignac-Fanconi syndrome biochemically by the presence of renal glycosuria, amino-aciduria, low serum phosphate, and low serum urate.

Question A child has glycosuria when his blood sugar level is 120 mg/100 ml but no amino-aciduria, and his serum phosphate and urate levels are normal. Do you think it is likely that he has Lignac-Fanconi syndrome?

Answer 1. Yes. Go on to **15.12**.
2. No. Go on to **15.16**.

15.15 Your answer – the dose of Calciferol is 500 units a day.
You are guessing. Read **15.20** again, carefully this time, then choose the correct answer.

15.16 Your answer – the child is *not* suffering from Lignac-Fanconi syndrome.
Correct. A more detailed study of distal tubular function in Lignac-Fanconi syndrome reveals an impairment of concentrating ability out of proportion to the reduction in glomerular filtration rate. Acidification of the urine is impaired: in spite of a persistent systemic acidosis the urinary pH is above 5.2 – often 6.0–7.0 i.e., the patient has distal renal tubular acidosis, a syndrome which will be discussed later in the chapter. Potassium conservation is impaired, possibly due to the loss of potassium in the ion-exchange of sodium for potassium during distal sodium reabsorption; in the normal person hydrogen ion as well as potassium is available for exchange with sodium whereas in the syndrome of renal tubular acidosis little or no hydrogen ion is available for the exchange, so that one potassium ion is lost for every sodium ion reabsorbed distally.

Question In a patient suffering from Lignac-Fanconi syndrome with a severe systemic acidosis, would you expect the urine pH to be more likely 4.6 or 6.0?

Answer 1. pH = 4.6. Go on to **15.18**.
2. pH = 6.0. Go on to **15.20**.

15.17 Your answer – the dose of calciferol is 250,000 units a day.
Correct. The prognosis in Lignac-Fanconi syndrome is bad: affected infants often die within a few months from dehydration or acidosis but affected children may live up to 10 or 15 years of age, particularly those who first present with rickets at the age of 2 years and have a generally milder course than the infantile form. It should be emphasised that this later childhood form is very similar to the infantile form, with cystine crystals deposited throughout the reticulo-endothelial system, cornea and conjunctiva and although the prognosis is somewhat better (a survival for several years being common) survival beyond puberty is exceptional. These infantile and childhood forms of Lignac-Fanconi syndrome are totally different from the adult disease in which cystine deposits are conspicuously absent.

Question Are cystine deposits found in the form of Lignac-Fanconi syndrome which presents in early childhood with rickets?

Answer 1. Yes. Go on to **15.19**.
2. No. Go on to **15.21**.

15.18 Your answer – the urine pH would be more likely 4.6.

No. In Lignac-Fanconi syndrome there is frequently a distal tubular abnormality of urine acidification, so that although the patient is severely acidotic the urine pH is fairly high. This is described in **15.16**. Go back and read it carefully.

15.19 Your answer – cystine deposits are found in patients with Lignac-Fanconi syndrome of childhood.

Good. The adult form of Fanconi syndrome is a most interesting but rare disease. Cystine is *not* deposited in the tissues in the adult form of Fanconi syndrome, although there are many other similarities. Some patients with the adult Fanconi syndrome have an inherited form of the disease but it may be *acquired* as in dysproteinaemias such as myelomatosis. The inherited form is recessive in its mode of inheritance, i.e., it occurs in siblings of one generation but not in successive generations in the same family.

Question Is the inherited form of adult Fanconi syndrome inherited by a dominant or recessive gene?

Answer 1. Dominant. Go on to **15.23**.
         2. Recessive. Go on to **15.25**.

15.20 Your answer – the urine pH is more likely to be 6.0.

Correct. The treatment of Lignac-Fanconi syndrome is entirely symptomatic. It is necessary to give copious fluids to prevent dehydration; the renal tubular acidosis requires treatment with Shohl's solution (a sodium citrate-citric acid mixture) and the hypokalaemia requires potassium therapy such as potassium citrate. For the rickets, treatment with large doses of calciferol, 250,000 units a day, will usually be adequate and result in healing. There is the ever present danger of hypercalcaemia due to vitamin D intoxication; consequently, the serum calcium level should be measured at frequent intervals and if levels above 11 mg/100 ml are encountered the calciferol should be temporarily suspended until normocalcaemia has been re-established.

Question What dose of calciferol would you prescribe for the treatment of rickets due to Lignac-Fanconi syndrome?

Answer 1. 500 units a day. Go on to **15.15**.
         2. 250,000 units a day. Go on to **15.17**.

15.21 Your answer – cystine deposits are not found in patients with the childhood form of Lignac-Fanconi syndrome.

You are wrong. Go back to **15.17** and read the paragraph again so that you pick up other facts which you may have missed. Then answer the question correctly.

15.22   Your answer – the cause of the bony pain is psychological.
   Unfortunately, the diagnosis of psychogenic pain is made for years before it is realized that organic disease is present and that the bone pain is due to osteomalacia; at this stage the urine is tested and glycosuria is detected without associated hyperglycaemia, so the patient is referred from the psychiatrist or orthopaedic surgeon to the physician. Now read **15.25** again. Then choose the correct answer.

15.23   Your answer – the inherited form of adult Fanconi sydrome is inherited as a dominant.
   No. It is inherited as a recessive. You have not read **15.19** with enough attention. Read it carefully again.

15.24   Your answer – the bone pain is caused by osteomalacia.
   Correct. The treatment of adult Fanconi syndrome is symptomatic: the correction of acidosis by Shohl's solution; calciferol in doses of 50,000 – 250,000 units a day for osteomalacia; potassium salts for hypokalaemia; and adequate fluid intake. There is a slow and progressive decrease in renal function in hereditary adult Fanconi patients partly due to renal infection which is so commonly associated with hypokalaemia.

Question Is adult Fanconi syndrome rapidly or slowly progressive?

Answer 1. Rapidly. Go on to **15.27**.
            2. Slowly. Go on to **15.29**.

15.25   Your answer – it is inherited as a recessive.
   Good. In adult Fanconi syndrome the patients most frequently are referred from the orthopaedic or psychiatric department to which they have been sent because of aches and pains all over the body. Careful history taking and examination reveal that the pain is bone pain, and biochemical and radiological examination show that severe osteomalacia is present with reduced bone density, codfish vertebrae, and Looser's nodes. There are also proximal and distal tubular lesions similar to those in infantile Lignac-Fanconi syndrome: these include renal glycosuria, a generalised aminoaciduria with normal or low plasma amino acids, hypophosphataemia with a decreased tubular reabsorption of phosphate, hypouricaemia, hypokalaemia and reduction in concentrating and acidifying ability, the latter causing a renal tubular acidosis syndrome. This will be described later. In a few cases of adult Fanconi syndrome there is an associated cirrhosis of the liver; in this form tyrosine loss in the urine is heavy and may itself be the factor predisposing to the cirrhosis.

Question What is the cause of the bony pain in adult Fanconi syndrome?

Answer 1. Psychological. Go on to **15.22**.
2. Osteomalacia. Go on to **15.24.**

15.26 Your answer – amino-aciduria is present in Lowe's syndrome.

You are correct. Another amino-aciduria of interest from the point of view of renal disease is that of hereditary glycinuria. This very rare amino-aciduria is associated with a urinary glycine excretion of about 1 gram a day (five times normal); calcium oxalate stones were present in the family studied by de Vries and his colleagues but it is not proven that they were not coincidental.

Question What type of renal stones were found in a family with hereditary glycinuria?

Answer 1. Glycine stones. Go on to **15.30**.
2. Calcium oxalate stones. Go on to **15.32.**

15.27 Your answer – adult Fanconi syndrome is rapildy progressive.

No. It is slowly progressive, taking many years before renal failure sets in. Read **15.24** again before choosing the correct answer.

15.28 Your answer – amino-aciduria is not present in Lowe's syndrome.

You are wrong. One of the important and characteristic features of Lowe's syndrome is amino-aciduria, in which lysine and tyrosine are predominant. Go back over **15.29** more carefully. Then answer the question correctly.

15.29 Your answer – adult Fanconi syndrome is slowly progressive.

You are correct. Lowe's syndrome is a rare disease; it is also known as cerebro-oculo-renal dystrophy, and is inherited as a sex-linked recessive. The disease affects infants at birth, the affected infants have cataracts and buphthalmos (congenital glaucoma) which may lead to total or partial blindness. They are severely mentally retarded, and muscular hypotonia is evident. The renal anomaly is a diffuse tubular anomaly – renal glycosuria, amino-aciduria with increase in lysine or tyrosine particularly, organic aciduria, hypophosphataemia and decreased tubular reabsorption of phosphate, inability to concentrate the urine and a defect of urinary acidification. Nephrocalcinosis may occur. The patients die of intercurrent infections or renal failure in infancy or childhood.

Question Is amino-aciduria present in Lowe's syndrome?

Answer 1. Yes. Go on to **15.26**.
2. No. Go on to **15.28.**

15.30 Your answer – glycine stones are found in hereditary glycinuria.

No. The stones found in hereditary glycinuria are calcium oxalate stones. Read **15.26** again before answering the question.

15.31 Your answer – the disease presents as osteo-arthritis in children.

No. It presents in adults in middle age as severe osteo-arthritis. In infants and children it presents as rickets. Go back and choose the correct answer in **15.34**.

15.32 Your answer – calcium oxalate stones are found in hereditary glycinuria.

Correct. Phosphate reabsorption in the proximal tubule is also depressed in *vitamin D resistant rickets*. This is inherited as a *sex-linked dominant* and affects more females than males. Affected males transmit the disease to all their daughters, but none of their sons is affected. Affected females transmit the disease to half their sons and half their daughters.

Question Is Vitamin D resistant rickets transmitted as a dominant or as a recessive?

Answer 1. Dominant. Go on to **15.34**.
2. Recessive. Go on to **15.36**.

15.33 Your answer – the disease presents as rickets in infants and children.

You are correct. The most readily recognisable biochemical abnormalities are the low serum inorganic phosphorus concentration and a raised serum alkaline phosphatase. The low level of serum inorganic phosphorus is caused by the loss of phosphate in the urine due to the reduction in renal tubular phosphate reabsorption. The alkaline phosphatase elevation is a reflection of the osteoblastic activity in the bone itself. Plasma calcium is usually normal.

Question What is the cause of the low serum inorganic phosphate level in vitamin D resistant rickets?

Answer 1. Hyperparathyroidism. Go on to **15.35**.
2. Low tubular reabsorption of phosphate. Go on to **15.37**.

15.34 Your answer – the disease is inherited as a dominant.

Correct. Vitamin D resistant rickets presents in two age groups: in infancy and childhood when rickets is the main manifestation; and in the middle-aged in which the disease presents as severe and crippling osteo-arthritis in a stunted or dwarfed adult.

Question How does the disease present in infancy and childhood?

Answer 1. As osteo-arthritis. Go on to **15.31**.
2. As rickets. Go on to **15.33**.

15.35 Your answer – the cause of the low serum inorganic phosphorus level is hyperparathyroidism.

No. The key biochemical abnormality in hyperparathyroidism is the raised serum calcium concentration. In vitamin D resistant rickets serum calcium is not elevated; sometimes it is normal and occasionally it is depressed. Do not guess answers: if you had read **15.33** carefully the correct answer would have been chosen. Choose the correct answer after reading the paragraph.

15.36 Your answer – vitamin D resistant rickets is inherited as a recessive.
No. The disease is inherited as a dominant, being manifest in generation after generation. Read **15.32** again and choose the correct answer.

15.37 Your answer – the cause of the low serum inorganic phosphorus level is the reduced renal tubular reabsorption of phosphate.
Good. The clinical manifestations of the disease are similar to those of nutritional rickets with epiphyseal changes, e.g. genu valgum or varum and resulting dwarfism, in spite of an apparently adequate intake of vitamin D, i.e., an intake of vitamin D sufficient to prevent rickets in a normal child. Muscular hypotonia and tetany are absent in vitamin D resistant rickets.

Question Can vitamin D resistant rickets develop if a child is given a dose of vitamin D sufficient to prevent the onset of ordinary rickets?

Answer 1. Yes. Go on to **15.39**.
        2. No. Go on to **15.41**.

15.38 If you are reading this you are not following the instructions. Attempting to read straight through without following the instructions is a waste of your time and effort.

15.39 Your answer – vitamin D resistant rickets can develop when the patient is being given a small dose of vitamin D adequate to prevent the development of ordinary rickets.
Good. The basic abnormality in vitamin D resistant rickets appears to be this remarkable resistance to the action of vitamin D, which can only be overcome by massive doses of vitamin D, or the order of 500,000 units of calciferol a day. The precise biochemical reason for this resistance to vitamin D is not known at present. It should be borne in mind that on dosage of this magnitude vitamin D may prove toxic, causing hypercalcaemia; accordingly patients on this dosage should have frequent serum calcium determinations.

Question What is the hazard in giving massive doses of vitamin D?

Answer 1. There is no hazard. Go on to **15.42**.
        2. Hypercalcaemia. Go on to **15.44**.

15.40 Your answer – I would accept a diagnosis of RTA if the urine pH fell to

You are wrong. The definition given in **15.44** was that the urine pH remained above 5.4 in spite of an adequate stress of acidosis. You should now choose the correct answer after reading **15.44**.

15.41 Your answer — vitamin D resistant rickets *cannot* develop while vitamin D is administered in a dosage sufficient to prevent the onset of ordinary rickets.

No. The difference between the two conditions which is at once striking is that the disease can develop when *small* doses of vitamin D are being given. Read **15.37** to make sure you have missed no other facts. Then choose the correct answer to the question.

15.42 Your answer — there is no hazard in giving massive doses of vitamin D.

You are wrong. There is always a hazard in giving large doses of vitamin D due to the production of vitamin D intoxication with hypercalcaemia. The hazard was mentioned in **15.39**. Go back and read that paragraph again; then choose the correct answer.

15.43 Your answer — I would reject a diagnosis of distal RTA if the urine pH fell to 4.6.

Correct. The normal person can produce a hydrogen ion concentration in the urine of 800 to 1,000 times that in the blood. Exactly why this cannot be done in the kidney of the patient with distal RTA is unknown, but an abnormality in hydrogen ion secretion appears to be the basic defect. The inability to lower the urinary pH leads to a reduction in total hydrogen ion excretion. You will remember from Chapter 2 that total hydrogen ion excretion is calculated as follows:

$H^+ = NH_3 + TA - HCO_3^-$ where H^+ = total hydrion excretion per minute.
NH_3 = ammonia excretion in mMols/min.
TA = titratable acidity in mEq/min.
HCO_3^- = bicarbonate excretion in mEg/min.

Now both TA and ammonia excretion are likely to be lower in conditions where the urinary pH is more than 5.4. The reasons for this are as follows:

Firstly, ammonia rediffuses back from the tubular lumen into the tubular cells unless the ammonia molecules are captured by hydrogen ions and converted into ammonium ions:

$$NH_3 + H^+ \longrightarrow NH_4^+$$

The ammonium ions, being charged, have great difficulty in diffusing back through the tubular cell wall from the tubular urine. Thus if more hydrogen ion is available, more ammonia will be 'captured' by hydrion and excreted in the urine as ammonium. More hydrogen ion is excreted therefore as ammonium when the urinary pH is low than when it is high.

Question Can ammonium ion diffuse back into the tubular cells from tubular lumen as readily as can ammonia molecules?

Answer 1. Yes. Go on to **15.46**.
2. No. Go on to **15.48**.

15.44 Your answer – the hazard in giving very large doses is hypercalcaemia.
Good. The next subject to be discussed is renal tubular acidosis (RTA). At the outset it should be made clear that this is not a disease sui generis, but a syndrome with many causes, which may be distal tubular in type and be characterised by – *the inability to produce a urine pH of below 5.4 under the stimulus of spontaneous metabolic acidosis or under the stress of a metabolic acidosis produced by the administration of ammonium chloride; or proximal in type with a urinary loss of bicarbonate at abnormally low levels of plasma bicarbonate; there is also a mixed form.*

Look at Fig. 15.44. It shows the urine pH at varying serum CO_2 levels in normal subjects and patients with proximal RTA. At a serum CO_2 level of 14 to 16 mEq/L the urine pH may still be 5.5, but it falls to less than 5 as the serum CO_2 falls to between 12 and 14 mEq/L. In distal RTA the pH remains above 5.1 irrespective of the plasma CO_2 level. In distal RTA the actual loss of bicarbonate in the urine is

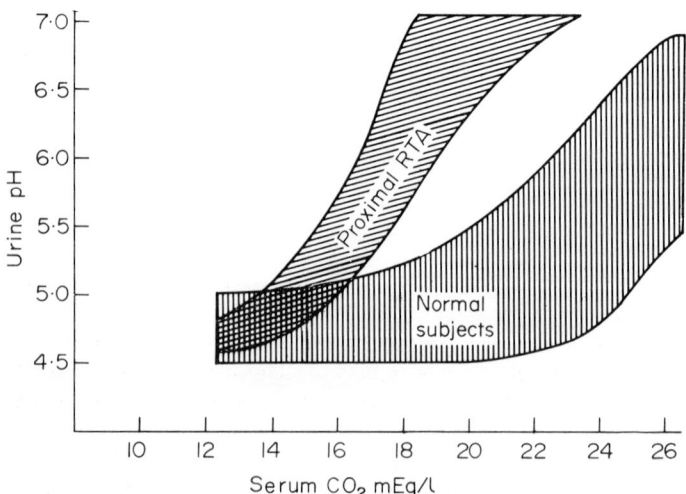

Fig. 15.44

small compared to the greater loss of bicarbonate in the urine in cases of proximal RTA.

Question If you gave a patient a metabolic acidosis using ammonium chloride and his urinary pH fell to 4.6 would you accept a diagnosis of distal renal tubular acidosis?

Answer 1. Yes. Go on to **15.40**.
2. No. Go on to **15.43**.

15.45 Your answer – at pH 4.6 there are urinary buffers of importance, other than phosphate.

Good. The acidosis of distal RTA is due mainly to an inability to acidify the urine rather than to destruction of tubules and glomeruli as seen in the acidosis of chronic renal failure, (although, contrary to other workers, we find a high proportion of the latter group are also unable to produce a highly acid urine). The common biochemical abnormalities in distal RTA are systemic acidosis with a paradoxically alkaline urine, low plasma bicarbonate, high plasma chloride and normal or low plasma phosphate. The plasma chloride is high in distal RTA because there is no general renal failure initially to cause retention of phosphate, sulphate, urate and organic acid such as is found in advanced renal failure with acidosis; so in distal RTA plasma chloride fills the gap left when plasma bicarbonate is lowered by the acidosis.

In proximal RTA the urine contains bicarbonate at a time when the plasma bicarbonate is below 25mM/L. You will recall that in normal people the $TmHCO_3$ is such that at levels of plasma bicarbonate below 25mM/L bicarbonate is completely reabsorbed from the tubular fluid and the urine is bicarbonate-free. In proximal RTA acidification of the urine to below 5.2 may occur. Look at Fig. 15.44 on the facing page.

Question Is plasma chloride high or low in distal RTA?

Answer 1. High. Go on to **15.47**.
2. Low. Go on to **15.49**.

15.46 Your answer – ammonium ion can diffuse as easily back into the cells as ammonia.

No. The cell membrane permits non-ionic diffusion much more readily than the diffusion of ions. Therefore ammonia will be able to diffuse back in much better than ammonium ion. Read **15.43** again before you choose the correct answer.

15.47 Your answer – plasma chloride is elevated in distal RTA.

Correct. The other biochemical abnormalities found in distal RTA reflect the clinical picture. Paralysis may occur because the serum potassium level is low; this is due to sodium reabsorption at the distal tubular exchange site, where H^+ or K^+ is available in the normal for exchange with Na^+ being reabsorbed. In distal RTA the H^+ is not available for secretion into the lumen – the apparent primary abnormality in this condition – and so for every sodium ion reabsorbed *at this site* a potassium ion is lost. There is also the possibility that secondary aldosteronism is present to stimulate further K^+ loss in the urine. A combination of these factors can cause severe potassium depletion, with muscular paralysis.

Question If no hydrogen ion can be secreted at the sodium-reabsorption site, how many potassium ions must be exchanged for each sodium ion exchanged here?

Answer 1. One. Go on to **15.52**.
          2. Two. Go on to **15.54**.

15.48 Your answer – ammonium ion cannot diffuse back into the cell as readily as ammonia.

Correct. Although ammonia is responsible for more than half the total hydrogen ion excreted, titratable acidity (TA) is responsible for most of the remaining hydrogen ion excretion. TA represents hydrogen ion mopped up by the urinary buffers – phosphate, creatinine, and, as the pH falls, the organic acids. If the pH is above 5.5, the organic acids and creatinine are of less importance as hydrogen ion acceptors whereas phosphate becomes the major hydrion acceptor.

Question At a pH of 4.6, are there any important urinary buffers other than phosphate?

Answer 1. Yes. Go on to **15.45**.
          2. No. Go on to **15.50**.

15.49 Your answer – plasma chloride is low in RTA.

You are correct only when renal failure has developed. In the majority of patients with RTA there is no generalised renal failure for years, and plasma chloride is elevated to fill the gap caused by the fall in HCO_3^-. Read **15.45** to get more details of this, then answer the question correctly.

15.50 Your answer – At pH 4.6 there are no other buffers of importance.

No. Read **15.48** again and you will see that as the urine pH falls below 5.5 the organic acids and creatinine have an increasingly important role as urinary buffers. Now answer the question in **15.48** correctly.

15.51 Your answer – the cause of the bone pain in RTA is psychological.

No. You are guessing. You have not read **15.58** properly. Read it again, carefully, then answer the question.

15.52 Your answer – one K^+ is exchanged for each Na^+.

Correct. Another striking biochemical finding is that of a low serum inorganic phosphorus level associated with decrease in tubular phosphate reabsorption; there is also a raised alkaline phosphatase. The cause of this lowered serum inorganic phosphorus level is a combination of secondary hyperparathyroidism and the systemic acidosis. The alkaline phosphatase elevation is associated with osteomalacia.

Question What causes the reduced tubular reabsorption of phosphate in RTA?

Answer 1. Hyperparathyroidism. Go on to **15.55**.
2. Acidosis. Go on to **15.56**.
3. Combination of hyperparathyroidism and acidosis. Go on to **15.58**.
4. Don't know. Go on to **15.60**.

15.53 Your answer – the cause of the bone pain in RTA is osteomalacia.

Correct. Many patients present with renal colic due to the passage of calculi. Look at Fig. 15.53. It is a plain X-ray of the abdomen of a man with distal RTA aged 51 and shows nephrocalcinosis with some areas of calcification which enlarge, enter the pelvis and may be passed as ureteric stones (causing renal colic) or pre-

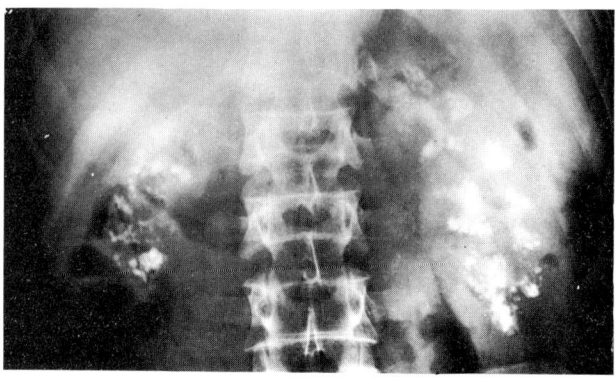

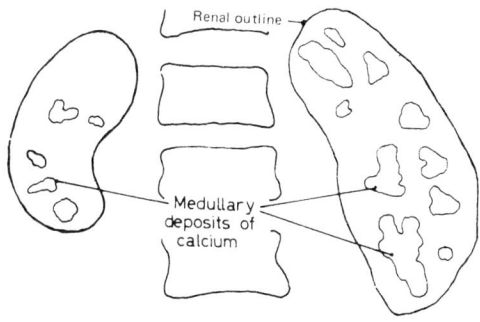

Fig. 15.53

cipitate an acute urinary infection such as pyelonephritis. The cause of the renal stones which are commonly found in RTA is probably related to the lowered urinary citrate excretion in this disease, a function of the acidosis. Citrate can chelate calcium and so keep it in solution.

Question What is the cause of nephrocalcinosis in RTA?

Answer 1. Pyelonephritis. Go on to **15.57**.
2. Low urinary citrate excretion. Go on to **15.59**.

15.54 Your answer — two K^+ are exchanged for each Na^+.

No. At the ion exchange site one ion of sodium is exchanged for one ion of potassium *or* one ion of hydrogen; if hydrogen is not available, then *one* ion of potassium is lost for each sodium ion absorbed *at this site*. Now choose the correct answer to the question in **15.47**.

15.55 Your answer — the cause is hyperparathyroidism.

You are probably correct, but the acidosis almost certainly plays some part. Go on to **15.58**.

15.56 Your answer — the cause is acidosis.

There is some evidence that acidosis is a factor but hyperparathyroidism is a more likely cause. Go on to **15.58**.

15.57 Your answer — the cause of the nephrocalcinosis is pyelonephritis.

No. Pyelonephritis frequently follows nephrocalcinosis but it is not likely to be the cause. Read **15.33** again, and answer the question correctly.

15.58 Your answer — the cause of the reduced tubular reabsorption of phosphate is the combination of hyperparathyroidism and acidosis.

You are correct. The clinical manifestations of the disease will now be described. Firstly, the patient may present with muscular paralysis due to hypokalaemia. Secondly, he may present with osteomalacia, bone pains, deformity and Looser's nodes. The cause of this is the hypophosphataemia described in the previous paragraph.

Question If a patient with RTA has bone pain what is the most likely cause?

Answer 1. Psychological. Go on to **15.51**.
2. Osteomalacia. Go on to **15.53**.

15.59 Your answer — the cause of the nephrocalcinosis is the low urinary citrate.

Good. The majority of the patients develop distal RTA, or have it recognised, in adolescence and early adult life. The ratio of males to females is 1:2, and the diagnosis is sometimes first made when females have the abdomen X-rayed for gynaecological or other reasons, and the nephrocalcinosis is then noticed.

Question Is the distal renal tubular acidosis of adults commoner in males or females?

Answer 1. Males. Go on to **15.62**.
2. Females. Go on to **15.64**.

15.60 Your answer – I don't know why tubular reabsorption of phosphate is reduced.

If you don't know you have not concentrated adequately while reading **15.52**. Do not continue reading if you are being distracted – you have to give particularly full attention to your reading in this chapter, much of it being difficult to absorb. Read **15.52** again and choose the correct answer this time.

15.61 Your answer – the concentrating defect may be useful.

Correct. There are many causes of distal RTA. There is first of all the rare inherited disease, probably inherited as an autosomal dominant. RTA syndrome may also be acquired in pyelonephritis, hydronephrosis, hypokalaemia and hypercalcaemia as well as in cystic medullary disease of the kidney. In all these diseases the medulla is the site of the major anatomical lesion, (and in particular the distal convoluted and collecting tubules), so that it is not surprising that there is an acidification defect in these patients which is responsible for the RTA syndrome.

Question Is the medulla or cortex the major site of disease in patients acquiring the distal RTA syndrome?

Answer 1. Medulla. Go on to **15.63**.
2. Cortex. Go on to **15.65**.

15.62 Your answer – adult distal type RTA is commoner in males than in females.

No. Females are twice as commonly affected as males. Read **15.59** again then choose the correct answer.

15.63 Your answer – the disease is mainly in the medulla.

You are correct. The treatment of this disease is straight forward. One gives a mixture of sodium and potassium citrate in a dosage of up to 8g/day, increasing until the plasma pH and serum potassium are within the normal range: hypertension may require treatment with guanethidine or other hypotensive drugs. Pyelonephritis should be treated with antibiotics.

Question How far should one push the dose of sodium and potassium citrate?

Answer 1. Until the patient is alkalotic. Go on to **15.67**.
2. Until the patient's pH and serum K are normal. Go on to **15.69**.

15.64 Your answer – adult distal type RTA is commoner in females.
Correct. Defects of urinary concentrating ability are found in distal RTA quite commonly, with difficulty in concentrating to an osmolality greater than that of plasma. This polyuria causes the symptoms of nocturia and severe thirst, but it may reduce the amount of calcium phosphate deposited as nephrocalcinosis.

Question May the concentrating defect of distal RTA be useful?

Answer 1. Yes. Go on to **15.61**.
2. No. Go on to **15.66**.

15.65 Your answer – the disease is mainly in the cortex.
No. You have missed the point made in **15.61**, that the diseases causing the RTA syndrome are primarily medullary – the site of final acidification of the tubular fluid being in the distal convoluted tubule and collecting tubules. Go back and read **15.61** again, then answer the question correctly.

15.66 Your answer – the concentrating defect is of no use.
No. It may keep calcium phosphate in solution which would otherwise have been deposited as nephrocalcinotic nodules. Read **15.64** again.

15.67 Your answer – push citrates until the patient is alkalotic.
No. The idea of therapy is not to make the patient alkalotic but to get the plasma pH in the normal range and adjust the ratio of sodium to potassium citrates until serum potassium levels are normal. Read **15.63** again.

15.68 Your answer – all the statements are false.
You are correct about statements 1 and 3 but incorrect about 2. Read from **15.47** to **15.87** then answer **15.81** again.

15.69 Your answer – give citrates until plasma pH and serum potassium are normal.
Good. The latter may require adjustment of the ratio of sodium citrate to potassium citrate, but this is usually simple. The prognosis is good for long term survival, i.e., many years, although surgical intervention may be needed to remove stones. The very slow renal destruction due to nephrocalcinosis may be accelerated by excessive calciferol therapy, pyelonephritis or hypertension. The prognosis of RTA syndrome secondary to pyelonephritis, hydronephrosis, etc. is that of the underlying disease.

Question What is the prognosis in RTA?

Answer 1. Years. Go on to **15.71**.
2. A few weeks. Go on to **15.73**.

15.70 Your answer − statement 1 is true, 2 and 3 false.

You are correct about statement 3 but incorrect about 1 and 2. Start at the beginning of the chapter and work on to **15.87** then answer the question in **15.81** again.

15.71 Your answer − the prognosis is measured in years.

Good. In infancy up to the age of $1\frac{1}{2}$ years, there is a form of RTA which differs from adult RTA. It is manifested by a failure to thrive, loss of appetite, constipation, dehydration and polyuria. There is a profound metabolic acidosis, with low plasma bicarbonate and hyperchloraemia; a high urinary pH (above 6.0), is usual. Nephrocalcinosis is present in one in every three cases; the majority of patients are males.

A proximal form of renal tubular acidosis (RTA) has been described by Edelman and his colleagues. In this form of RTA children are affected, but nephrocalcinosis and hypokalaemia do not occur. In contrast to RTA as described earlier these patients are able to acidify their urine normally in response to an acid load. They have an inappropriately large urinary bicarbonate leak, in *the absence of renal failure*, i.e., their urine contains large amounts of bicarbonate when its pH is less than 6. Edelman calls this disease 'proximal RTA' because the abnormalities are confined to those of proximal tubular function.

Question Does nephrocalcinosis occur in RTA of infancy?

Answer 1. Yes. Go on to **15.74**.
2. No. Go on to **15.75**.

15.72 Your answer − all the statements are true.

You are correct about statement 2 only. Go back and work through the chapter from **15.1** to **15.47** then from **15.81** to **15.87** again.

15.73 Your answer − the prognosis is a few weeks.

No. The prognosis for survival is excellent. Read **15.69** with more care.

15.74 Your answer − nephrocalcinosis *does* occur in infancy.

Correct. The treatment is to correct the sodium loss caused by vomiting and give alkalinising mixtures of sodium citrate to return the plasma pH to normal. The disease usually remits spontaneously and completely after months or years. The prognosis is therefore good.

Question What is the cause of the sodium depletion in infantile RTA?

Answer 1. Vomiting. Go on to **15.77**.
2. Salt loss in urine. Go on to **15.79**.

15.75 Your answer – nephrocalcinosis does not occur in RTA of infancy.
You are wrong. Do not guess. Read **15.71** again more carefully.

15.76 Your answer – statements 1 and 3 are true, 2 is false.
You are wrong about all 3 statements. Read the chapter again.

15.77 Your answer – sodium loss is due to vomiting.
Correct. The next subject to be discussed is idiopathic hypercalciuria, a condition in which over 400 mg of calcium are excreted a day in the urine. Hodgkinson and Pyrah showed that about 8 per cent of men excreted more than 300 mg of calcium in the urine daily (in females 250 mg a day) when on a normal diet. Idiopathic hypercalciuria is frequently associated with renal stones. Nordin has recently shown that as calcium intake is increased there is a steeper rise in urinary calcium excretion in idiopathic hypercalciuria when compared to the normal individual and there is evidence that a proportion of patients have occult primary hyperparathyroidism.

Question What is the usual urinary calcium excretion in the normal male on normal diet?

Answer 1. Less than 250 mg. Go on to **15.80**.
2. Less than 300 mg. Go on to **15.82**.
3. Less than 400 mg. Go on to **15.83**.

15.78 Your answer – statements 2 and 3 are true, 1 is false.
You are correct about 1 and 2; 3 is false, not true. Read on from **15.87** to the end of the chapter.

15.79 Your answer – Urinary salt loss is the cause of the sodium depletion.
No. You are guessing. In **15.74** it is mentioned that the sodium loss is due to vomiting. Read **15.74** again, then choose the correct answer.

15.80 Your answer – urinary calcium maximum is less than 250 mg in the normal male.
No. You are confusing the female maximum of 250 mg with the male. Read **15.77** again.

15.81 Your answer – the metabolic cause of oxalosis is *not* known with certainty.
Correct. Now look carefully at the statements below before you pick the appropriate answer.

Statement 1 In adult Fanconi syndrome, cystine deposits are widespread.

Statement 2 Hypokalaemia is common in adult distal RTA.

Statement 3 Salt losing nephritis responds to treatment with aldosterone.

Answer 1. All the statements are true. Go on to **15.72**.
2. All the statements are false. Go on to **15.68**.
3. Statement 1 is true, 2 and 3 false, Go on to **15.70**.
4. Statement 2 is true, 1 and 3 false. Go on to **15.85**.
5. Statement 3 is true, 2 and 1 false. Go on to **15.104**.
6. Statement 1 and 2 are true, 3 is false. Go on to **15.105**.
7. Statement 1 and 3 are true, 2 is false. Go on to **15.76**.
8. Statement 2 and 3 are true, 1 is false. Go on to **15.78**.

15.82 Your answer − less than 300 mg of calcium a day.

Correct. The problem of hypercalciuria is of great importance; one third of patients with renal stones have hypercalciuria and of these only one quarter have a known cause for the hypercalciuria, such as hypercalcaemia of any cause. In idiopathic hypercalciuria, the serum calcium level is *normal* but both uptake of calcium from the bowel and urinary calcium excretion are abnormally high.

In renal tubular lesions there is an increase in the excretion of lysozyme (mol wt = 14,000) and ribonuclease (mol wt = 17,000), their presence in the urine indicating that tubular damage is present. Similarly small globulins such as β microglobulin and γ microglobulin are found in the urine in renal tubular damage.

Question Is the serum calcium level normal or raised in idiopathic hypercalciuria?

Answer 1. Elevated. Go on to **15.84**.
2. Normal. Go on to **15.86**.

15.83 Your answer − less than 400 mg of calcium a day.
This is above the normal maximum and is hypercalciuria. Read **15.77** again.

15.84 Your answer − serum calcium is elevated in idiopathic hypercalciuria.
No. If serum calcium is elevated, then the diagnosis is not idiopathic hypercalciuria, but of one of the causes of hypercalcaemia. Read **15.82** again before answering the question.

15.85 Your answer − statement 2 is true, 1 and 3 are false.

You are quite correct. Before going on to the next chapter you may want to look up some of the following references.

Milne M.D. (1963) Chapter on renal tubular disorders in Strauss M. B. & Welt L. G. (eds) Diseases of the Kidney. Churchill, London. This chapter is excellent and should be read first before any other reference.

Crawhall J. C. et al. (1963) Brit. Med. J. **1**, 558 (Cystinuria).

Bickel H. et al. (1952) Acta. paediatrica. **42**, Supplementum **90**, 22 (Lignac Fanconi syndrome).

Milne M. D. et al. (1952) Quart. J. Med., **21**, 61 (adult Fanconi syndrome).

Stanbury S. W. & Mahler R. F. (1959) Quart. J. Med., **28**, 425 (salt losing nephritis).

Wrong O. M. & Davies H. E. F. (1959) Quart. J. Med., **28**, 259 (renal tubular acidosis).

Scowen E. F. et al. (1959) J. Path. Bact., **77**, 195 (oxalosis and primary oxaluria).

Henneman P. H. et al. (1958) J. Clin. Invest., **37**, 901 (uric acid stones).

de Lucca, H. F. (1969), New Eng. J. Med. 281, 1103 (Vitamin D).

de Vries et al. (1957) Am. J. Med., **23**, 408 (hereditary glycinuria).

Anon (1965) Editorial on idiopathic hypercalcinuria. Brit. med. J. **1**, 671.

Harrison, J. E. et al. Lancet 1968 **1**, 371 (Lysozyme).

Soriano et al. (1967) Paediat. Res. **1**, 81 (Proximal RTA).

Morris R. C. Jr. (1969). New Eng. J. Med. 281, 1405 (RTA).

Manuel, Y. Revillard J. P. and Betuel, H. Proteins in normal and patho-logical urine. S. Karger, 1970.

Morris, R. C., Renal acidosis Kidney International 1970, **1**, 322.

15.86 Your answer – serum calcium is normal.

Good. The only useful and practical therapy in idiopathic hypercalciuria is to *reduce absorption* of calcium from the bowel with sodium phytate and cellulose phosphate. The latter is preferable as it does not cause diarrhoea (unlike phytate) and should be given in a dose of 5 g t.d.s. These drugs cause a sharp fall in urinary calcium excretion in idiopathic hypercalciuria.

Question What is the effect on faecal calcium absorption of sodium phytate or cellulose phosphate?

Answer 1. Increased. Go on to **15.88**.
2. Decreased. Go on to **15.90**.

15.87 Your answer – 40 mEq a day.

Correct. Some patients have a much larger 'salt leak' and they are referred to as suffering from 'salt-losing nephritis.' These patients may lose vast amounts of sodium in the urine – up to 100–200 mEq/day – and so reach states of extreme salt depletion with a clinical picture like that of untreated Addison's disease – pigmentation, with low blood pressure, hypovolaemia, hyponatraemia, severe dehydration going on to shock, and a urine paradoxically rich in sodium. Unlike Addison's disease there is no decrease in urinary sodium concentration on adminis-tration of aldosterone, DOCA or fludrocortisone (9α fluorohydrocortisone), the renal tubules being refractory to these drugs; parenteral saline therapy may be required to restore lost sodium.

Question Does the urinary sodium excretion decrease in salt losing nephritis when aldosterone is administered?

Answer 1. No. Go on to **15.91**.
2. Yes. Go on to **15.93**.

15.88 Your answer – faecal calcium absorption is increased.

No. The point of giving phytate is to *decrease* faecal calcium absorption. Read **15.86** again.

15.89 Your answer – 200 mEq of sodium a day.

No. This is a massive loss and is quite rare. Read **15.90** again.

15.90 Your answer – faecal calcium absorption is decreased.

Correct. The next subject to be discussed is salt losing nephritis. This has already been mentioned in the chapter on chronic renal failure. Many uraemic patients have some renal tubular inability to conserve sodium, an obligatory salt loss of 40 ot 50 mEq/day being commonplace and of little importance unless the patient is given a low salt diet or has salt deficiency induced by vomiting.

Question What is the size of the salt leak usually found in chronic renal failure?

Answer 1. 40 mEq/day of sodium. Go on to **15.87**.
2. 200 mEq/day of sodium. Go on to **15.89**.

15.91 Your answer – urinary sodium excretion is unaffected.

Correct. The patients usually have a *severe degree of renal failure* even when the salt loss is corrected and must take additional salt supplement to balance urinary salt loss and thus prevent recurrence of a low salt state. The aetiology of the syndrome of 'salt-losing nephritis' is usually chronic pyelonephritis and very rarely cystic disease of the medulla.

Question When the salt loss is corrected is renal function normal in 'salt losing nephritis' apart from the tubular handling of sodium?

Answer 1. Yes. Go on to **15.92**.
2. No. Go on to **15.95**.

15.92 Your answer – renal function is normal in salt losing nephritis.

No. Most of the patients have advanced renal disease. Go back to **15.91** and read the paragraph again.

15.93 Your answer – urinary Na excretion decreases.

No. The renal tubules are refractory to the action of salt retaining drugs such as DOCA, aldosterone and fludrocortisone. Read **15.87** again, then answer the question correctly.

15.94 Your answer – not all gouty patients have uric acid stones.

Correct. Uric acid stones are found more commonly in hot countries where fluid intake is not enough to give a high urine flow. There is a racial predisposition to uric acid stones: they are frequent among Jews and Italians. Uric acid stones are radio-translucent and do not show up on plain X-rays.

Question Are uric acid stones radio-opaque or radio-translucent?

Answer 1. Radio-translucent. Go on to **15.96**.
2. Radio-opaque. Go on to **15.98**.

15.95 Your answer – renal function is abnormal in salt losing nephritis.
Correct. Uric acid stones are of renal and metabolic interest and so will be discussed next. Uric acid stones are seen in about 1 in 6 patients suffering from gout. Many patients have uric acid stones *without* clinical gout, although hyperuricaemia is common in patients with uric acid stones.

Question Do all gouty patients have uric acid stones?

Answer 1. Yes. Go on to **15.97**.
2. No. Go on to **15.94**.

15.96 Your answer – uric acid stones are radio-translucent.
Correct. Uric acid is much less soluble in acid urines, and this appears to be a major cause of stone formation, because it has been shown that uric acid stone formers produce an acid urine day and night, with a pH of less than 6 and without the normal alkaline tides. Treatment of the stones is by alkalinising the urine with 100 mEq of sodium bicarbonate a day, and increasing the urine volume to 3 litres a day by increased fluid intake. This therapy will not only prevent stones from forming but it will dissolve stones already formed. It is a curious fact that 10% of urate stone formers have hyperparathyroidism.

Question Do uric acid stone formers naturally tend to have an acid or alkaline urine?

Answer 1. Acid. Go on to **15.99**.
2. Alkaline. Go on to **15.101**.

15.97 Your answer – all gouty patients have uric acid stones.
No. Only 1 in 6 has clinical evidence of stone. Read **15.95** again.

15.98 Your answer – uric acid stones are radio-opaque.
No. They are invisible on plain X-rays. Read **15.94** again with more care.

15.99 Your answer – the urine is naturally acid.
Correct. The last subject in this chapter is the rare cause of renal stones known as primary hyperoxaluria or oxalosis. This is associated with nephrocalcinosis, hyperoxaluria and calcium oxalate stones, but remember however that calcium

oxalate stones are common and this disease is very rare. The urinary oxalate excretion is about ten times normal (up to 400 mg/day) in primary hyperoxaluria; it is a disease which starts in infancy and causes death from renal failure before adult life.

Question Do all patients with calcium oxalate stones suffer from primary hyperoxaluria with oxalosis?

Answer 1. Yes. Go on to **15.100**.
2. No. Go on to **15.102**.

15.100 Your answer – all patients with oxalate stones suffer from oxalosis.
No. Calcium oxalate stones are common; oxalosis is a very rare metabolic disease. Read **15.99** again.

15.101 Your answer – the urine is usually alkaline.
No. The very cause of the urate precipitation is the *constantly* acid urine of these patients. Go back to 15.96 and re-read it.

15.102 Your answer – not all patients with oxalate stones suffer from oxalosis.
Correct. At autopsy in cases of oxalosis, widespread deposits of oxalate are found throughout the kidneys, arteries, heart, gonads, and metaphyseal ends. The cause of the oxalosis and primary oxaluria is unknown but probably involves the metabolism of glyoxylate. There is no effective therapy.

Question Is the cause of oxaluria known with certainty?

Answer 1. No. Go on to **15.81**.
2. Yes. Go on to **15.103**.

15.103 Your answer – the metabolic defect in oxalosis is known with certainty.
No. It is unknown. Read **15.102** again.

15.104 Your answer – statement 3 is true, 2 and 1 are false.
You are correct about statement 1 only. Read from **15.47** on through the rest of the chapter.

15.105 Your answer – statements 1 and 2 are true, 3 is false.
You are correct about 2 and 3 but wrong about 1. Read from the beginning of the chapter to **15.47**.

Time for this chapter: 30 minutes

Chapter 16
Congenital and inherited diseases of the kidney

16.1 The commoner congenital and inherited diseases of the kidney will be described in this chapter. First of all let us discuss *polycystic disease of the kidneys*. Polycystic disease is a common anomaly. Its rate of occurrence in the general population is unknown precisely, but autopsy series suggest that it occurs with a frequency of between 1 in 300 and 1 in 1000. The disease has quite different clinical presentations in infancy and in adult life: the infantile form may obstruct labour or lead to death from renal failure in the first few weeks or months of life. Adults on the other hand usually survive into middle age.

Question Which has the better prognosis – infantile or adult polycystic disease?

Answer 1. Infantile. Go on to **16.3**.
2. Adult. Go on to **16.5**.

16.2 Your answer – the straight collecting tubules originate from the mesonephric bud.
Correct. Now what has this to do with polycystic kidneys? There is no certain proof how polycystic kidneys originate. Some authorities consider that there is an abnormality in the fusion of the mesonephric (straight) collecting tubules, and the metanephric (curved) collecting tubules. Other authorities suggest that there is a malformation of some of the tubules so that link-up between the collecting tubular lumens is impossible. Against all these theories is the histological evidence of three types of cysts – glomerular, tubular secretory and excretory cysts. The glomerular cysts are closed, whereas the tubular secretory cysts are open and may communicate with the renal pelvis. The collecting duct cells are hypertrophied in the adult form of polycystic disease, and some authors attribute the cyst formation to distal obstruction of the collecting duct by the cellular hypertrophy. The infantile form has only the closed, non-communicating and therefore non-draining cysts. The adult cysts are of all three types.

Question Are the cysts in the infantile form of polycystic disease communicating or closed?

Answer 1. Closed. Go on to **16.6**.
2. Communicating. Go on to **16.8**.

16.3 Your answer – infantile polycystic disease has the better prognosis.

No. Infantile polycystic disease is responsible for early death in contrast to the better prognosis in adults. Read **16.1** again and answer the question correctly.

16.4 Your answer – the straight collecting tubules originate in the metanephros.

No. The adult nephron up to and including the *curved* parts of the collecting tubules, comes from the metanephros, but the mesonephric bud forms the ureter, pelvis, calyces, and straight collecting tubules. Now choose the correct answer after reading **16.5** again.

16.5 Your answer – adult polycystic disease has the better prognosis.

Correct. The embryology of the kidneys has to be understood before the aetiology of polycystic kidneys can be comprehended. The ureter is formed from a bud from the mesonephros, the cephalic tip of which grows into the the metanephric tissue and stimulates the formation of the nephrons in the metanephros. The metanephric part of the nephrons comprises glomeruli, proximal and distal tubules, and the curved proximal part of the collecting tubules. The straight part of the collecting tubules, calyces, pelvis and ureter is from the mesonephric bud.

Question What is the embryological origin of the straight collecting tubules?

Answer 1. Mesonephric bud. Go on to **16.2**.
         2. Metanephros. Go on to **16.4**.

16.6 Your answer – the cysts are closed.

Correct. The kidneys in polycystic disease may attain enormous size, filling the abdomen and compressing the other viscera. The cut surface of the large kidneys is studded with cysts of all sizes. Some of the cysts are filled with blood from old or recent haemorrhage into the cysts, a common occurrence; the majority however, are filled with urine, and cystic nephrons may still be functional from the point of view of urine formation. Some cysts may be filled with opaque yellow material (pus from episodes of infection) and stones are frequent.

Question Are cystic nephrons ever capable of urine formation?
Answer 1. Yes. Go on to **16.10**.
         2. No. Go on to **16.12**.

16.7 Your answer – there *are* symptoms in the first stage of polycystic disease.
No. There are no symptoms at all. Read **16.10** again.

16.8 Your answer – the cysts are communicating.
No. You are guessing. Go back and read **16.2** again; then choose the correct answer.

16.9 Your answer — there are *no* symptoms in the first stage of polycystic disease.

Correct. In the second stage symptoms appear, *not* due to uraemia but due to the complications of polycystic disease itself, namely —

(1) Haemorrhage into the cysts. This causes pain in the loin and haematuria, with ureteric colic.

(2) Urinary tract infections. These are very common in polycystic kidney disease. They are responsible for pyrexia, dysuria, malaise and frequency. Microscopy of the urine discloses pus cells and organisms.

(3) Stone. Renal calculus occurs in 1 in 10 patients with polycystic disease and is a cause of ureteric colic.

(4) Pain in the abdomen and general discomfort due to the size of the kidneys.

Question What is the probable cause of haematuria in a man with polycystic kidneys?

Answer 1. Haemorrhage into a cyst. Go on to **16.11**.
2. Acute urinary tract infection. Go on to **16.13**.

16.10 Your answer — cystic nephrons are capable of urine formation.

Correct. The clinical features of adult polycystic disease are as follows:

In the first stage, which may last up to the fourth or fifth decade, there are no symptoms, although the polycystic kidneys may be seen on a plain X-ray of the abdomen carried out for other reasons. There are *no* symptoms referable to the genito-urinary tract or due to pressure from the kidneys.

Question Are there any symptoms in the first stage of adult polycystic kidney disease?

Answer 1. Yes. Go on to **16.7**.
2. No. Go on to **16.9**.

16.11 Your answer — the cause of the haematuria is bleeding into cysts.

Correct. Haematuria presumably occurs because the cyst is communicating with the renal pelvis.

Hypertension is present in about *half* the adult patients with polycystic kidneys, and this may contribute to the increased incidence of subarachnoid haemorrhage and 'berry' aneurysms in polycystic kidney disease. The hypertension is usually benign hypertension, with a diastolic blood pressure below 130 mm Hg.

Question In what proportion of patients with polycystic kidneys does hypertension occur?

Answer 1. In all. Go on to **16.14**.
2. In half. Go on to **16.16**.
3. In only a few. Go on to **16.18**.

16.12 Your answer – the cystic nephrons are not capable of urine formation.

No. They are capable of urine formation: this is one of the factors which make Rovsing's operation of cyst puncture undesirable, for even if the cyst is large it may yet be a part of a functioning nephron, and every functioning nephron is important to the patient with advanced renal disease. Now go back to **16.6**.

16.13 Your answer – the cause of the haematuria is an acute urinary tract infection.

Although haematuria may be caused by an acute urinary tract infection, it is usually caused by haemorrhage into a communicating cyst. Read **16.9** to make sure you have not missed any other facts, then answer the question correctly.

16.14 Your answer – hypertension occurs in all patients with adult polycystic disease.

No. Only about half are affected with hypertension. Go back to **16.11** and read it again to ensure that you have not missed any of the other facts it contains. Then answer the question correctly.

16.15 Your answer – The progress of renal failure is rapid.

No. The progress in polycystic disease is remarkably slow, unless there is a superimposed urinary tract infection. Read **16.16** again carefully.

16.16 Your answer – hypertension occurs in about half of the cases of polycystic disease.

You are correct. The third stage of polycystic disease is the stage of chronic renal failure, which is noteworthy because of its very slow rate of deterioration. Patients may survive for several years with a GFR below 3 ml/min. The anaemia of uraemia in polycystic renal disease is sometimes remarkably mild, and on occasion, absent. Some patients with polycystic kidney disease have renal polycythaemia, thought to be caused by renal erythropoietin produced in the cystic kidneys.

Question Is the deterioration of renal function in polycystic renal disease rapid or slow?

Answer 1. Rapid. Go on to **16.15**.
2. Slow. Go on to **16.17**.

16.17 Your answer – The progress of renal failure is slow.

Correct. The physical signs characteristic of polycystic renal disease are the cystic kidneys themselves. Both kidneys are considerably enlarged and are palpable in 80 per cent of cases; and sometimes they are over 50 cm long and can be seen as huge masses in the loins. 1 in 4 patients has only one kidney enlarged. 3 out of 4 patients have proteinuria, and 1 in 2 have a urinary tract infection.

Question Is unilateral enlargement of the kidneys ever found in polycystic disease?

Answer 1. Yes. Go on to **16.19**.
2. No. Go on to **16.21**.

16.18 Your answer – hypertension occurs in only a few patients with polycystic disease.
   No. Do not guess. Hypertension is common in polycystic disease. Read **16.11** again.

16.19 Your answer – unilateral enlargement of the kidneys does occur in polycystic disease.
   Correct. There is no curative therapy in this disease. Rovsing's operation of multiple cyst puncture is of doubtful value since there is evidence of a permanent deterioration in renal function after the cyst puncture has been carried out. There is, however, evidence that pain from distended cysts may be considerably relieved by Rovsing's operation. Otherwise, the treatment is that of chronic renal failure, discussed in Chapter 9.

Question What is the effect of Rovsing's operation on renal function?

Answer 1. Deterioration. Go on to **16.22**.
2. Improvement. Go on to **16.20**.
3. No effect. Go on to **16.24**.

16.20 Your answer – Rovsing's operation causes an improvement in renal function.
   No. The operation has the opposite effect. Read **16.19** more carefully.

16.21 Your answer – unilateral enlargement is not found in polycystic kidney disease.
   You are wrong. Read **16.17** again with greater care.

16.22 Your answer – this operation causes a deterioration in renal function.
   Correct. The prognosis of adult polycystic disease is fairly good. Some patients survive up to the age of eighty, but there are many deaths in the fourth and fifth decades, either from renal failure, renal infection, or renal hypertension. The prognosis in congenital or infantile polycystic disease is bad. Some infants have massive kidneys, so that they cause an obstructed labour and may be born dead; others die of renal failure or other congenital abnormalities within a short time of birth.

Question Is the life expectancy in adult polycystic disease longer than that in the congenital or infantile form?

Answer 1. Yes. Go on to **16.25**.
         2. No. Go on to **16.27**.

16.23   Your answer – the cysts are found in the cortex.
    No. Not only are you guessing, but you are not guessing intelligently, for the name of the disease implies some disease of the medulla. Read **16.25** again, more carefully this time.

16.24   Your answer – Rovsing's operation has no effect on renal function.
    You are guessing. Read **16.19** more carefully this time. Then answer the question.

16.25   Your answer – life expectancy is longer in the adult form of polycystic kidney disease.
    You are correct. The next subject to be dealt with is *medullary sponge kidney*. This is a rare disorder of middle aged and elderly people, and is characterised by a cystic condition of the renal pyramids. In addition to the cysts proper, there are dilated tubules which are lined by several layers of epithelium, the cysts being lined by a single layer of cuboidal epithelium.

Question In medullary sponge kidney what parts of the kidney are involved by the cysts?

Answer 1. Cortex. Go on to **16.23**.
         2. Medulla. Go on to **16.28**.
         3. Pyramids. Go on to **16.30**.

16.26   Your answer – more frequently in a retrograde pyelogram.

    No. The retrograde pyelogram only occasionally fills the cyst cavities: read **16.30** again.

16.27   Your answer – life expectancy is shorter in the adult form than in the congenital or infantile form.
    No. Read **16.22** more carefully. You should have learned this point earlier in this chapter.

16.28   Your answer – the cysts are found in the medulla.
    You are correct in so far as you have gone, but you should be able to localise the area of medulla involved with greater precision after reading **16.25** again: then choose the correct answer.

16.29 Your answer — the diagnosis can be more frequently made from intravenous pyelogram.

Correct. The clinical features are associated primarily with the *calculi* which are responsible for:

(1) Ureteric colic due to passage of a stone.
(2) Haematuria due to passage of a stone or urinary tract infection.
(3) Pyelonephritis with frequency, dysuria, pyrexia, pyuria and a significant bacteriuria.

Many patients have no renal symptoms at all until they approach middle age, when the calculi cause symptoms. Formal testing shows impaired ability to concentrate the urine, (as would be expected when the pyramids are damaged and the counter current multiplier system interfered with), and an acidification defect.

Question What are the symptoms of medullary sponge kidney due to primarily?

Answer 1. Calculi. Go on to **16.32**.
2. Renal tract infection. Go on to **16.34**.

16.30 Your answer — the cysts are found in the pyramids.

Correct. They may be shown on IVP as clusters of grape-like cystic swellings adjoining the calyces. They do not fill in 75 per cent of cases on retrograde pyelography. The diagnosis may be inferred from a plain X-ray of the abdomen, in which radio-opaque calculi can be seen in clusters in the positions of the renal pyramids.

Question Would you expect to see the diagnostic features of medullary sponge kidney more frequently in an intravenous pyelogram than in a retrograde pyelogram?

Answer 1. More frequently in a retrograde pyelogram. Go on to **16.26**.
2. More frequently in an intravenous pyelogram. Go on to **16.29**.

16.31 Your answer — the prognosis is worse in medullary sponge kidney.

No. The reverse is true. You have not concentrated well enough when reading **16.32**. Read it again and then choose the correct answer.

16.32 Your answer — the symptoms are due to renal calculi.

Correct. The prognosis of medullary sponge kidney is good, in striking contrast to that in *cystic disease of the medulla*, in which death occurs in uraemia in adolescence or early adult life. Histologically in cystic disease of the medulla, the entire medulla from the cortico-medullary junction to the tips of the pyramid, is honeycombed with cysts, lined with a single layer of flattened epithelium. The disease is very rare, and the patients develop renal failure with salt wasting and inability to excrete acid adequately; the chronic renal disease causes renal osteomalacia and renal hyperparathyroidism.

Question Is the prognosis worse in medullary sponge kidney or in cystic disease of the medulla?

Answer 1. Medullary sponge kidney. Go on to **16.31**.
2. Cystic disease of the medulla. Go on to **16.36**.

16.33 Your answer – give salt supplements.

You are correct in that this will remedy the salt leak but it will do nothing for the acidosis. Read **16.36** again and read how Shohl's solution is useful for both sodium loss and acidosis. Then choose the correct answer.

16.34 Your answer – the symptoms are due to renal tract infection.

No. Renal tract infections certainly occur in medullary sponge kidney, but they are associated with renal calculi which are the indirect cause of all the symptoms. Read **16.29** before choosing the correct answer.

16.35 Your answer – the extra ureter always drains into the bladder.

No. Often it drains into the posterior urethra and sometimes into the vagina. Read **16.38** again, then answer the question.

16.36 Your answer – the prognosis is worse in cystic disease of the medulla.

Correct. The only treatment for this disease is symptomatic – salt supplements to prevent salt depletion because of the salt-wasting. If the patient is acidotic as well the sodium can be given as Shohl's solution which will both correct the acidosis and provide sodium. The chronic renal failure should be treated on the lines discussed in the Chapter 9 on 'Chronic Renal Failure.'

Question If you have a patient with cystic disease of the medulla who has a large 'salt leak' and also is acidotic, what would you give him?

Answer 1. Salt supplements. Go on to **16.33**.
2. Shohl's solution. Go on to **16.38**.

16.37 Your answer – the extra ureter does not always drain into the bladder.

Correct. The clinical features of duplex kidney or ureter are those of the complications: these are:

(1) Pyelonephritis.
(2) Hypertension.
(3) Renal calculus.

The anomaly is not rare and can be picked up frequently during an IVP during investigation of the symptoms just listed. The pyelonephritis is often chronic with recurrent attacks of urinary tract infections which cannot be eradicated until the diseased renal tissue forming the extra kidney and pelvis is itself excised.

Question If a patient with duplex ureters and kidneys develops a urinary tract infection, is it likely to recur?

Answer 1. Yes. Go on to **16.40**.
2. No. Go on to **16.42**.

16.38 Your answer – use Shohl's solution.

Correct. The subject of duplex kidney and ureter is of considerable interest, not only because this is a common anomaly, but also because the complications are important. In duplex kidney one or both kidneys may be duplicated, the kidney being rarely separated from its ipsilateral fellow. Usually the two kidneys are continuous, the major diagnostic feature being two separate pelves. Look at Fig. 16.38.

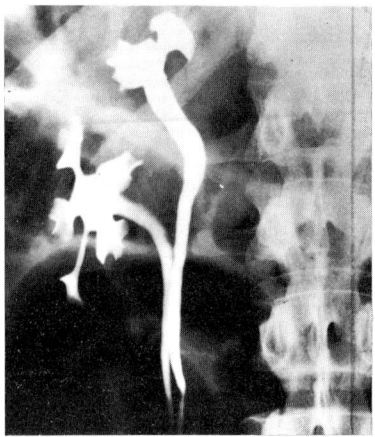
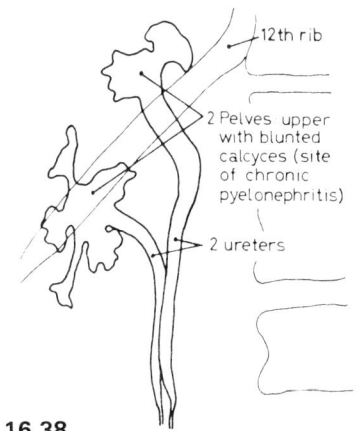

Fig. 16.38

Sometimes only the ureter is duplicated, there being a joint renal pelvis. The extra ureter may end in the bladder or it may terminate distal to the internal sphincter of the bladder, giving rise to dribbling incontinence. In some women the extra ureter ends in the vagina, causing urinary incontinence.

Question Does the extra ureter in the case of the duplex ureters always drain into the bladder?

Answer 1. Yes. Go on to **16.35**.
2. No. Go on to **16.37**.

16.39 Your answer – hypertension responds to excision of the kidney.

No. The hypertension can be readily controlled by medical means – the standard method of treatment. Read **16.40** again, more carefully this time, then answer the question correctly.

16.40 Your answer – the infection will usually recur.

You are correct. There is a high incidence of recurrent urinary tract infections because of the urinary stasis in one of the renal pelves. The treatment of double ureter, if asymptomatic, is to leave it alone. If there is evidence of unilateral chronic pyelonephritis in one of the pelves of the kidneys and also hypertension, nephrectomy of the affected kidney may be indicated. Sometimes this will involve removal of the affected half of the kidney and its associated pelvis, but in others, for technical reasons, both pelves and kidneys on the same side might have to be removed. The hypertension usually responds adequately to medical treatment which is the therapy of choice. Urinary tract infections should be treated with adequate dosage of the appropriate antibiotic depending on the antibiotic sensitivities of the organisms isolated from the urine.

Question Does the hypertension associated with duplex kidneys and ureter respond only to surgical excision of the affected kidney?

Answer 1. Yes. Go on to **16.39**.
2. No. Go on to **16.43**.

16.41 Your answer – females are more severely affected in hereditary haematuric nephritis.

No. In the majority of affected families the opposite is true. Males die younger than females, dying from uraemia, and are much more severely affected than females. Read **16.43** again.

16.42 Your answer – the infection will not recur.

No. The anatomical abnormality in the duplex ureters may be responsible for some urinary stasis in one renal pelvis, and so recurrent infections may occur. Read **16.37** again.

16.43 Your answer – hypertension does not respond only to surgical excision of the kidney.

Correct. The next subject to be discussed is familial nephritis, i.e., the occurrence of nephritis in more than one member of a family. If one considers an epidemic with type 12 streptococci, it is possible that several affected members of the same family may develop acute glomerulonephritis, and we deliberately differentiate this form of simultaneous acute post-streptococcal glomerulonephritis from the other forms of nephritis referred to as 'familial nephritis.' This latter group is not related to streptococcal infections, and in different members of the same family may be manifest as a pyelonephritis with positive urine cultures or as a haemorrhagic glomerulonephritis. This type of familial nephritis is associated with nerve deafness, haematuria and 'foam cells' in the urine, hence one of the names for this disease is hereditary haematuric nephritis with deafness. Another synonym is 'Alport's syndrome.' The disease usually affects males more severely than females, many males dying of uraemia before the age of 30. In a few families, however, the males and females are equally affected. In some families deafness is not found.

Question Are females or males more likely to be severely affected by hereditary haematuric nephritis?

Answer   1. Females. Go on to **16.41**.
           2. Males. Go on to **16.45**.

16.44 Your answer: all are true. No. 3 is false. Go back and read on from **16.43**.

16.45 Your answer – males are more severely affected than females.

You are correct about the majority of families. The attacks of haematuria start in childhood, often about the age of 4 or 5 and last a few days at a time; they may be precipitated by upper respiratory tract infections, by measles and other childhood exanthemata, or they may arise without obvious precipitating cause. In other families haematuria is absent, and the patient may present with proteinuria, hypertension or chronic renal failure. The proteinuria may be considerable and foam cells may appear in the urine. The origin of these foam cells is thought to be tubular cells filled with lipid. They are found in nephrotic syndrome of any cause and are in no way specific to familial nephritis.

Question Are foam cells found in any disease other than familial nephritis?

Answer   1. Yes. Go on to **16.47**.
           2. No. Go on to **16.49**.

16.46 Your answer – all the statements are false.

No. Only 3 is false. Go back to **16.1**, work through to **16.43**, then answer the question in **16.57** again.

16.47 Your answer – foam cells are found in other diseases as well as in familial nephritis.

Correct. The inheritance of familial nephritis is complicated by the fact that there are several different clinical types of the disease and therefore, not unexpectedly, the form of inheritance also varies from one type to another. In many families the disease occurs in several generations, and is inherited as an autosomal dominant, but in other families this is not the case. In this latter group of families there are more females than males, suggesting some linkage or association of the familial nephritis gene with the sex chromosomes. The gene for nerve deafness appears to be a quite separate gene segregating in the same families.

Question Is the mode of inheritance of familial nephritis identical in all families?

Answer Yes. Go on to **16.51**.
         No. Go on to **16.53**.

16.48 Your answer – statement 1 is true, 2 and 3 are false.
   You are correct about 1 and 3 but not about 2. Go back to **16.28**, and read on from there to **16.43**, then answer the question in **16.57** again.

16.49 Your answer – foam cells are not found in any other disease.
   No. Foam cells are not confined to familial nephritis; they are found whenever there is a considerable proteinuria, and are thought to be due to the toxic affects of reabsorbed protein on the tubular cells. Read **16.45** again.

16.50 Your answer – statement 2 is true, 1 and 3 are false.
   You are wrong about statement 1. Read from **16.1** to **16.28**, then answer the question in **16.57** correctly.

16.51 Your answer – the mode of inheritance of familial nephritis is identical in all families.
   No. Read **16.47** again more carefully then answer the question.

16.52 Your answer – statements 1 and 2 are true, 3 is false.
   You are correct. Before leaving this Chapter you may care to look at the following references:

Polycystic kidneys: Dalgaard O. Z. (1957) Acta. med. Scand. **158**, supplement 328.
Medullary sponge kidney: Anon (1965) Presse Medicale, number 6.
Cystic disease of renal medulla: Strauss M. B. (1963) in Strauss M. B. & Welt L. G. (eds) Diseases of the Kidney, Churchill, London.
Familial nephritis: Perkoff G. T. et al. (1951) Arch. int. Med. **88**, 191; (1958) ibid. **102**, 733.
Graham J. B. 1959. Amer. J. Human Genetics, **11**, 333.
Perkoff G. T. (1967) New. Eng. J. Med. **277**, 77–129 (Hereditary Renal Diseases – A Review).

16.53 Your answer – the mode of inheritance is *not* identical in all families.
   Correct. There are several forms of nephritis affecting infants and neonates which are inherited as recessives, and which have an extremely bad prognosis, with death in a few months. Thus there is a congenital form of the nephrotic syndrome apparently of immunologic origin; there is a congenital type of glomerulonephritis and also lastly a rare disease termed 'nephronophthisis' by Fanconi and his colleagues. This is probably identical with medullary cystic disease. The clinical features of this are progressive renal failure in a child in whom the urine contains no gross abnormality. There is no curative therapy for any form of inherited nephritis. Treatment is symptomatic, and is identical with that used in any other form of chronic renal failure.

Question Is the prognosis good or bad in congenital nephrotic syndrome?

Answer 1. Bad. Go on to **16.57**.
2. Good. Go on to **16.55**.

16.54 Your answer − statement 3 is true, 1 and 2 false.
No. You are quite wrong. Go back and read the chapter again.

16.55 Your answer − the prognosis is good.
No. The prognosis is bad in all forms of congenital nephritis. Read **16.53** again.

16.56 Your answer − 1 and 3 are true, 2 is false.
You are correct about 1 only. Go back to **16.28** and read on from there to the end of the chapter.

16.57 Your answer − the prognosis is bad in congenital nephrotic syndrome.
Correct. Before answering the present question study the statements below carefully, and choose the correct answer. Choice of the wrong answer indicates faulty knowledge, and therefore you may find yourself reading the chapter from the beginning again.

Statement 1 In the majority of patients with polycystic disease of the kidneys both kidneys are affected.

Statement 2 The diagnosis of medullary sponge kidney is more readily made on IVP than on retrograde pyelography.

Statement 3 In familial nephritis, females are usually more severely affected than males.

Answer All the statements are true. Go on to **16.44**.
2. All the statements are false. Go on to **16.46**.
3. Statement 1 is true, 2 and 3 false. Go on to **16.48**.
4. Statement 2 is true, 1 and 3 false. Go on to **16.50**.
5. Statement 3 is true, 1 and 2 false. Go on to **16.54**.
6. Statements 1 and 2 are true, 3 false. Go on to **16.52**.
7. Statements 1 and 3 are true, 2 false. Go on to **16.56**.
8. Statements 2 and 3 are true, 1 false. Go on to **16.58**.

16.58 Your answer − 2 and 3 are true, 1 is false.
You are correct about 2 only. Read from **16.1** to **16.28** then from **16.43** to the end of the chapter.

Time for this chapter: 30 minutes

Chapter 17
Focal nephritis and miscellaneous nephritides

17.1 The term 'focal nephritis' is applied to a specific histological picture which is caused by several different disease processes. The histological appearance is of the involvement of some of the glomeruli only, the others being normal. The affected glomeruli have 'local' involvement i.e., only some lobules are affected by cellular infiltration with the remaining lobules quite normal. Look at Fig. 17.1.

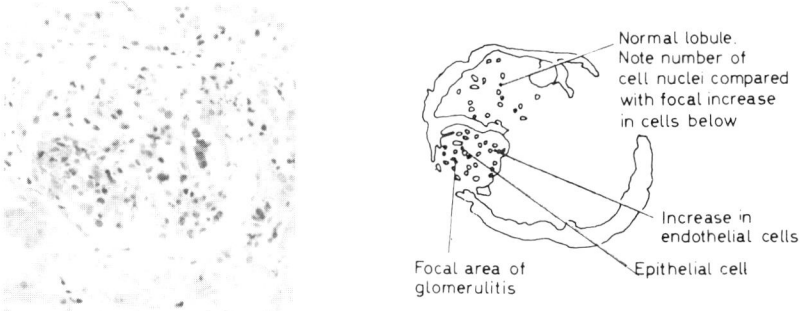

Fig. 17.1

The first form of 'focal nephritis' to be considered is that which occurs at the height of a febrile illness such as lobar pneumonia, and is a clinical syndrome consisting of haematuria at the *height of* the febrile attack. The haematuria usually lasts a day or two, and complete recovery is usual, providing the primary (non-renal) disease is not fatal. There is also a form of recurrent haematuria coming on shortly after a febrile illness in whom focal nephritis is found on biopsy and where IgA is found on immunofluorescent studies in the glomerulus. The prognosis of this IgA type focal nephritis, as Richet calls it, is quite good.

Question What is the clinical manifestation of focal nephritis occuring during lobar pneumonia?

Answer 1. Renal failure. Go on to **17.5**.
    2. Haematuria. Go on to **17.3**.

17.2 Your answer – children have a greater chance of developing subacute or chronic glomerulonephritis.

335

No. Adults have a worse prognosis; go back to **17.9** again and read it through more carefully.

17.3 Your answer – the usual clinical manifestation is haematuria.
Correct. There are many other types of focal nephritis, many of them associated with hypersensitivity phenomena, an example of which is Henoch-Schönlein purpura. This disease is of unknown aetiology, in spite of its alternative names of allergic or anaphylatoid purpura. It is associated with polyarthritis, skin purpura, and abdominal pains due to purpura in the bowel resulting in gastrointestinal bleeding and melaena. Renal involvement occurs in less than half the patients, and may be identical with that of acute poststreptococcal glomerulonephritis, or there may be focal nephritis. In the focal form the lesion is focal *within* the kidney, and local within the glomerulus. This means that some glomeruli are involved, the remainder being normal This is quite different from the acute glomerulonephritic form in which all the glomeruli are involved. In the focal form the inflammatory and exudative changes are confined to a few lobules only of each affected glomerulus i.e. most of the lobules of the affected glomeruli are normal.

Question In the focal nephritis of Henoch-Schönlein purpura are all the glomeruli involved?
Answer 1. Yes. Go on to **17.6**.
2. No. Go on to **17.9**.

17.4 Your answer – in rheumatic fever there is focal nephritis.
No. You are choosing an answer by guesswork. Go back and read **17.7** again.

17.5 Your answer – focal nephritis occurring during an attack of pneumonia is manifested clinically by renal failure.
No. The sole manifestation in the majority of cases is haematuria. Go back to **17.1** and read it carefully.

17.6 Your answer – all the glomeruli are involved.
No. The term focal nephritis implies a lesion which is 'focal' in the kidney, so that only some of the glomeruli are involved. Read **17.3** again.

17.7 Your answer – adults have a greater chance of developing subacute or chronic glomerulonephritis.
Correct. In some patients with focal nephritis there is no abdominal pain or melaena but skin purpura and polyarthropathy are both common, the manifestation of renal involvement being haematuria and proteinuria. Histologically the lesions consist of focal glomerulitis indistinguishable from the focal form of Henoch-Schönlein purpura. The precise relationship between this syndrome and Henoch-Schönlein nephritis is obscure. Histological forms of focal nephritis are

found at renal biopsy in many diseases, particularly frequently in collagen diseases such as systemic lupus erythematosis and sometimes in polyarteritis nodosa.

Question In what form of collagen disease is focal nephritis found on histological examination?

Answer 1. Systemic lupus. Go on to **17.10**.
2. Rheumatic fever. Go on to **17.4**.

17.8 You should not be reading this paragraph if you are following the instructions correctly.

17.9 Your answer — Not all the glomeruli are involved.

Good. The form of Henoch-Schönlein nephritis which is similar to if not identical with acute post-streptococcal glomerulonephritis has a histological picture identical with that of acute glomerulonephritis and in some patients develops into the subacute or chronic types of glomerulonephritis. In the acute form and in the focal nephritic form the features are haematuria, proteinuria, oedema and hypertension. The majority of the patients have complete healing of the renal lesion, although a smaller proportion of affected adults escape the sequelae of progression to subacute or chronic glomerulonephritis when compared with the disease in children; hypertension is found to be less common than in post-streptococcal glomerulonephritis. Progression to the subacute phase is manifested by failure of the haematuria to clear up, with persistence of proteinuria of such an extent that nephrotic syndrome develops. There is no curative therapy in Henoch-Schönlein nephritis; steroids do not prevent the steady deterioration of renal function in those patients who go on to the subacute or chronic phases.

Question Do children or adults have a greater chance of developing subacute or chronic glomerulonephritis with Henoch-Schönlein purpura?

Answer 1. Children. Go on to **17.2**.
2. Adults. Go on to **17.7**.

17.10 Your answer — in systemic lupus there is a focal nephritis.

Correct. Goodpasture's syndrome is a rare and usually fatal disease of unknown cause in which there is a combination of acute glomerulonephritis and intrapulmonary haemorrhage probably due to necrotising alveolitis. The histological changes in the kidney are similar to those in post-streptococcal acute glomerulonephritis with proliferative changes in and necrosis of glomeruli but on electronmicroscopy no humps are seen i.e. there is no antigen-antibody complement complex. Look at Fig. 17.10.

The pulmonary changes are those of a haemorrhagic exudate into the alveoli with numerous siderophages and red blood cells; some workers have demonstrated

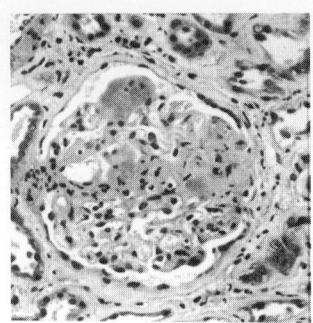 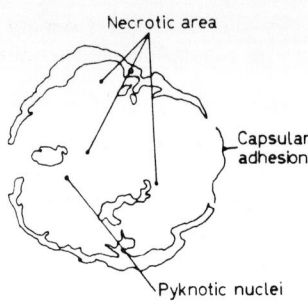

Fig. 17.10

changes in the alveolar wall. An antibody-antigen reaction is probably responsible for the acute glomerulonephritis in this disease because fluorescein labelled anti IgG is selectively taken up by the glomerular basement membrane in this disease giving rise to a *linear* fluorescence, suggesting that the basement membrane is itself coated with IgG; the alveolar basement membrane has a similar antigenicity to the glomerular basement membrane, and it is likely that an antibody, in the form of a IgG, attacks the basement membranes of both the pulmonary alveoli and the glomeruli.

Question What substance has been demonstrated to be present on the basement membrane in Goodpasture's syndrome?

Answer 1. IgG. Go on to **17.11**.
2. Anti IgG. Go on to **17.13**.

17.11 Your answer – IgG is present on the basement membrane.

Correct. The clinical features of Goodpasture's syndrome are striking and diagnostic. First let us look at the pulmonary features, which have much in common with pulmonary haemosiderosis. The patient develops dyspnoea on exertion, cough, and haemoptysis. He is found to have a severe iron deficiency anaemia, with a very low serum iron of the order of 10 μg/100 ml. The anaemia does not respond to oral iron therapy: the anaemia is due to haemoglobin being sequestered in the lungs, as shown by ^{59}Fe studies. Examination of the rusty sputum shows red blood cells and numerous siderophages. X-ray of the chest is likely to show multiple opacities. The anaemia varies, with exacerbations and spontaneous remissions, but the serum iron remains depressed in spite of oral iron administration.

Question Where do ^{59}Fe studies demonstrate the iron to be sequestered in Goodpasture's syndrome?

Answer 1. Sputum. Go on to **17.14**.

2. Lungs. Go on to **17.16**.
3. Kidneys. Go on to **17.18**.

17.12   Your answer – the patient is likely to survive a few weeks.

Correct. The treatment of Goodpasture's syndrome is unsatisfactory; in addition to frequent transfusions which are required because of the anaemia, the therapy is empirical and controversial, centering on whether immunosuppressive drugs such as azathioprine (Imuran) and prednisone should be given or withheld. Our practice is to give both these drugs in immunosuppressive dosage, because the majority of the recorded cases which have recovered have been on corticosteroids. The haemoptysis frequently clears up early when a course of adequate steroid dosage is given, but the disease is so rare that no adequate controlled trial of therapy has yet been carried out.

Question Does the haemoptysis clear up if the patient is given corticosteroids in adequate dosage?

Answer 1. No. Go on to **17.15**.
2. Yes. Go on to **17.17**.

17.13   Your answer – Anti IgG is present on the basement membrane.

You are correct in that this can be demonstrated by putting fluorescein conjugated anti IgG onto a biopsy section and showing that fluorescence of the glomerular basement membrane can then be demonstrated. But in order for anti IgG to adhere firmly to any tissue there must be IgG present there initially. Now answer the question in **17.10** again.

17.14   Your answer – the iron is sequestered in the sputum.

No. There is certainly iron in the sputum, but most of it is sequestered in the lungs, where it is *not* immediately available for transport to the blood forming organs, so that a severe iron deficiency state develops. Go back and read **17.11** again.

17.15   Your answer – the haemoptysis does not clear up when adequate dosage of corticosteroids is given.

No. Do not choose your answer at random. Go back and read **17.12** with care.

17.16   Your answer – the iron is sequestered in the lungs.

Correct. At the onset there may be no evidence of renal involvement, and a diagnosis of idiopathic pulmonary haemosiderosis may be made; later, however renal involvement appears, initially as proteinuria but within a few days or weeks the patient has oliguria, haematuria, hypertension and oedema; then he becomes anuric and dies of renal failure within a few weeks of the onset of signs of renal involvement. Other patients develop evidence of pulmonary and renal involvement simultaneously and so the diagnosis can be made early. In a few patients the renal disease regresses and the patient makes a partial or complete recovery. The haemoptysis usually lessens or disappears on prednisone and immunosuppressive therapy but there is no consistent improvement in the anaemia which varies spontaneously and unpredictably.

Question In the majority of cases, once renal involvement has appeared, how long does the patient with Goodpasture's syndrome survive?

Answer 1. A few weeks. Go on to **17.12**.
         2. A few years. Go on to **17.19**.

17.17 Your answer – the haemoptysis clears up when adequate steroid dosage is given.

Correct. The next subject to be discussed is much less exotic and far more frequent – the renal involvement in subacute bacterial endocarditis (SABE) which is still responsible for a high proportion of deaths in this disease in spite of antibiotics. Broadly speaking, there are three groups of renal involvement in SABE –

(1) Infarction of renal tissue due to large emboli.
(2) Focal embolic nephritis.
(3) Diffuse acute glomerulonephritis similar to that found in post-streptococcal glomerulonephritis.

Let us first deal with *infarction of renal tissue.* Parts of the vegetations on the heart valves in SABE composed of fibrin and organisms, break off and are swept down the aorta and into the renal artery which may itself be occluded or, alternatively, one of its branches may become occluded. This results in infarction of the whole or part of the kidney. This presents clinically as dull or sharp loin pain, with tenderness over the kidney on deep palpation, and haematuria. In the occasional case severe hypertension follows lodgment of an embolus which occludes the renal artery. Intravenous pyelography shows no secretion of radio-opaque material unilaterally in the case of complete occlusion of one main renal artery with infarction of one kidney. Smaller infarcts may be ultimately diagnosed by a local thinning of cortex and medulla with distortion of the calyceal pattern in this area.

Question Is IVP helpful in the diagnosis of complete renal artery occlusion due to embolisation in SABE?

Answer 1. Yes. Go on to **17.21**.
         2. No. Go on to **17.23**.

17.18 Your answer – the iron is sequestered in the kidneys.

No. You are guessing. Go back to **17.11** and read it through more carefully.

17.19 Your answer — the patient is likely to survive a few years.

No. Few patients survive more than a few weeks after renal involvement develops, the majority dying rapidly. Read **17.16** with greater care.

17.20 Your answer — all the statements are true.

You are correct about statements 1 and 3 but 2 is wrong. Go back to **17.17** and read on to **17.34**. Then answer the question in **17.36** again.

17.21 Your answer — IVP is helpful.

Correct. The scintillogram using ^{203}Hg labelled chlormerhydrin is a useful way of diagnosing small infarcted areas of the kidney; clinically they are frequently painless, but there may be macroscopic or microscopic haematuria: the latter is also a feature of both focal 'embolic' and diffuse glomerulonephritis and is *not* in itself diagnostic. In focal 'embolic' nephritis there are focal and local lesions which may be embolic although the evidence for this is not conclusive: the area of inflammation in the glomeruli is often necrotic, and this is probably an immune complex nephritis, but may be due to micro-emboli lodging in the glomerular capillary tufts and causing ischaemic necrosis of some of the glomeruli. Microscopic haematuria is constant, but the diagnosis can only be made with certainty in life by renal biopsy.

Question Is microscopic haematuria diagnostic of focal 'embolic' nephritis?

Answer 1. Yes. Go on to **17.25**.
2. No. Go on to **17.27**.

17.22 Your answer — all the statements are false.

Your are correct about statement 2 only. You should go back to **17.1** and read to **17.16** inclusively. Then go on to **17.34** and finish the chapter.

17.23 Your answer — IVP is not helpful.

No. It is extremely useful in the diagnosis of renal artery obstructon but is much less useful in the diagnosis of occlusion of branches of the renal artery. Read **17.17** again.

17.24 Your answer — statement 1 is true, 2 and 3 are false.

Your are correct about 1 and 2 but wrong about 3. Read on from **17.34** to the end of the chapter.

17.25 Your answer — microscopic haematuria is diagnostic of focal embolic nephritis.

No. It may be found in all forms of renal involvement in SABE. Read **17.21** again, then answer the question correctly.

17.26 Your answer — statement 2 is true, 1 and 3 false.

You are quite wrong. Start at the beginning of the chapter again and work through it again.

17.27 Your answer – microscopic haematuria is not diagnostic of focal embolic nephritis in SABE.

Correct. The diffuse glomerulonephritis which is found in SABE is thought to be due to immune complex disease produced by the production of antibodies to the bacteria in the diseased heart valves combining with bacterial antigen to form an antibody-antigen complex with IgG and C^1_3 laid down in the glomerular capillaries. It is usually manifested not by the typical oliguria, haematuria, and oedema of acute post-streptococcal nephritis but rather by a more insidious course, with microscopic haematuria, proteinuria, increasing blood urea levels and finally terminal renal failure. The histology is that of a proliferative diffuse glomerulonephritis. Look at Fig. 17.27.

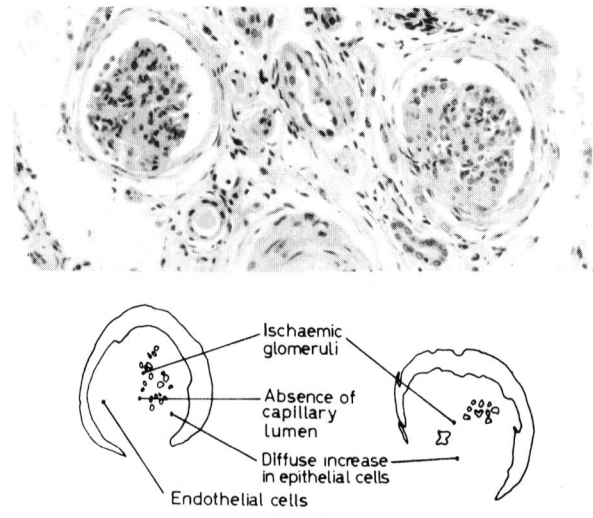

Fig. 17.27

Although its frequency of occurrence is probably reduced by antibiotics, many patients still die of renal failure caused by diffuse glomerulonephritis which may have developed before antibiotic treatment commenced.

Question If a patient with SABE develops progressive renal failure what is the likely cause?

Answer 1. Diffuse glomerulonephritis. Go on to **17.29**.
2. Focal glomerulonephritis. Go on to **17.31**.

17.28 Your answer – statement 3 is true, 2 and 1 are false.
You are wrong about statement 1. Read from **17.1** to **17.17**.

17.29 Your answer – renal failure indicates diffuse glomerulonephritis in SABE.
Correct. The next group of nephritides to be discussed is the interstitial nephritis group. Interstitial nephritis occurs to a greater or lesser extent in all cases of glomerulo*nephritis*, thus it is common in acute post-streptococcal nephritis and in SLE. It also occurs in pyelonephritis and in the drug induced nephritis of phenacetin, and in patients taking phenindione (phenylindanedione or Dindevan). Phenacetin causes a chronic interstitial infiltration with a severe pyelonephritis; papillary necrosis may develop. The phenacetin usually has to be taken in a large dosage i.e. 6 tablets of tab. codeine Co (NF) daily for a long period of time, before renal involvement occurs, and prompt withdrawal of the drug may be lifesaving, with improvement in renal function. There is a body of opinion which suggests that an impurity in the phenacetin is the cause of the renal damage, while yet others implicate aspirin which is known to cause an increase in tubular epithelial cell excretion in the urine. This will be discussed further in Chapter 20.

Question Can renal function ever improve after phenacetin withdrawal in patients suffering from phenacetin nephritis?

Answer 1. Yes. Go on to **17.32**.
2. No. Go on to **17.34**.

17.30 Your answer – the urine osmolality will be 300 mOsm/kg.
No. The odd thing about the urine osmolality in this condition is that it may be 600 mOsm/kg. This is remarkable because the urine in severe oliguric renal failure in the majority of other diseases is about the level of plasma osmolality i.e. approximately 300 mOsm/kg to 400 mOsm/kg. Read **17.32** again.

17.31 Your answer – renal failure suggests focal glomerulonephritis.
Renal failure rarely results if a nephritis remains focal i.e. if only a few glomeruli are affected. It is not certain how frequently the focal glomerulonephritis of SABE develops into diffuse glomerulonephritis. For renal failur to develop the vast majority of the nephrons must be damaged severely, i.e. by a diffuse process. Now answer the question in **17.27** again.

17.32 Your answer – renal function can improve after phenacetin withdrawal.
Correct. Phenindione or phenylindanedione (Dindevan) is an anticoagulant in common usage which occasionally causes hypersensitivity reactions involving (1) the skin – causing erythematous rashes and even exfoliative dematitis; (2) the liver – causing hepatic necrosis; and (3) the kidneys – causing an acute interstitial nephritis. The interstitial nephritis is quite remarkable for two reasons:

(1) The cells infiltrating the renal parenchyma may be largely eosinophils, and
(2) The patients develop severe oliguria with urine osmolalities of about 600 mOsm/kg, the only recognised cause of a renal oliguria associated with a urine osmolality of this level.

Treatment consists of withdrawal of the drug and administration of corticosteroids.

Question What is the value of urine osmolality that you might expect with acute oliguria due to phenindione (phenylindanedione) hypersensitivity?

Answer 1. 300 mOsm/kg. Go on to **17.30**.
2. 600 mOsm/kg. Go on to **17.36**.

17.33 Your answer – statements 2 and 3 are true, 1 is false.

You are correct about statement 3 only. Go back to the beginning of the chapter and work through it again.

17.34 Your answer – renal function never improves after phenacetin withdrawal.

No. There is always the possibility that renal function may improve if the drug is stopped, or that deterioration will not be maintained. Of course if sufficient damage has been done to cause necrosis of papillae there is little chance of improvement of renal function and the best that can be hoped for is that no further deterioration will occur. Read **17.29** again before selecting the correct answer.

17.35 Your answer – statements 1 and 3 are true, 2 is false.

Your are correct. Before leaving the chapter you may wish to look up some references on this subject.

Focal nephritis: Heptinstall R. H. & Jockes A. M. (1963) in Strauss M. B. & Welt L. G. (eds) Diseases of the Kidney. Churchill, London. Ross J. H. (1960) Quart. J. Med. **29**, 391.
Goodpasture's syndrome; Rusby & Wilson C. (1960) Quart. J. Med. **29**, 501. Also A. J. Prosky et al, Am J. Med. (1970) **48**, 162.
Berlyne G. M. Chapter on Kidney and Systemic Disease in Black DAK Renal Disease 2nd Edition. Blackwell Scientific Publications, Oxford 1967.
Henoch-Schönlein nephritis: Gairdner D. (1948) Quart. J. Med. **17**, 95.
SABE Gutman R. A. et al Medicine (Balt) (1972), **51**, 1.

17.36 Your answer – the urine osmolality will be 600 m0sm/kg. Correct.

Now look at the following statements and think carefully before choosing the correct answer.

Statement 1 Renal involvement occurs in about half the cases of Henoch-Schönlein nephritis.

Statement 2 Goodpasture's syndrome has an excellent prognosis.

Statement 3 Phenindione sensitivity can cause an interstitial nephritis.

Answer 1. All the statements are true. Go on to **17.20**.
2. All the statements are false. Go on to **17.22**.
3. Only statement 1 is true, 2 and 3 false. Go on to **17.24**.
4. Statement 2 is true, 1 and 3 are false. Go on to **17.26**.
5. Statement 3 is true, 1 and 2 are false. Go on to **17.28**.
6. Statements 1 and 2 are true, 3 is false. Go on to **17.37**.
7. Statements 2 and 3 are true, 1 is false. Go on to **17.33**.
8. Statements 1 and 3 are true, 2 is false. Go on to **17.35**.

17.37 Your answer: statement 3 is false, 1 & 2 are true.

You are wrong about statements 3 & 2. Read on from **17.10** to the end of the chapter.

Time for this chapter: 20 minutes

Chapter 18
Surgical diseases of the kidney

18.1 In this chapter we shall briefly discuss surgical lesions of the kidney which may present to the physician. More detailed consideration of these topics will be found in textbooks of urology. The topics covered in this chapter are tumours of the kidney, tuberculosis and hydronephrosis.

The commonest renal tumour is the hypernephroma (renal cell carcinoma or adenocarcinoma). These tumours are malignant adenomas; they are usually encapsulated at first. Histologically they consist of clear cells reminiscent of the adrenal cortex, with an admixture of dark granular cells. The cells lie in a papillary or acinar arrangement. There is frequently necrosis and bleeding into the tumour. The tumour spreads into the surrounding kidney and into the renal veins. Tumour tissue may grow along the renal vein into the inferior vena cava (IVC); and locally it may grow through the renal capsule into the perinephric tissues and adjacent viscera.

Question How does a hypernephroma reach the inferior vena cava?

Answer 1. Direct spread. Go on to **18.3**.
2. Spread along renal vein. Go on to **18.5**.

18.2 Your answer – I would do a nephrectomy.
You are partially correct. If a solitary metastasis is found it may well be worthwhile to remember the metastasis as well.
Answer the question in **18.5** again.

18.3 Your answer – the tumour spreads directly into the IVC.
No. It spreads commonly down into the renal vein, along into the lumen of the inferior vena cava. Read **18.1** again, and answer the question correctly.

18.4 Your answer – I would do a lobectomy.
No. This would be pointless unless you also remove the primary tumour. Answer **18.5** again.

18.5 Your answer – it spreads along the renal vein.
You are correct. Metastases are most common in the renal venules but also are found in the lungs, where they give rounded 'cannon ball' shadows on X-ray of the chest. The liver, lymph nodes, peritoneum and brain are also frequently invaded by metastases of hypernephroma. The metastases in the brain and lungs have been

occasionally reported to regress after the primary hypernephroma has been removed. The metastases are often very slow in growing and sometimes are present in the same site for years before the patient dies. Metastases are sometimes solitary, so that it may be worthwhile to remove the primary tumour and a solitary secondary in the lung or cerebellum.

Question If you had a patient with a hypernephroma and visible evidence of a hypernephroma metastasis in the form of a solitary 'cannon ball' deposit in the right lower lobe, what would you advise?

Answer 1. Nephrectomy. Go on to **18.2**.
2. Right lower lobectomy. Go on to **18.4**.
3. Nephrectomy and right lower lobectomy. Go on to **18.7**.

18.6 Your answer — it is necessary to perform an IVP in *every* patient with unexplained haematuria.

Correct. There may be no abnormal physical signs unless the tumour is large or metastases are present. Sometimes the tumour mass is readily palpable as a large mobile kidney mass. Examination of the urine shows haematuria, macroscopic or microscopic. There may be anaemia or polycythaemia. Eosinophilia sometimes is found. Diagnosis is usually made on IVP. The tumour may have calcification in it, (Fig. 18.6a). The diagnosis on IVP is made by the finding that the calyceal pattern is distorted by a radio-translucent mass, occupying part of the kidney. Tomography may show the renal outline to be distended by the mass, but

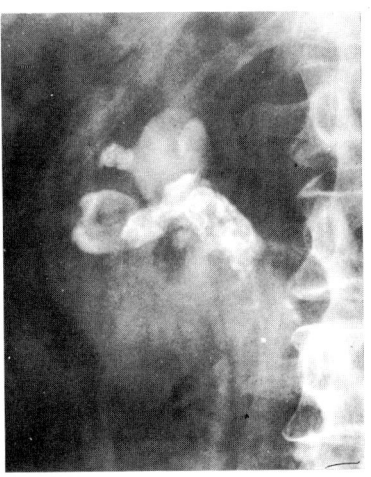
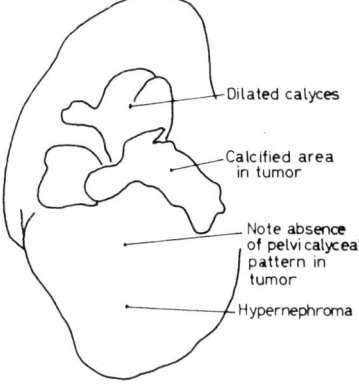

Fig. 18.6

IVP and tomography may not differentiate between a simple renal cyst and a hypernephroma because both distort the calyceal pattern and may give a similar localised space occupying lesion on tomography. The differential diagnosis may be made more certainly by selective renal arteriography, which may show tumour vessels in hypernephroma (see Fig. 18.6 b) although this is not constant. Simple renal cysts are avascular on arteriography.

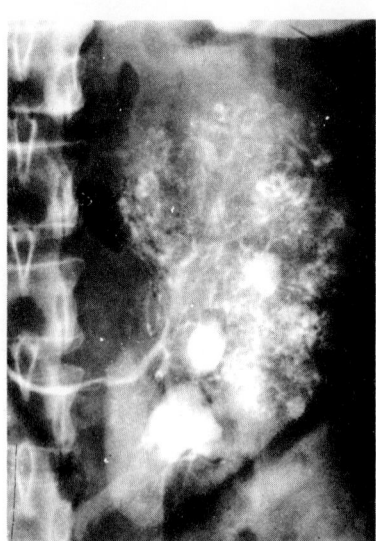 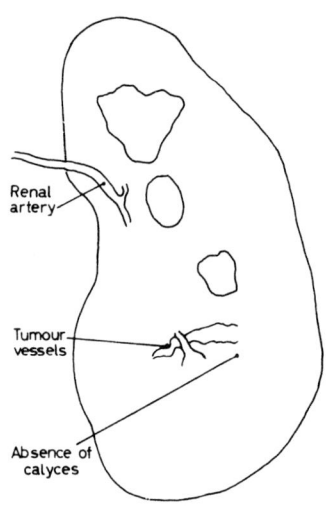

Fig. 18.6b

Question Can a definite diagnosis of hypernephroma always be made on intravenous pyelography?

Answer 1. Yes. Go on to **18.8**.
2. No. Go on to **18.10**.

18.7 Your answer − I would do a lobectomy and a nephrectomy.

Correct. The symptoms of hypernephroma will now be considered. Hypernephroma may be symptom-free until metastases develop. Commonly there is haematuria in more than half the patients as the presenting symptom. The haematuria is often transitory and is painless. For this reason *all patients with unexplained haematuria should have an IVP*. Pain occurs in 1 in 4 patients as an early symptom. It is usually in the loin of the affected side but may be in the site of a metastasis. There are the usual symptoms of malignancy; anorexia, weight loss, fatigue, lassitude, and anaemia. Sometimes the tumour presents as a pyrexia of undetermined origin (PUO). Occasionally the tumor has endocrine secretion, causing Cushing's syndrome or hyperparathyroidism. Some patients present with polycythaemia due to excessive renal erythropoietin production but the normochromic anaemica of malignancy is more frequent.

Question Is it necessary to carry out an IVP examination in *every* patient with unexplained transitory haematuria?

Answer 1. Yes. Go on to **18.6**.
2. No. Go on to **18.9**.

18.8 Your answer – a definite diagnosis of hypernephroma can always be made on IVP.

Very often it is impossible to be certain that a filling defect on IVP is a hypernephroma rather than a simple cyst. Read **18.6** carefully again then choose the correct answer.

18.9 Your answer – it is *not* necessary to do an IVP in *every* patient with haematuria.

Your are wrong. You will miss the occasional patient with hypernephroma or other tumour of the renal tract. You may also miss deformities of the calcyes due to chronic pyelonephritis and occasionally due to tuberculosis. Go back to **18.7** read through the paragraph, and then choose the correct answer.

18.10 Your answer – a definite diagnosis of hypernephroma *cannot* always be made on IVP.

Good. The treatment of hypernephroma is nephrectomy, with care not to miss tumour which may be growing along the renal vein. Solitary metastases may be removed simultaneously. Post-operative irradiation improves the 5 years survival rate. Metastases may also prove radio-sensitive. Even without operation or radio-therapy the tumour may grow so slowly that the patient may survive for several years.

Question What is the preferred treatment for a hypernephroma without metastases?

Answer 1. Nephrectomy. Go on to **18.12**.
2. Irradiation. Go on to **18.13**.
3. Nephrectomy and post-operative irradiation. Go on to **18.14**.

18.11 You should not be reading this paragraph as it is not included in the instructions

18.12 Your answer – the treatment of hypernephroma is nephrectomy.

You are correct but post-operative irradiation improves the 5 year-cure rate. Go on to **18.14**.

18.13 Your answer – the treatment of hypernephroma is irradiation.
No. Some surgeons use irradiation pre-operatively to shrink a huge tumour; otherwise irradiation is more commonly used post-operatively. Go on to **18.14**.

18.14 Your answer – the treatment of hypernephroma is nephrectomy and post-operative irradiation.
Correct. Carcinoma of the renal pelvis is usually a papillary tumour. It is best to consider that *all* papillary tumours of the ureters and renal pelvis are malignant. They are frequently multiple, and give rise to haematuria and flank pain. They may cause an obstructive hydronephrosis. If bilateral, renal failure may ensue. Some tumours are squamous and associateed with stones of the renal pelvis. Patients who work with carcinogens such as benzidine and β naphthylamine may develop malignant papilloma of the renal pelvis, ureters or bladder. The urine in these patients as well as those with other types of the malignant papilloma, contains malignant cells identifiable by microscopy of the urinary sediment in 90 per cent of patients.

The treatment of a papillary carcinoma of the renal pelvis is nephro-ureterectomy, followed by repeated cystoscopy to fulgurate new papillomata as they arise in the bladder. Villous papillomas of the bladder give rise to symptoms of haematuria, attacks of cystitis, and pain at the end of micturition. They should be destroyed by fulguration. If the malignancy has spread from the papilloma into the bladder wall, total or partial cystectomy may be necessary. Some surgeons utilise intra-vesical irradiation for malignant bladder tumours. In infants and early childhood a Wilms tumour (embryoma) may develop. This presents as a swelling in the abdomen with haematuria and abdominal pain. Treatment is nephrectomy and post-operative irradiation. Only 1 in 4 survive 5 years.

Question Is cytological examination of the urine of any value in the diagnosis of carcinoma of the renal pelvis or ureter?

Answer 1. Yes. Go on to **18.16**.
2. No. Go on to **18.18**.

18.15 Your answer – advise him to empty his rectum as frequently as possible.
Good. Tuberculosis of the kidneys is a common disease. It is usually a blood borne infection coming usually from a pulmonary focus. A miliary tubercle starts in a glomerulus and grows into a sloughing caseous renal lesion which excretes M. tuberculosis into the urine. Several tubercles may coalesce and ulcerate into a calyx at which time there may be X-ray evidence of calyceal distortion and cavitation. Later the entire kidney may be involved with the renal tissue being replaced by a caseous mass which later calcifies. (See Fig. 18.15). The symptoms

are dysuria and frequency due to bladder involvement, with painless haematuria and sometimes an ache in the flank. In adults epididymitis is common. *The finding of sterile pyuria should always lead to a careful search for tubercle bacilli in the urine.* Sterile pyuria should never be ignored until a diagnosis of tuberculosis of the kidneys has been positively excluded. The treatment of tuberculosis of the kidneys is long term drug therapy for at least two years with streptomycin, isoniazid and PAS.

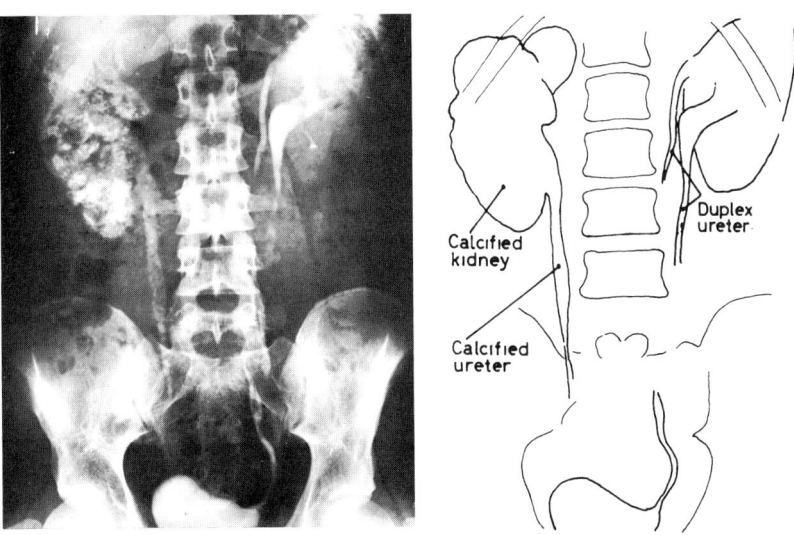

Fig. 18.15.

Question Would you investigate any further if a patient with dysuria was found to have white cells in excess numbers in the urine but it is sterile on routine agar culture?

Answer 1. Yes. Go on to **18.20**.
2. No. Go on to **18.22**.

18.16 Your answer – microscopy of the urine *is* of value in making a diagnosis of carcinoma of the pelvis of the kidney.

Correct. In patients who have the bladder removed the ureters may be implanted into the sigmoid colon. This is known as uretero-sigmoidostomy, which is associated with several complications;

(1) *Recurrent pyelonephritis* due to reflux of faecal material up the ureters due to the high colonic pressure during defaecation.

(2) *Hydropelvis and hydroureter*. This occurs in up to $\frac{2}{3}$ patients and may be caused by stenosis of the ureters at their site of implantation in the colon or to reflux of colonic contents up the ureters.

(3) *Hypokalaemia with hyperchloraemic acidosis*. This interesting metabolic disturbance occurs in half to three quarters of patients with ureterosigmoidostomy. The cause of this is due to the colon secreting a fluid of high bicarbonate content and low chloride content. Thus if a solution of normal saline is instilled into the normal colon then it becomes after 5 or 6 hours, alkaline, with a high HCO_3^- content, a low Cl^- content and a high K^+ content. Similarly, if urine which is being secreted by the kidneys is low in bicarbonate and potassium and high chloride ion, and remains in the colon for a few hours in a patient with a ureterosigmoidostomy, there will be an increase in its HCO_3^- and K^+ content and reabsorption of Cl^-. Thus the patient develops a hyperchloraemic acidosis with hypokalaemia. The preventive therapy of this condition is to ensure that the patient empties the urine out of the colon *as often as possible* – at hourly or two hourly intervals. In addition one may need to give sodium and potassium citrate in sufficient quantity to restore HCO_3^- and K^+ levels to normal. Failure to treat the acidosis may lead to the development of renal osteomalacia.

Question If a patient with ureterosigmoidostomy has a hyperchloraemic acidosis what would you advise him to do if he refuses drug therapy?

Answer 1. Keep the urine in his colon for as long as possible. Go on to **18.17**.
2. Pass the urine from the colon as frequently as possible. Go on to **18.15**.

18.17 Your answer – advise him to keep the urine in his colon as long as possible. This is the worst possible advice because the disorder is due to the colon secreting bicarbonate and potassium into the colonic urine and reabsorbing chloride from it. The shorter the time urine is in the colonic lumen the better. Answer **18.16** again after careful re-reading of the paragraph.

18.18 Your answer – microscopy of the urine is of no value in the diagnosis of carcinoma of the renal pelvis.

Wrong. In 90 per cent of patients a positive cytological diagnosis can be made. Read **18.14** again more carefully this time. Then answer the question correctly.

18.19 Your answer – distal tubular defects develop in hydronephrosis.

Correct. Now answer the questions below after reading the statements carefully.

Statement 1 Hypernephroma tissue may grow along the renal vein.

Statement 2 Sterile pyuria may indicate renal tuberculosis.

Statement 3 In ureterosigmoidostomy a hyperchloraemic acidosis may develop.

Answers 1. All the statements are true. Go on to **18.23**.
2. All the statements are false. Go on to **18.24**.
3. Statement 1 is true, 2 and 3 false. Go on to **18.25**.
4. Statement 2 is true, 1 and 3 false. Go on to **18.26**.
5. Statement 3 is true, 1 and 2 false. Go on to **18.27**.
6. Statements 1 and 2 are true, 3 false. Go on to **18.28**.
7. Statements 1 and 3 are true, 2 false. Go on to **18.29**.
8. Statements 2 and 3 are true, 1 false. Go on to **18.30**.

18.20 Your answer — I *would* investigate it further.

Correct. Hydronephrosis may be unilateral or bilateral. The sequential changes in the IVP as hydronephrosis develops are seen in Chapter 4. Bilateral hydronephrosis may be congenital, due to obstruction in the urethra i.e. phimosis, pinhole meatus, urethral valves, — or acquired, due to prostatic adenoma, carcinoma or urethral structure. Sometimes there is congenital dilatation of the urinary tract (mega-ureter and mega-cystis) in patients with Hirschprung's disease. Bilateral hydronephrosis also occurs in pregnancy as a physiological phenomenon. This is discussed in the chapter on the Kidney and Pregnancy. Unilateral hydronephrosis may be congenital; it may also be caused by ureteric structure, stone or tumour. Uretero-pelvic anomalies such as neuromuscular defects are frequently diagnosed but the diagnosis is hypothetical, for we have little idea of the cause of hydronephrosis in these patients. Bands and aberrant arteries have also been blamed for hydronephrosis but this may well be due to the swelling kidney pushing up against a blood vessel or band, rather than the latter acting as the primary source of obstruction. Advanced bilateral hydronephrosis leads to renal failure but there are specific disorders of distal tubular function leading to renal diabetes insipidus and the syndrome of renal tubular acidosis in the occasional patient. Retroperitoneal tumour or periureteric fibrosis may be the cause of unilateral or bilateral hydronephrosis. All patients with suspected retroperitoneal fibrosis (features of back and loin ache, hydronephrosis, raised ESR, renal failure) should be asked if they have migraine, because methysergide, a drug used to treat migraine, causes retroperitoneal fibrosis. The diagnosis of hydronephrosis is made by IVP and, if there is severe renal failure, retrograde pyelogram. The latter may introduce infection into a sterile hydronephrosis and should only be done under antibiotic cover. The treatment of hydronephrosis is removal of the obstruction although plastic operations on the pelvis may be undertaken in those patients without obvious cause for the hydronephrosis.

Question Do some patients with hydronephrosis develop distal tubular abnormalities?

Answer 1. Yes. Go on to **18.19**.
2. No. Go on to **18.21**.

18.21 Your answer – distal tubular defects do not develop in hydronephrosis. No. Read **18.20** again paying more attention this time.

18.22 Your answer – I would not investigate it any further.
You are wrong. The whole purpose of **18.15** was to point out that sterile pyuria often meant tuberculosis of the kidneys. Go back to **18.15** and read it carefully before you answer the question again.

18.23 Your answer – all the statements are true.
You are correct. Chapters worth reading on these subjects are to be found in most textbooks of urology, to which the reader is referred for further information.

18.24 Your answer – all the statements are false.
No. You are wrong. Go back to **18.1** and read through the chapter again.

18.25 Your answer – statement 1 is true only.
No. Because this is a short chapter read it through again from **18.1**.

18.26 Your answer – statement 2 is true only.
No. Because this is a short chapter, read it through again from the beginning.

18.27 Your answer – statement 3 is true only.
No. Because this is a short chapter, read it again from the beginning.

18.28 Your answer – statement 3 is false.
No. This is a short chapter, so read through it again.

18.29 Your answer – statement 2 is false.
No. Read this short chapter through from the beginning.

18.30 Your answer – statement 1 is false.
No. Read this short chapter through again from **18.1**.

Time for this chapter: 20 minutes

Chapter 19
The bones and the kidney

19.1 In this chapter hyperparathyroidism and bone diseases associated with kidney disease will be discussed. Primary hyperparathyroidism is a rare disease due usually to adenoma of the parathyroid glands. It is associated with the following clinical features:

Bony lesions. These are the characteristic lesions associated with osteitis fibrosa cystica in which there is a generalised demineralisation of bone associated with the presence of bone cysts. The histological picture is of an increase in fibrous tissue in the woven bone, the lamellae of which are eroded by an increased number of osteoclasts. The osteoclasts erode the bone away. The cysts may be the site of pathological fracture. Clinically, there is bone pain with swelling and deformity over the cysts.

Question What is the cell type which erodes the bone in excessive amounts in hyperparathyroidism?

Answer 1. Fibrous tissue. Go on to **19.3**.
2. Osteoclasts. Go on to **19.5**.
3. Osteoblasts. Go on to **19.7**.

19.2 Your answer – the serum alkaline phosphatase level is raised.

Correct. Renal involvement is common in primary hyperparathyroidism and takes two forms:

(1) Renal calculi.
(2) Non-calculous renal failure.

Let us consider the renal calculi first. In patients with primary hyperparathyroidism on a high calcium intake renal stones are common. The frequency of hyperparathyroidism in renal stone patients varies from 2 per cent to 10 per cent in different series. Because hyperparathyroidism is curable, all patients with renal stones should have their serum calcium, inorganic phosphorus and alkaline phosphatase estimated to exclude hyperparathyroidism. In 10% of urate stone patients hyperparathyroidism is present. In primary hyperparathyroidism there is usually a serum calcium of greater than 10.5 mg/100 ml, a serum inorganic phosphorus of 2.5 mg/100 ml or less, and a serum alkaline phosphatase of greater than 17 KA units/100 ml. The single most useful investigation is repeated measurement of serum calcium. Tubular reabsorption of phosphate is reduced but this test is frequently difficult to interpret. If radioimmunoassay of parathyroid hormone is available, it is found that PTH levels are frequently but not always elevated in peripheral venous blood in primary hyperparathyroidism. The renal stones may sometimes be associated with generalised nephrocalcinosis.

Non-calculous renal failure may occur due to hypercalcaemia. This acts by a direct nephrotoxic action, there being precipitation of calcium in the renal tubules and a fall in GFR. It also causes distal tubular dysfunction, with polyuria, renal diabetes insipidus and inability to acidify normally; this may cause renal tubular acidosis. In addition hypercalcaemia causes vomiting and salt depletion and thus extra-renal uraemia.

Question Does hypercalcaemia cause renal failure?

Answer 1. Yes. Go on to **19.6**.
2. No. Go on to **19.8**.

19.3 Your answer – fibrous tissue.

You are correct only in so far as there is an excess of fibrous tissue present. The fibrous tissue does not erode the bone. This is done by osteoclasts. Read **19.1** again then answer the question correctly.

19.4 Your answer – the serum alkaline phosphatase level is not raised.

No. You are incorrect. Read **19.5** again then answer the question.

19.5 Your answer – osteoclasts erode the bone.

Correct. The osteoclasts are strikingly prominent in primary hyperparathyroidism but the osteoblasts, although less noticeable, are very active and consequently bone turnover is increased. This is reflected in the high serum

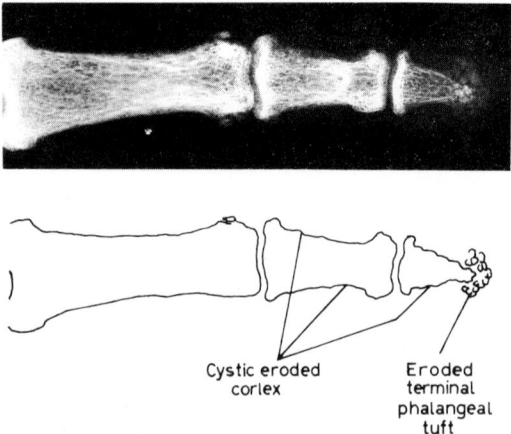

Fig. 19.5

alkaline phosphatase of hyperparathyroidism where bone disease is present. Bone changes, including generalised demineralisation and cystic changes are sometimes totally absent, particularly in patients on a high calcium intake. An early and consistent sign of bony involvement is erosion of the cortex of the terminal phalanges of the fingers seen on X-ray (see Fig. 19.5) due to osteoclastic activity.

Question In hyperparathyroidism is the serum alkaline phosphatase level raised?

Answer 1. Yes. Go on to **19.2**.
2. No. Go on to **19.4**.

19.6 Your answer – hypercalcaemia causes renal failure.

You are correct. Estimation of urinary calcium excretion on a normal calcium intake is by itself an unreliable method for the diagnosis of hyperparathyroidism because an increase in urinary calcium excretion is more commonly due to idiopathic hypercalciuria. It is essential therefore to seek other evidence of hyperparathyroidism.

Question Is an increased urinary calcium excretion adequate to make a diagnosis of hyperparathyroidism?

Answer No. Go on to **19.9**.
Yes. Go on to **19.10**.

19.7 Your answer – osteoblasts erode the bone.

No. You are confusing osteoblasts, the cells which form bone, with osteoclasts, the cells which erode bone. Read **19.1** more carefully. Then answer the question correctly.

19.8 Your answer – hypercalcaemia does not cause renal failure.

You are incorrect. Hypercalcaemia has a direct nephrotoxic action and also causes extra-renal uraemia. Read **19.2** again. Then answer the question.

19.9 Your answer – hypercalciuria is not by itself adequate to make a diagnosis.

Correct. In patients who have primary hyperparathyroidism death may occur from hypercalcaemia causing cardiac arrest, or from renal failure. Peptic ulceration is frequent and pancreatitis sometimes occurs. The diagnosis of primary hyperparathyroidism is based on the clinical triad of bone pains, abdominal pains (due to peptic ulcer or pancreatitis) and renal colic from renal stones coupled with radiological and biochemical evidence. (Renal or ureteric colic is a very severe pain which may last for hours, radiating from the loin along the line of the ureter and passing to the tip of the penis or to the pubis). The other symptoms of hyperparathyroidism are due to hypercalcaemia and include anorexia, dysphagia, constipation, nausea and vomiting, itching, polyuria, and sometimes a metallic taste in the mouth.

Question Does peptic ulceration ever complicate primary hyperparathyroidism?

Answer 1. Yes. Go on to **19.11**.
2. No. Go on to **19.13**.

19.10 Your answer – an increased urinary calcium excretion is adequate to diagnose hyperparathyroidism.

No. It is one of the pieces of evidence in favour of hyperparathyroidism but by itself is inadequate to make a diagnosis. Read **19.6** again.

19.11 Your answer – peptic ulceration complicates primary hyperparathyroidism.

Correct. We have given a thumb-nail sketch of primary hyperparathyroidism which is only of relevance to this book in so far as the disease is a cause of renal stones and renal failure. The subject of 'renal osteodystrophy' will now be considered. In Britain bony disease *commonly* complicates slowly progressive chronic renal failure and this association of renal failure with bony changes is referred to as 'renal' or azotaemic osteodystrophy. Its incidence is variable from country to country. Thus renal osteodystrophy is slightly less frequently seen in the U.S.A. The reason for this geographic variation in incidence is unknown but the virtual absence of renal osteodystrophy in Israel is likely to be caused by the low P content of the normal Israeli diet associated with a moderately low protein intake. Possible causes are variation in the amount of vitamin D synthesised in the skin in countries with differing amounts of sunshine, dietary vitamin D and calcium intake, and racial factors.

There are 4 major types of renal osteodystrophy.

(1) Renal rickets or renal osteomalacia.
(2) Renal hyperparathyroidism.
(3) Osteoporosis.
(4) Osteopetrosis or increase in bone density.

Histological examination of the bone in advanced chronic renal failure often shows both osteomalacia and hyperparathyroidism to be present simultaneously. It is common to find clinically that one of the two diseases predominates, however.

Question In a patient with renal osteodystrophy can both osteomalacia and hyperparathyroidism occur simultaneously?

Answer 1. Yes. Go on to **19.14**.
2. No. Go on to **19.16**.

19.12 Your answer — there is a true fracture of the bone at a Looser's node.

No. A Looser's node is radiotranslucent because the bone is demineralised but the bone matrix is continuous across the area. Read **19.14** again.

19.13 Your answer — peptic ulcer does not complicate primary hyperparathyroidism.

You are wrong. Peptic ulceration in combination with renal stones or bone pains is one of the clinical syndromes caused by primary hyperparathyroidism. Read **19.9** again.

19.14 Your answer — renal osteomalacia and hyperparathyroidism can occur simultaneously.

Correct. Let us consider renal osteomalacia first. Pathologically it is similar to nutritional rickets due to insufficient vitamin D, with irregularity and broadening of the epiphyses in children due to irregular growth of the cartilage. In both children and adults there is an increased width of osteoid (non-calcified bone) round the bony lamellae and a calcification front is absent. Clinically this failure to calcify bone results in weakness of the long weight-bearing bones with resultant genu valgum or varum. The epiphyses are swollen in children. There is usually tenderness over the long bones on direct pressure. X-ray of the long bones shows the broadened irregular epiphyses of rickets in children. In adults and children

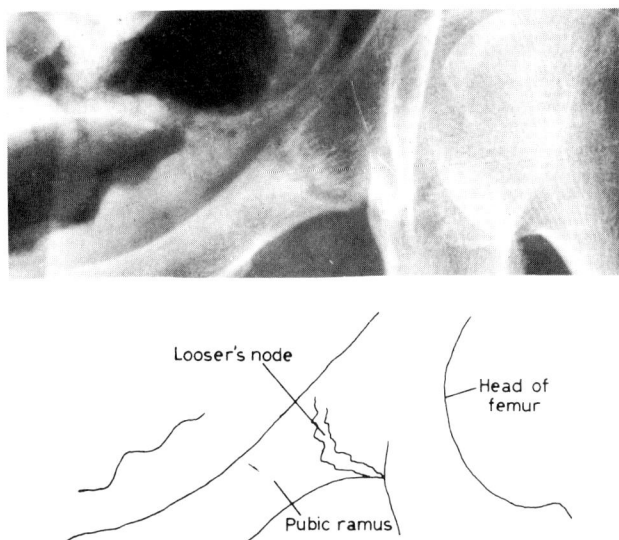

Fig. 19.14

there are radiolucent areas in the bones which look like fractures but which are areas of decalcification of the bone. The bone matrix is continuous across these areas, in spite of their radiolucency (see Fig. 19.14). They are called Looser's nodes. They commonly occur in the pelvis, particularly on the pubic rami, but also frequently occur in the femur, scapula, ribs, and humerus. Diagnosis of Looser's nodes is solely by X-ray examination.

Question Is there a true fracture of bone at the site of the Looser's nodes?

Answer 1. Yes. Go on to **19.12**
2. No. Go on to **19.17**.

19.15 Your answer – renal osteodystrophy associated with a decreased formation of 1:25 dihydroxy D_3.

Correct. The serum inorganic phosphorus level is usually very high in chronic renal failure, figures of 9–15 mg/100 ml not being exceptional. Patients with renal osteomalacia have similar high serum inorganic phosphate levels but their serum calcium concentrations are usually reduced; serum calciums of 6–7 mg/100 ml are common. The serum calcium X serum phosphorus product is usually above 70 in renal hyperparathyroidism. In renal osteomalacia the serum calcium X serum phosphorus product is less than 70 in most cases. The serum alkaline phosphatase is frequently elevated in both osteomalacia and hyperparathyroidism. Patients with renal osteomalacia tend to have lower serum calcium levels than those with renal hyperparathyroidism. The clinical diagnosis of renal osteomalacia is made by the combination of clinical, biochemical and radiological data: i.e., tender bones, bony deformities, raised alkaline phosphatase, rachitic epiphyseal changes (in children), and Looser's nodes. However in many cases there are histological changes on bone biopsy with normal clinical, biochemical and radiological findings.

Question Is the serum alkaline phosphatase usually normal or elevated in renal osteomalacia?

Answer 1. Normal. Go on to **19.20**.
2. Elevated. Go on to **19.18**.

19.16 Your answer – renal osteomalacia and hyperparathyroidism do not occur simultaneously.

No. They are frequently found together. You should read **19.11** again with more care.

19.17 Your answer – there is no true fracture of the bone at a Looser's node.

Correct. Callus does not form at a Looser's node: should you be in doubt about whether a translucency is a fracture or not this is a way of finding out.

The types of disease which cause renal osteomalacia are slowly progressive renal diseases such as chronic glomerulonephritis, chronic pyelonephritis, polycystic disease and hypoplastic kidneys (in which the kidneys are tiny and shrunken and a certain nosological diagnosis cannot be made).

Renal osteomalacia is probably due to an increased resistance to the action of vitamin D which occurs in uraemia. There is an abnormality in the metabolism of the polar metabolite 25-hydroxycholecalciferol with reduced circulating levels of this compound. The stools contain almost all the ingested calcium and little calcium is excreted in the urine. On giving large doses of vitamin D (e.g. 50,000 units/day) by mouth, the faecal calcium falls and urinary calcium excretion increases. The bones heal slowly although they remain painful for 3 to 4 weeks. The Looser's nodes disappear. Vitamin D is poorly absorbed in chronic renal failure. If a very large amount of calcium is given orally, i.e. 20 G of calcium lactate a day, healing of renal osteomalacia can be seen in the absence of additional vitamin D. This is due to the absorption of calcium due to the high concentrations of calcium in the intestine, as has been demonstrated by De Wardener and colleagues. Remember that when small amounts of calcium are present in the diet — i.e. 1 G or so/day, there is virtually no absorption of calcium from the gut, due to resistance to vitamin D in renal failure.

The cause of vitamin D resistance is partly understood at the present. The kidneys, as Kodicek has shown are the sole organs capable of coverting the relatively inactive 25 hydroxy vitamin D_3 (which was hydroxylated in the liver) to 1:25 dihydroxy vitamin D_3, the latter being the active hormone at bony level. It seems that the hydroxyl group at the 1 position is essential for the full metabolic action of Vitamin D_3. In renal failure the kidneys are incapable of converting adequate amounts of 25 hydroxy vitamin D_3 to the 1:25 dihydroxy form. Rassmussen has shown that the presence of parathyroid hormone enhances the hydroxylation by the kidney to the 1:25 dihydroxy form, and that thyrocalcitonin inhibits the conversion. 1:25 $(OH)_2$ D_3 also promotes intestinal absorption of calcium.

Question Is renal osteodystrophy associated with excess or reduced production of 1:25 dihydroxy Vitamin D_3?

Answer 1. Excess. Go on to **19.19**.
2. Reduced. Go on to **19.15**.

19.18 Your answer — the serum alkaline phosphatase level is usually high in renal osteomalacia.

Correct. The treatment of osteomalacia is vitamin D, 50,000 units/day, increasing cautiously, if there is no response in 3 to 4 weeks, to larger doses up to 250,000 units/day. The great danger of using these large doses of vitamin D is the development of vitamin D intoxication, causing hypercalcaemia and rapid deterioration in the already impaired renal function. Initially serum calcium levels should be estimated weekly, then later at monthly intervals.

Question A patient being treated for renal osteomalacia with vitamin D has a serum calcium of 12.5 mg/100 ml. What would you do?

Answer 1. Stop vitamin D. Go on to **19.21**.
2. Do nothing. Go on to **19.23**.

19.19 Your answer – renal osteodystrophy is associated with excess production of 1:25 dihydroxy vitamin D_3.

No. You have not followed the argument in **19.17** properly. You should reread it at least twice before answering the question again.

19.20 Your answer – the serum alkaline phosphatase level is usually normal.

No. It is elevated. Read **19.15** again to find out if you have missed any other facts, before you choose the correct answer.

19.21 Your answer – stop vitamin D administration.

You are correct. Secondary hyperparathyroidism commonly occurs in chronic renal failure. Bricker has pointed out that there is an increase in parathyroid hormone secretion (PTH) early in renal failure when the GFR is around 75 ml/min. and that PTH levels progressively increases as renal failure increases. This has been shown experimentally in the dog, both by direct measurement of PTH levels and also by the measurement of tubular reabsorption of phosphate (TRP). The TRP falls as PTH increases. This is shown in Fig. 19.21a. Eventually in end stage renal failure there is frank hyperparathyroidism with renal osteodystrophy and hyperplastic or occasionally adenomatous parathyroid glands. He propounded the theory that early on in renal failure the minimal fall in GFR was associated with a slight rise in plasma inorganic phosphorus levels. This causes a slight fall in plasma ionized calcium level the latter triggering off parathyroid hormone secretion at a higher level. This results in a decreased TRP and more P is excreted in the urine. This causes a slight fall towards normal of plasma P level and a restoration of ionized calcium in the plasma to normal. With further decrease in GFR there is a further increase in parathyroid secretion and this is sufficient to keep P levels normal until GFR drops to 25–30 ml/min. It has been shown that if dietary P is reduced then the stimulus to parathyroid secretion is less and PTH levels remain much lower and TRP remains at normal until much lower levels of GFR are reached. Thus hyperparathyroidism starts early in renal failure. In these patients the pathology of the bone lesions is similar to that of primary hyperparathyroidism with osteoclasts eroding the bony lamella and fibrous tissue occupying the enlarged spaces between the lamellae. Bone cysts may develop. The striking telescoping of the terminal phalanges (Fig. 19.21 b) gives an appearance of clubbing, referred to as pseudo-clubbing. It is caused by resorption of the distal parts of the terminal phalanges. In addition there may be large swellings arising in the soft tissues due to masses of metastatic calcification. X-ray of the spine may

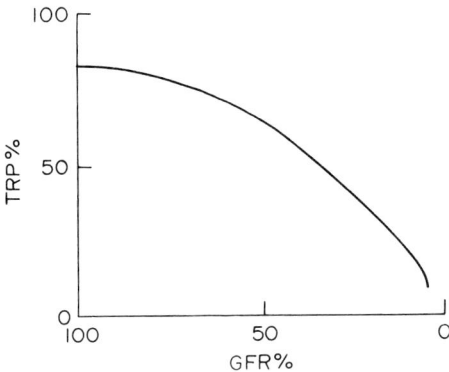

Fig. 19.21a

show banded sclerosis, the typical 'rugger jersey' spine of hyperparathyroidism due to alternate bands of osteosclerosis and osteoporosis. The ends of the clavicle may be eroded, causing pain in the shoulder girdle. Metastatic deposition of calcium may occur in the arteries. Look at Fig. 19.21c. This is a plain X-ray of the leg. The arteries are calcified.

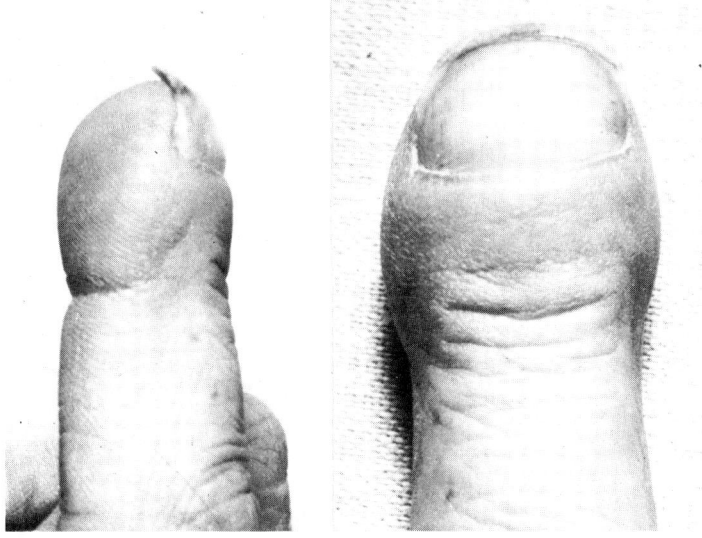

Fig. 19.21b

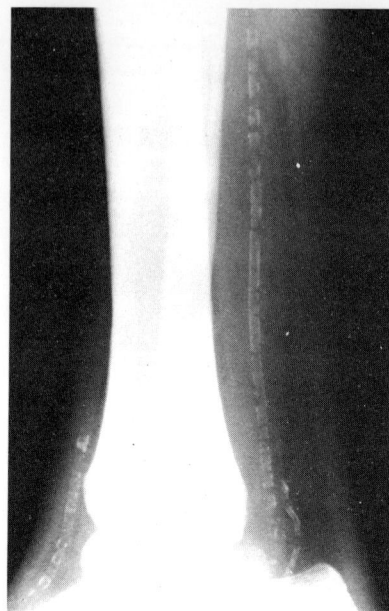

Fig. 19.21c

Question What is the cause of pseudo-clubbing in hyperparathyroidism caused by renal failure?

Answer 1. Bone resorption in terminal phalanges. Go on to **19.24**.
2. Concomitant chest disease. Go on to **19.26**.

19.22 Your answer – parathyroidectomy.
You are partially correct, but because of the hazards of this operation it is better to try to reduce the metastatic calcification by reducing serum inorganic phosphate levels. This can be done by aluminium hydroxide to bind phosphate in the bowel. Read **19.23** again.

19.23 Your answer – do nothing.
No. The danger of vitamin D intoxication is the hypercalcaemia it produces. This can be best treated at this level by stopping vitamin D administration. Read **19.18** again and answer the question correctly.

19.24 Your answer – pseudo-clubbing is due to bone resorption.
Correct. Sometimes the patients develop conjunctival soreness and injection

('red eyes') due to deposits of metastatic calcification in the conjunctiva (see Fig. 19.24a). More commonly the eyes are white, with crystals of calcium phosphate which can be seen with a slit lamp, lying superficially in the conjunctiva and as a band at the limbus. Look at figure 19.24b. The treatment of renal hyperparathyroidism is firstly to reduce metastatic calcification by giving 200 ml of aluminium hydroxide gel or 6g of aluminium hydroxide dried gel (BP) a day by mouth. This combines with phosphate in the bowel, and lowers the serum inorganic phosphorus level; gradually the metastatic calcification is resorbed. If the bone pains persist and the patient is intolerant of the aluminium hydroxide treatment (usually because of nausea and vomiting), parathyroidectomy may be carried out as a last resort. The parathyroids in renal secondary hyperparathyroidism are usually all hypertrophied, with a mixed cellular hyperplasia, although occasionally adenomas may be present. This operation has a moderate mortality but in selected patients the response is dramatic. The serum calcium falls, itching and bone pain disappear, the metastatic calcification disappears and the bones recalcify, the pseudo-clubbing disappearing. In patients with untreated renal hyperparathyroidism the serum calcium tends to be higher than in patients with renal osteomalacia. The serum phosphorus levels are high but fall on treatment with aluminium hydroxide therapy. The serum alkaline phosphatase level is usually elevated in renal hyperparathyroidism.

Question What treatment would you give for a patient with metastatic calci-

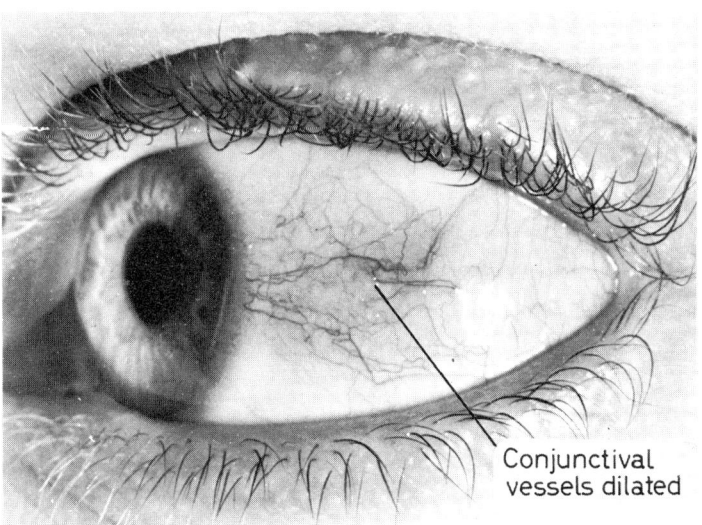

Fig. 19.24a

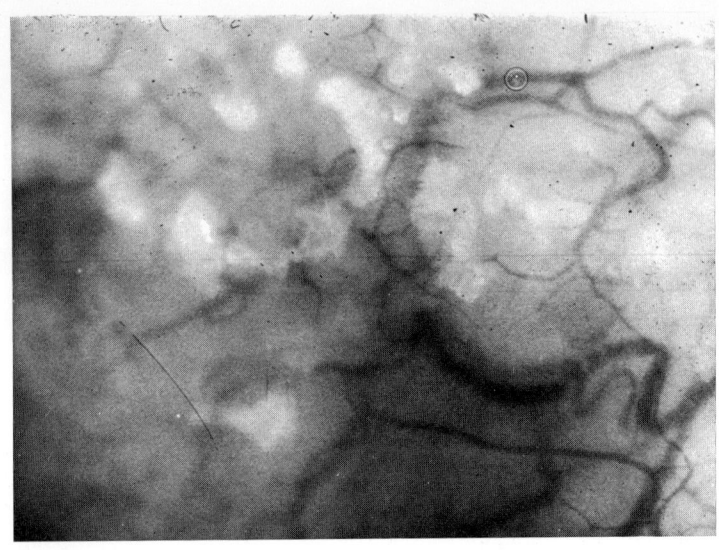

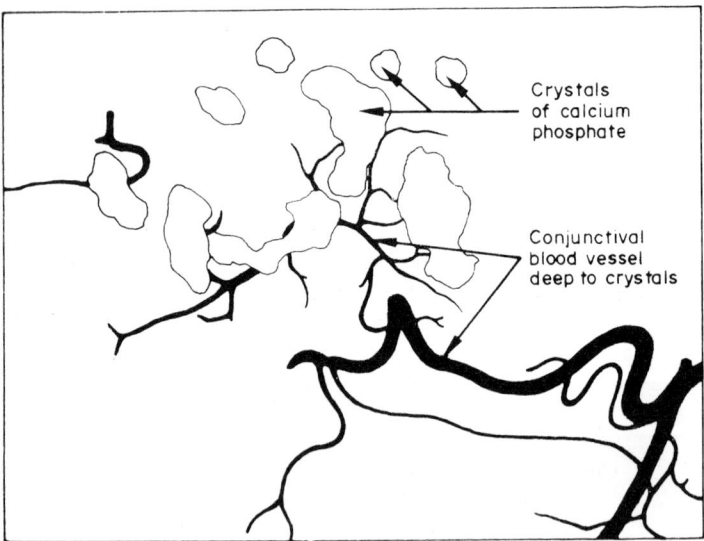

Fig. 19.24b

fication and the following results?
Serum calcium 11.5 mg/100 ml.
Serum inorganic phosphorus, 7.0 mg/100 ml.
Blood urea 200 mg/100 ml.
Alkaline phosphatase 30 KA units/100 ml.

Answer 1. Parathyroidectomy. Go on to **19.22**.
2. Aluminium hydroxide. Go on to **19.25**.

19.25 Your answer – aluminium hydroxide.

You are correct. The lowering of the plasma inorganic phosphate reduces the value of the serum Ca-P product and so helps cause resorption of the metastatic calcification. In hyperparathyroidism secondary to renal disease it is unusual to get radiographic evidence of renal stones unless they were there to begin with as the primary disease. Nephrocalcinosis is likewise rare unless initially present.

Patients with renal osteomalacia and renal hyperparathyroidism usually have a blood urea of at least 100 mg/100 ml on a normal diet, and many are above 150 mg/100 ml. In renal osteodystrophy there is a curious waddling gait due to a proximal myopathy. This responds to vitamin D therapy.

Question If a man on a normal diet has a blood urea of 60 mg/100 ml and hyperparathyroidism, do you think the latter is primary or secondary to renal disease.

Answer 1. Primary. Go on to **19.29**.
2. Secondary to renal disease. Go on to **19.27**.

19.26 Your answer – pseudo-clubbing is due to concomitant chest disease.

You are wrong. There is no point in guessing. The answer is given in **19.21** which you should read again.

19.27 Your answer – he has secondary hyperparathyroidism.

No. It is most unusual to find a patient with renal disease causing secondary hyperparathyroidism and a blood urea of only 60 mg/100 ml (when he is eating a normal protein diet). Usually a blood urea of 60 mg/100 ml and hyperparathyroidism implies renal damage *secondary to the hypercalcaemia* of primary hyperparathyroidism. Now read **19.25** again and then answer the question.

19.28 Your answer – I would give citrates.

You would be disappointed by the response. This is not surprising if you consider that the demineralisation of the bone may be the result of years of loss of bone salts neutralising the acid which is not being adequately excreted. Correction of the acidosis with oral citrates can stop the further loss of bone mineral; vitamin D helps to recalcify the bone. Now read **19.31** again.

19.29 Your answer – he has primary hyperparathyroidism.
Correct. Unfortunately, if the blood urea is 160 mg/100 ml it is more difficult to differentiate primary hyperparathyroidism from secondary renal hyperparathyroidism. In that case one must rely on the past history of renal disease to suggest secondary hyperparathyroidism, unless the renal disease is calculous in type. If renal calculi have been noticed or there are symptoms of peptic ulcer or pancreatitis, primary hyperparathyroidism is more likely. If the kidneys are large on tomography a diagnosis of primary hyperparathyroidism is probable. Small kidneys are indicative of long standing renal disease and are therefore evidence in favour of secondary (renal) hyperparathyroidism being present. Renal biopsy disclosing microscopic nephrocalcinosis without other renal disease is suggestive of primary hyperparathyroidism.

Question A man is found to have a blood urea of 200 mg/100 ml. He has large kidneys on tomography and nephrocalcinosis on biopsy; serum calcium is 13.0 mg/100 ml and he has a raised alkaline phosphatase. X-rays suggest active bone disease of hyperparathyroidism. Is the hyperparathyroidism primary or secondary to renal disease?

Answer 1. Primary. Go on to **19.31**.
2. Secondary to renal disease. Go on to **19.33**.

19.30 Your answer – all the statements are true.
You are correct, about statements 1 and 3 but not about 2. Read from **19.14** to **19.23** and then answer the question in **19.34** again.

19.31 Your answer – Primary hyperparathyroidism is probably present.
Correct. In renal tubular acidosis (RTA) and in adult Fanconi syndrome renal osteomalacia is often found. The pathology of the renal rickets is similar to that of nutritional rickets. The patients in both RTA and adult Fanconi syndrome do not necessarily have chronic renal failure of severe degree. The blood urea is often only slightly elevated. The cause of the osteomalacia is uncertain but it may be due to the severe acidosis in both these diseases. In the presence of severe acidosis the bone salts have been shown to titrate large amounts of dietary and metabolically produced acid each day and ultimately the mineral content of the bone is reduced. Whether this loss of mineral salt can result in demineralisation without loss of the matrix or whether the matrix also is destroyed is uncertain. The presence of histological osteoid in these patients could be explained either by loss of mineral with exposure of demineralised matrix, due to acidosis, or due to some resistance to the action of vitamin D. The osteomalacia of RTA and Fanconi syndrome requires vitamin D for *initial* healing, although *maintenance* therapy with alkalinising sodium and potassium citrate is probably adequate once remineralisation of the bone has taken place with the help of vitamin D.

Question If you were asked to treat the severe osteomalacia in a patient with RTA would you give citrates or would you give vitamin D?

Answer 1. Citrates. Go on to **19.28**.
2. Vitamin D. Go on to **19.34**.

19.32 Your answer – all the statements are false.
No. You are correct about 2 only. Start from the beginning of the chapter and work through it to **19.34**.

19.33 Your answer – the hyperparathyroidism is secondary.
No. Evidence of nephrocalcinosis and large kidneys suggest a rapidly progressive disease not like that associated with renal hyperparathyroidism, which is found in slowly progressive advanced chronic renal failure with small kidneys. Read **19.29** again.

19.34 Your answer – I would give vitamin D.
Correct. Now look carefully at the statements before choosing the answer.

Statement 1 Primary hyperparathyroidism is associated with renal stones.
Statement 2 Looser's nodes are true fractures.
Statement 3 Metastatic calcification can be treated by aluminium hydroxide gel.

Answer 1. All the statements are true. Go on to **19.30**.
2. All the statements are false. Go on to **19.32**.
3. Statement 1 is true, 2 and 3 false. Go on to **19.40**.
4. Statement 2 is true, 1 and 3 false. Go on to **19.35**.
5. Statement 3 is true, 1 and 2 false. Go on to **19.36**.
6. Statement 1 and 2 are true, 3 false. Go on to **19.37**.
7. Statement 2 and 3 are true, 1 false. Go on to **19.38**.
8. Statement 1 and 3 are true, 2 false. Go on to **19.39**.

19.35 Your answer – statement 2 is true, 1 and 3 false.
You are incorrect about all. Start at **19.1** and read through the rest of the chapter.

19.36 Your answer – statement 3 is true. 1 and 2 false.
You are wrong about statement 1 only. Start at **19.1** and read through to **19.14**.

19.37 Your answer – statements 1 and 2 are true, 3 is false.
You are correct about statement 1 only. Read the chapter from **19.14** onwards again.

19.38 Your answer – statements 2 and 3 are true, 1 is false.

You are correct about statement 3 only. Read from **19.1** to **19.23** again, then answer the question in **19.28**.

19.39 Your answer – 1 and 3 are true, 2 is false.

You are correct. Articles recommended for further information on this subject are:

Stanbury S. W. & Lumb G. A. (1966) Quart. J. Med. N.S. **35**, 1.
Stanbury S. W. (1967) Chapter on bony complications of renal disease, in Black D. A. K. (ed.) Renal Disease, Blackwell Scientific Publications, Oxford.
Stanbury S. W. & Lumb G. S. (1962) Medicine, Baltimore **41**, 1.
Dent C. E. et al. (1961) Quart. J. Med. N.S. **30**, 1.
Divalent Ion Metabolism, Osteodystrophy and chronic renal disease. Arch Int. Med. Symposia Volume 3. 261. Editor Charles R. Kleeman.
M. Cochran et al. Brit. Med. J. 1970, **1**, 135.
De Luca, H. F. 1969 New Eng. J. Med. 1969, **281**, 1103.
Stanbury S. W. Chapter on Bone Disease in Strauss & Welt, The Kidney Disease 2nd Edition 1972.
De Lucca H. F. 1972. Leading article on Vitamin D metabolism. New England J. Med. **287**, 926.
Rasmussen, H. J. Clin. Invest. Sept, 1972. Short communication.
Brickman A. S. et al. Use of 1:25 $(OH)_2D_3$ in Uraemic man, New Eng. J. Med. **287**, 891.
Omdahl J. L. and De Luca, H. F. Regulation of Vitamin D Metabolism and Function – Physiology. Rev. 1973, **53**, 327–372.
De Luca H. F. Review of Vit D. New Eng. J. Med. 1973 **289**, 359–365.

19.40 Your answer – statement 1 is true, 2 and 3 false.

You are wrong about statement 3 only. Read on from **19.23** to the end of the chapter.

Time for this chapter: 30 minutes

Chapter 20
Drugs and the kidney

20.1 In this chapter two groups of drugs are considered:
1. Those drugs which are nephrotoxic.
2. Those drugs whose main route of excretion is via the kidneys, and in whom the dosage has to be modified in renal failure.

The nephrotoxic drugs include drugs taken therapeutically and various poisons. The drugs taken therapeutically include:

Phenacetin

Phenacetin ingestion in large doses (i.e. 1 G or more) over long periods leads to a specific type of renal failure caused by interstitial nephritis and a severe acute or chronic pyelonephritis. Necrotising papillitis is particularly frequent, and is thought to be due to damage to the arterial blood supply to the medulla. If rats are given a regular dose of aspirin, phenacetin and caffeine pro rata equal to that taken by addicts of these drugs, papillary necrosis develops in 55 per cent after 6–9 months. Bluemle and his colleagues have demonstrated that there is a high concentration of phenacetin in the medulla. This concentration is much higher than in the cortex and would suggest an active transport mechanism on the lines of the counter current system for urine concentration. The preferential concentration in the pyramids might explain the selection of these regions for medullary necrosis, presumably caused by the direct toxic action of high concentrations of phenacetin or its metabolites on the papillary cells. The phenacetin is taken by addicts for chronic pain, such as headaches. In some factories in Scandinavia the workers were encouraged to take a phenacetin powder for this purpose.

The clinical features of analgesic nephropathy are:

1. Silent pyelonephritis, chronic in type, with or without positive urine cultures.

2. Necrotising papillitis with insidious renal failure or severe acute or subacute pyelonephritis with haematuria, dysuria and the passage of lumps of renal tissue, – the papillae. The disease progress rapidly into severe renal failure.

Renal function tests show abnormalities of distal tubular function including impairment of the urine concentrating ability, defects of urinary acidification, increase in ammonia excretion and hypocitraturia.

It has also been documented that phenacetin nephropathy, or analgesic nephropathy as it is better termed, is in its earlier stages reversed if the drug ingestion is stopped. If, however, renal failure is already advanced, sufficient vascular damage has occurred that the renal damage is usually not reversible.

The identity of drugs responsible for analgesic nephropathy has been the subject of some debate. Phenacetin as generally prepared contains a toxic contaminant, but it has now been shown that even in the absence of toxic contaminants, phenacetin can cause lesions in rat kidneys if ingested in large enough dosage for long enough. It is worth remembering that analgesic abuse in man also has been shown to be a predisposing cause of renal pelvic carcinoma.

Question Does the nephritis of analgesic abuse always present as renal failure of insidious onset?

Answer 1. Yes. Go on to **20.3**.
2. No. Go on to **20.5**.

20.2 Your answer – phenacetin is the only analgesic causing renal damage.

You are wrong. Paracetamol (Panadol) has also been implicated as a cause of renal damage. Read **20.5**.

20.3 Your answer – it always presents as insidious renal failure.

Wrong. The nephritis of phenacetin abuse may present insidiously, on the other hand it may present as acute or chronic pyelonephritis or as necrotising papillitis. Read **20.1** again with more care.

20.4 Your answer – phenacetin is concentrated in the renal papilla.

You are correct. Troxidone (Tridione) and penicillamine are recorded as having caused nephrotic syndrome. Tolbutamide, potassium perchlorate and probenacid have been recorded as causing nephrotic syndrome. Many of these drugs give a reversible renal lesion, but others, such as troxidone, are recorded as having given irreversible changes. Amino-nucleoside causes nephritis with nephrotic features on experimental administration in rats and also in humans to whom it has been administered therapeutically for Chaga's disease.

Question Is the nephrotic syndrome induced by troxidone always reversible?

Answer 1. Yes. Go on to **20.9**.
2. No. Go on to **20.11**.

20.5 Your answer – it does not always present as renal failure of insidious onset.

Correct. It has been suggested that the phenacetin kidney is not a result of the action of pure phenacetin, but rather due to the presence of a chemical contaminant formed during manufacture. However paracetamol has also been implicated in the production of renal failure like those of phenacetin. The X-ray appearance of phenacetin kidney is that of chronic pyelonephritis, (Chapter 7) and that of necrotising papillitis with characteristic ring shadows on IVP.

Question Is phenacetin the only analgesic likely to cause renal damage?

Answer 1. Yes. Go on to **20.2**.
         2. No. Go on to **20.7**.

20.6 Your answer – phenacetin is not concentrated in the renal papilla. Wrong. You have not read **20.5** carefully. Read it again.

20.7 Your answer – Renal failure may be caused by analgesics other than phenacetin.

Correct. The precise pathogenesis of 'analgesic' or 'phenacetin' nephropathy is unknown. It is possible that the papillae suffer primarily because phenacetin is concentrated in the papillae: when compared to the cortical phenacetin concentration that in the papillae may be more than ten times as great.

Question Is phenacetin concentrated in the renal papillae?

Answer 1. Yes. Go on to **20.4**.
         2. No. Go on to **20.6**.

20.8 Your answer – Alkalinisation of the urine causes more sulphonamide crystals to appear in the urine. Wrong. The opposite is true. To choose this answer you must have been concentrating poorly. Start again reading **20.12** and do not let your attention wander.

20.9 Your answer. The nephrotic syndrome of troxidone is always reversible.
You are wrong. Usually troxidone nephritis is reversible, but occasional cases are irreversible. Read **20.4** again.

20.10 Your answer. It causes anuria by oxalate crystal obstruction. You are incorrect, Propylene glycol is not metabolised to oxalate. You are confusing it with ethylene glycol. Read **20.15** again and then answer the question again.

20.11 Your answer: the nephrotic syndrome of toxidone is not reversible always.
You are correct. Doubtless as new drugs are introduced further nephrotoxic side-effects will be discovered. The next group of nephrotoxic drugs are the organic solvents – carbon tetrachloride, ethylene glycol and propylene glycol.

Carbon tetrachloride causes acute tubular necrosis with necrosis of the proximal tubular cells and an intact basement membrane. When recovery occurs, it is complete, but there may be a prolonged period of oliguria. Death is usually due to hepatic necrosis caused by carbon tetrachloride, rather than renal damage.

Question In carbon tetrachloride poisoning is anuria irreversible?

Answer 1. It is irreversible. Go on to **20.13**.
         2. It is not irreversible. Go on to **20.15**.

20.12 Your answer – it causes anuria by intravascular haemolysis. Correct. The sulphonamide group of drugs have long had a bad reputation as a cause of renal failure either by precipitation of the drug or its acetyl derivative in the renal tubules causing obstruction, or obstruction in the renal pelves. In some there is an interstitial hypersensitivity-type nephritis. Sulphacetamide and sulphadimidine have relatively solube urinary products. In patients given sulphonamides it is essential to give copious fluids and sodium bicarbonate to alkalinise the urine to reduce the chance of crystallization in the urinary tract.

Question Does alkalinisation of the urine produce more or less sulphonamide crystals in the urinary tract?

Answer 1. More. Go on to **20.8**.
2. Less. Go on to **20.14**.

20.13 Your answer – it is irreversible. No. It is reversible, although the recovery period may be prolonged, with a correspondingly protected oliguria period. Read **20.11** again before answering the question.

20.14 Your answer – alkalinisation of the urine causes less sulphonamide crystals to appear in the urine.

You are correct. Several antibiotics are noted for their nephrotoxic properties. Streptomycin, kanamycin, vancomycin and neomycin are poorly absorbed when taken by mouth, but on parenteral administration are slowly excreted by glomerular filtration, and so maintain high plasma levels for a long time. Of these four antibiotics neomycin is particularly nephrotoxic, but in the presence of renal failure plasma levels are particularly high because of the delay in excretion, and all are liable to exacerbate renal damage as well as damaging the eighth cranial nerve. With kanamycin 20 per cent of people with hitherto normal kidney function develop proteinuria, haematuria and cast formation.

Colistin, polymyxin and bacitracin are all nephrotoxic on parenteral administration causing proteinuria and cast formation initially, then a higher blood urea and renal failure. Amphotericin B is particularly nephrotoxic and fatal renal failure has been reported following Amphotericin B therapy.

Question Is streptomycin more or less nephrotoxic than neomycin?

Answer 1. More nephrotoxic. Go on to **20.17**.
2. Less nephrotoxic. Go on to **20.19**.

20.15 Your answer – it is not irreversible. You are correct. The glycols cause two different types of poisoning – ethylene glycol (anti freeze) is metabolised to oxalate which is deposited in crystals in the tubules and causes a proximal tubular dilation and obstruction. There may be a superimposed pyelonephritis. Propylene glycol, on the other hand, causes renal failure by inducing intravascular haemolysis. It is not metabolised to oxalate.

Question How does propylene glycol cause anuria?

Answer 1. By oxalate crystal obstruction in the tubules. Go on to **20.10**.
2. By intravascular haemolysis. Go on to **20.12**.

20.16 Your answer – Tetracycline is not dangerous in renal disease. No. it is dangerous. You are wrong. Read **20.19** again. You are not concentrating on what you are reading.

20.17 Your answer – streptomycin is more nephrotoxic than neomycin.
You are wrong. Streptomycin is less nephrotoxic than neomycin; if it were more nephrotoxic it would be unsafe to use in the treatment of tuberculosis. Read **20.14** again, slowly and carefully. It contains many important facts.

20.18 Your answer – 250 mg of ampicillin 6 hourly.
Wrong. This is a normal dosage schedule and is likely to result in very high blood levels of ampicillin with a 60 per cent chance of developing a toxic rash, therefore the doage schedule should be altered. Read **20.21** again.

20.19 Your answer – streptomycin is less nephrotoxic than neomycin.
You are correct. Tetracycline is an antibiotic which deteriorates on storage in warm and moist conditions to form breakdown products – anhydrotetracycline and epianhydrotetracycline; these cause proximal tubular damage with a reversible Fanconi syndrome – renal glycosuria, amino aciduria, low plasma phosphate, increased TRP, low plasma urate, hypokalaemia, polyuria and acidosis. Imuran (azathioprine) has been reported as inducing Fanconi syndrome in grafted kidneys. Tetracycline induced Fanconi syndrome is slowly reversible. Tetracyline does not cause renal damage if it is fresh and stored in cold dry conditions. However in renal failure tetracycline is dangerous, causing a deterioration in renal function which may prove fata. *Tetracyclines should not be given to patients with impaired renal function.*

Question Is tetracycline dangerous in patients with renal disease?

Answer 1. Yes. Go on to **20.21**.
2. No. Go on to **20.16**.

20.20 Your answer – I would not use chlortetracycline.
Correct. Chloramphenicol is rapidly broken down, in renal failure, into inactive metabolites and can be given in full dosage, as if the patient has no renal disease whatever. It is, it should be remembered, a potentially toxic drug, causing aplastic

anaemia. It should only be given in strictly limited dosage e.g. 250 mg 6 hourly for 7 to 10 days.

Kanamycin, streptomycin, polymyxin B, gentamycin and colistin should be avoided if possible. If the organism is sensitive solely to one of these antibiotics, then these drugs be given with one initial injection, followed by a half dose every 3–4 days, and preferably with monitoring of serum levels of the antibiotic.

Question Is chloramphenicol given in reduced dosage in renal failure?

Answer 1. Yes. Go on to **20.22**.
2. No. Go on to **20.24**.

20.21 Your answer – Tetracycline is dangerous in renal disease.

Correct. In renal failure the administration of drugs has to be very carefully controlled so that the impairment of excretion does not lead to high plasma levels which may be toxic. Kunin and Richet have reviewed the majority of antibiotics and other commonly used drugs in respect of their dosage schedules in renal failure. They take into account the mode of excretion and metabolism before excretion, plasma levels, toxicity of high plasma levels, and recommend dosage accordingly. Let us first consider the antibiotics in common usage.

The penicillins and related compounds are removed mainly by the kidney but also by the liver. Their blood levels can reach very high levels before toxicity develops – skin rashes and convulsions (excluding allergic reactions). The following data refer to patients with a GFR of less than 10ml/min. Methicillin and cloxacillin require no change in normal dosage schedules. Penicillin G should be given in half the usual dosage at 8–10 hourly intervals. Cephalexin should be given in half dosage once every 24 hours. Do not use Cephaloridine. It causes renal failure itself. Ampicillin should be used in a normal dosage but administered only once a day instead of 6 hourly. In peritoneal dialysis not more than 50 mg should be given intraperitoneally with each liter of dialysate, or, as Lee has shown, there is a 60 per cent incidence of toxic skin rashes.

Question A patient with a GFR of 3 ml/min requires ampicillin treatment for a urinary tract infection. Which dosage schedule would you advise?

Answer 1. 250 mg 6 hourly. Go on to **20.18**.
2. 250 mg daily. Go on to **20.23**.
3. 500 mg 6 hourly. Go on to **20.25**.

20.22 Your answer – chloramphenicol is given in reduced dosage in renal failure.

You are wrong. Chloramphenicol is rapidly metabolised in renal failure and the metabolites which accumulate in renal failure are apparently inactive metabolically. You have not read **20.20** with enough care. Read **20.20** again before answering the question.

20.23   Your answer – 250 mg daily.

You are correct. Erythromycin can be given in normal dosage. The tetracycline group, however, require special consideration. Apart from the potential damage caused by tetracycline which has deteriorated and caused Fanconi syndrome, there is a major problem in using all the tetracyclines in renal failure. All of them are excreted through the kidney and the liver, and if given in normal dosage would cause toxic plasma levels which give rise to liver damage, increase in blood urea levels due to renal damage, and riboflavinuria. Thus the dosage has to be modified so as to prevent these side-effects. Again you should bear in mind that the patients we are considering have a GFR of 10 ml/min or less. Chlortetracycline is rapidly metabolised but in spite of this its metabolic effects persist, and we have found it causes a rapid increase in blood urea; chlortetracycline should not be used in renal failure. The other tetracyclines, after 500 mg has been given as the loading dose, should be given every 3–4 days in a dose of 250 mg if there is no alternative safer antibiotic to which the organism is sensitive. Doxycycline should be given in normal dosage in renal failure.

Question   Would you use chlortetracycline in renal failure?

Answer   1. Yes. Go on to **20.28**.
2. No. Go on to **20.20**.

20.24   Your answer – chloramphenicol is given in normal dosage in renal failure.

Correct. Nitrofurantoin is best avoided in renal failure in view of the possibility of the development of peripheral neuropathy. It has been shown that there is virtually no urinary excretion of nitrofurantoin when the GFR is less than 20 ml/min. PAS and Isoniazid dosage should be controlled by monitoring the serum levels, there being little available data on which to base empiric dosage. Nalidixic acid also has delayed excretion in renal failure and its use should be restricted to hospitals with laboratory facilities for monitoring serum levels of the drug. It takes about 2 days to reach a high enough concentration in the urine.

Apart from antibiotics there are many other drugs whose excretion is delayed in renal failure so that their dosage has to be modified accordingly. These include digoxin (whose action is potentiated by hypoklalemia), quinine, phenobarbitone, opiates, atropine, α-methyldopa, guanethidine, pempidine, cortico-steroids and phenylbutazone. Doses of these drugs should be the minimum required to produce the maintain the pharmacological effect.

Although sulphonamides can be safely given in non-anuric renal failure, trimethoprim is retained, so that the normal 4:1 ratio of these 2 drugs in Septrim has to be altered.

Question   Would you be cautious about administration of guanethidine in renal failure, or would you increase the dose as rapidly as in a patient with healthy kidneys.

Answer 1. Be cautious. Go on to **25.26**.
2. Increase the dose as in the normal. Go on to **20.38**.

20.25 Your answer — 500 mg 6 hourly.
You are wrong. With a dosage like this you would get extremely high blood levels and toxic side effects are likely, in particular skin rashes. Read **20.21** again this time concentrate on it; it contains many important facts which you need to know.

20.26 Your answer — be cautious.
You are correct. The radio-opaque organic iodine contrast media from time to time produce an allergic hypotensive reaction in which acute tubular necrosis occurs. This is particularly liable to occur in patients with obstructive jaundice. The reactions usually follow attempted intravenous pyelography or renal arteriography. Oliguric renal failure has been reported frequently in patients with multiple myeloma who are having an IVP with dehydration. The danger of this procedure has been described in Chapter 4.

In non-myelomatous patients IVP has occasionally proved dangerous because of hypotension causing acute tubular necrosis. In renal arteriography acute tubular necrosis may develop as the result of very high concentrations of organic iodine compounds perfusing the kidneys and causing acute tubular necrosis *without* hypotensive change, presumably a direct toxic effect on the tubular cells.

Phenylindanedione is remarkable in causing an allergic interstitial nephritis in which the patient has haematuria and oliguria often with a relatively high urine osmolality.

Question What is the cause of acute tubular necrosis after renal arterography?

Answer 1. Hypotension. Go on to **20.29**.
2. Direct toxic effect. Go on to **20.32**.

20.27 Your answer — the kidneys are asymmetrically contracted.
You are wrong. They are symmetrically uniformly shrunken. Read **20.30** again. Then answer the question correctly.

20.28 Your answer — I would use chlortetracycline.
You are wrong. Although chlortetracycline undergoes rapid degradation to breakdown products it appears from our experience and those of others that the drug still retains harmful metabolic activity and is therefore best avoided. Read **20.23** again carefully.

20.29 Your answer — hypotension causes ATN after renal aortography.
You are wrong. Hypotension is not the factor in ATN — rather it is the direct

toxic effect of a large dose of an organic iodide perfusing the kidney tissues directly. Read **20.26** again, this time with more care.

20.30 Your answer – Gout is more frequent in lead poisoning.

You are correct. The pathological findings are contracted kidneys with loss of cortical tissue which is both diffuse and symmetrical. The histological picture is non-specific, although there is a tendency of some of the glomeruli to be spared and remain relatively large. Electron microscopy showed intranuclear inclusion bodies in the proximal tubules.

Question Is the kidney of chronic lead poisoning symmetrically shrunken or asymmetrical with spared areas?

Answer 1. Symmetrical. Go on to **20.31**.
2. Asymmetrical. Go on to **20.27**.

20.31 Your answer – the kidneys are symmetrically shrunken.

You are correct. Cadmium poisoning may be acute, (in which case it gives rise to Fanconi syndrome), or chronic. Chronic cadmium poisoning, usually found in alloy and battery workers, may present as proteinuria usually developing after at least 8 years' exposure to cadmium. The proteinuria is more readily demonstrated on precipitation by salicylsulphonic acid rather than boiling, has a molecular weight 20,000–30,000 and on paper electrophoresis there is a tubular proteinuria pattern with α_2 and β globulins. Some patients develop the feature of a chronic Fanconi syndrome. There is no particularly specific histological picture in this disease.

Question What type of proteinuria is found in chronic cadmium poisoning?

Answer 1. Glomerular. Go on to **20.33**.
2. Tubular. Go on to **20.35**.

20.32 Your answer – it acts by direct toxic effect.

You are correct. We shall now consider various metallic intoxications. Lead is responsible for renal damage in both acute and chronic lead poisoning. The characteristic response of the kidney to mental poisoning is the development of Fanconi syndrome. Histologically acute lead poisoning gives rise to atrophy of the epithelial cells of the proximal tubules, with signs of regeneration, and thickening of tubular basement membranes with increase in interstitial connective tissue. In addition there is a characteristic type of intranuclear inclusion bodies in the cells of the proximal convoluted tubes. Glomerular changes are not visible on light microscopy. Chronic lead poisoning usually presents as chronic renal failure, although malignant hypertension is uncommon. Proteinuria is insufficient to cause nephrotic syndrome. Gout is found in 50 per cent of cases of chronic renal failure due to lead, and there is an increase in plasma urate levels in lead nephropathy compared to renal failure of non-plumbic origin. Extra-renal clinical features will not be considered here.

Question Is gout more frequent in renal failure due to lead than due to other causes?

Answer 1. More frequent in lead poisoning. Go on to **20.30**.
2. More frequent in non-lead causes. Go on to **20.34**.

20.33 Your answer – cadmium poisoning gives glomerular proteinuria.
You are wrong. The proteinuria is tubular. Read **20.31** more carefully. Then answer the question.

20.34 Your answer – Gout is more frequent in non-lead types of renal failure.
You are wrong. Gout is more common in lead poisoning, and there is a higher mean plasma urate level in lead poisoning than in other types of renal failure of comparable severity. Read **20.32** again, and answer the question.

20.35 Your answer – cadmium poisoning gives a tubular proteinuria.
Correct. Mercury poisoning is quite strikingly different from that found in lead and cadmium poisoning. In acute mercury poisoning the picture is that of acute renal failure with anuria within 24 hours. The anuria persists for about 10 days. Simultaneously there is frequently necrosis of the intestinal epithelium. Acute mercury poisoning is usually caused by inorganic mercuric salts; the occasional case of poisoning from organic mercurial diuretics is found in those patients with pre-existing renal failure. The pathological picture is necrosis of the proximal tubules with calcification of the epithelium, the calcification being characteristic of mercurial poisoning.

Question Do mercurial diuretics usually cause renal failure in people with hitherto normal renal function?

Answer 1. Yes. Go on to **20.37**.
2. No. Go on to **20.39**.

20.36 Your answer – the dimercaprol-mercury complex is excreted in the bile.
You are wrong. The major route of excretion is via the urine. In this patient anuria is present and this is not therefore possible as a route of excretion. The dimercaprol-mercury complex has to be dialysed from the patient. Read **20.39** again. Then answer the question.

20.37 Your answer – mercurial diuretics usually cause renal failure in people with hitherto normal renal function.
Wrong. The patient usually has pre-existing renal disease. This is one of the reasons for taking an elevated blood urea as a contra-indication to mercurial

diuretics. It is doubtful if with the modern diuretics now available, that mercurial diuretics should ever be prescribed. Read **20.35** again with more care. Then answer the question correctly.

20.38 Your answer – increase the dose as in the normal.
Wrong. Guanethidine excretion is impaired in renal failure. Thus the serum concentration will gradually increase and the patient will have a sudden and possibly disastrous fall in blood pressure. Read **20.24** again, more carefully.

20.39 Your answer – they usually have abnormal renal function.
You are correct. The treatment of acute renal failure due to mercury poisoning is divided into two parts – the first being non-specific treatment with diet and dialysis mentioned in Chapter 8 (Acute Renal Failure), the second being dimercaprol (BAL) which complexes the mercury so reducing its toxicity. In anuria it has to be dialysed off the patient. Penicillamine has also been used in mercury poisoning. EDTA causes further renal damage and is not recommended. Chronic mercury poisoning gives rise to proteinuria but there is little proof of any well described renal picture in chronic mercury poisoning. Nephrotic syndrome occurs in children taking teething powders, organic mercurial drugs, ointments and on exposure to mercury vapour. The nephrotic syndrome remits on withdrawal of the patient from exposure to mercury. Dimercaprol (BAL) may speed recovery.

Question If dimercaprol (BAL) is used to treat acute renal failure due to mercuric chloride, and the patient is anuric, how is the dimercaprol-mercury complex removed from the body?

Answer 1. Excreted in the bile. Go on to **20.36**.
2. By dialysis. Go on to **20.41**.

20.40 Your answer – only statement 1 is true. You are partly correct. Statement 3 is also true. Read on from **20.35**.

20.41 Your answer – the dimercaprol-mercury complex can be removed by dialysis.
You are correct. Gold may cause an acute nephropathy with proteinuria and haematuria, but Fanconi syndrome does not develop. The proteinuria if massive may give rise to nephrotic syndrome. Because the gold is usually given for patients with rheumatoid arthritis, who often have other renal lesions (see Chapter 10), it is impossible to be dogmatic about the aetiological relationship of gold in the genesis of an individual case of proteinuria. Remission sometimes occurs spontaneously so that the apparent efficacy of dimercaptrol is unconfined. Uranium intoxication causes a Fanconi type syndrome in laboratory animals and in a few human cases so far reported.

Question Is gold undoubtedly responsible for the development of proteinuria in rheumatoid arthritis treated with gold?

Answer 1. Yes. Go on to **20.43**.
2. No. Go on to **20.45**.

20.42 Your answer – all the statements are false.
You are correct about statement 2 only. 1 and 3 are true. Start again at **20.5** and read on from there to **20.12**, and then on from **20.35**.

20.43 Your answer – gold is undoubtedly responsible for the development of proteinuria in RA.
You are wrong. There is considerable doubt about the implication of gold in the genesis of proteinuria. You should read **20.41** again, then answer the question.

20.44 Your answer – all the statements are true.
You are correct about 1 and 3, but 2 is not true. Go back to **20.12** and read on from there to **20.35**.

20.45 Your answer – gold is not undoubtedly responsible for the proteinuria of RA. You are correct. Good.

Copper poisoning causes haematuria and acute renal failure with oliguria. There is a severe haemolytic anaemia which makes it difficult to distinguish between the haemoglobinuria and shock causing renal failure and a direct nephrotoxic action of copper. Chronic copper poisoning causes a severe haemolytic anaemia, haemoglobinuria and renal damage caused by haemoglobinuria. In Wilson's disease or hepato-lenticular degeneration there is an increased quantity of copper loosely bound to albumin and a reduced amount of ceruloplasmin. Copper absorption by the bowel is increased; copper excretion in the urine is also increased. The deposition of the copper in the tubular epithelium causes Fanconi syndrome, a generalised amino aciduria paralleling the excretion of copper. Glycosuria is rarely present, but T_mG is reduced. In Fanconi syndrome of Wilson's disease, hypercalcuria and osteomalacia are frequently found. These are rare in Fanconi's syndrome due to other metals. Bismuth causes acute oliguric renal failure, followed by the development of Fanconi syndrome.

Question How does the Fanconi syndrome of Wilson's Disease differ from that caused by metals other than copper?

Answer 1. Increased incidence of hypercalciuria and osteomalacia. Go on to **20.47**.
2. Decreased incidence of glycosuria. Go on to **20.49**.
3. Increased hypercalciuria and decreased glycosuria. Go on to **20.51**.

20.46 Your answer − statements 1 and 3 are true, 2 is false.

You are correct. If you want to refer to more detailed work on this subject the following references will prove useful:

Reidenberg, M. M. Renal Function and Drug Action. Saunders 1971.
Richet, G. (1960), Journal d'Urologie et Nephrologie **72**, No. 4 (In French).
Kunin, C. M. (1967). Annals Int. Med. **67**, 151.
Milne, M. D. Chapter 22. Drugs, Poisons and the Kidneys, in Renal Disease, edited by D. A. K. Black. 2nd Edution, 1967 Blackwells Scientific Publications, Oxford.
Emmerson, B. T. Chapter 23. Metals and the Kidney. Ibid.
Eastwood, J. R. et al. 1970. Lancet **2**, 39.
Weinstein L. and Kaplan K. The cephalosporins Annals Int. Med. 1970, **72**, 729.
Kunin C. & Finkelberg 2. Annals Int. Med. 1970, **72**, 349.
Bell D., et al. 1969. Brit. Med. J. **2**, 378.

20.47 Your answer − increased incidence of hypercalciuria and osteomalacia. You are partly correct.

There is also a lower incidence of glycosuria. Read **20.45** again, more carefully. Then pick the correct answer.

20.48 Your answer − only statement 2 is true.

You are quite wrong. Start at the beginning of the chapter and read through again.

20.49 Your answer − there is a decreased incidence of glycosuria.

You are partly correct. There is also an increased incidence of long bone involvement. Read **20.45** again, more carefully. Then choose the correct answer.

20.50 Your answer − only statement 3 is true.

You are partly correct. Statement 1 is also true. Go back and read from **20.5** to **20.12**.

20.51 Your answer − there is a decreased incidence of glycosuria and an increased incidence of hypercalciuria. You are correct.

Digoxin plasma levels are higher in renal failure, and any given dose of digoxin is made more toxic by a low serum potassium level, less toxic by high serum potassium levels. In the uraemic patient, after the original loading dose of digoxin has been given, it is necessary to give only about 8 per cent of the total loading dose daily to maintain full digitilisation. In haemodialysis and peritoneal dialysis of patients taking digoxin it is necessary to ensure the maintenance of normal serum K levels to prevent cardiotoxicity of the drug which occurs with potassium depletion. In advanced renal failure the promazines readily accumulate and cause an extra pyramidal syndrome with trismus and limb spasms. Dosage should be markedly reduced and the patient observed carefully.

Statement 1. Necrotising papillitis is a complication of phenacetin abuse.

Statement 2. Acidification of the urine reduces the chance of sulphonamides crystallising in the urine.

Statement 3. Mercurial diuretics are more commonly nephrotoxic in patients with pre-existing renal disease.

Now choose the appropriate answer.

Answer
1. All the statements are true. Go on to **20.44**.
2. All the statements are false. Go on to **20.42**.
3. Only statement 1 is true. Go on to **20.40**.
4. Only statement 2 is true. Go on to **20.48**.
5. Only statement 3 is true. Go on to **20.50**.
6. Statement 1 and 2 are true, 3 is false. Go on to **20.53**.
7. Statement 1 and 3 are true, 2 is false. Go on to **20.46**.
8. Statements 2 and 3 are true, 1 is false. Go on to **20.52**.

20.52 Your answer – statements 2 and 3 are true, 1 is false.

You are correct about 3 only. Go back and read from **20.5** to **20.35**.

20.53 Your answer – statement 1 and 2 are true, 3 is false.

You are correct only about statement 1. Go back to **20.12** and read on from there.

Time for this chapter: 20 minutes

Chapter 21
Renal transplantation

21.1 Transplantation of the kidney has an important place in the treatment of advanced renal failure. The majority of the biochemical and surgical difficulties have now been overcome and the major problems to require complete solution are of an immunological nature. The types of kidney which are commonly transplanted are either from related live donors (i.e. siblings, parents, or children) or from cadavers. The chance of a kidney grafted from a live sibling donor surviving for a year is 9 out of 10. In cadaver grafts the chance of survival is about six out of ten in the first year. Now answer the question.

Question Which has the better chance of survival – related live donor or cadaver grafts?

Answer 1. Cadaver graft. Go on to **21.3**.
2. Related live donor graft. Go on to **21.5**.

21.2 You should not be reading this section. Follow the instructions or stop reading. Never fool yourself.

21.3 Your answer – Cadaver graft has a better survival. You are wrong. The cadaver graft is from an unrelated donor and is extracted after death from the donor's body. It may even be diseased or damaged by ischaemia. Read **21.1** again but this time follow the contents more closely. Then answer the question correctly.

21.4 Your answer – platelets share antigens with the kidney. You are not concentrating. Read **21.5** again.

21.5 Your answer – a related live donor has a better chance of survival. Good. There is at present a fairly limited comprehension of the immunological mechanisms involved in rejection. It appears that there are two components to the rejection phenomenon – humoral and cellular. The humoral components are antibodies produced by the host in response to antigens in the donor kidney which the host plasma and lymphoid cells recognize as foreign cells. Cellular components from the host also invade the graft and contribute to its destruction. The cellular antigens on the surface of kidney cells are thought to be virtually identical with the antigens present in the lymphocytes of the peripheral blood. The antigens on the lymphocyte are far more difficult to identify or type than those on the red cell. There are several systems of nomenclature but at the moment it is apparent that a group of antigens known as HL-A are extremely important, and that if the donor has antigens in this group which are not shared by the recipient, rejection of the graft is more likely. Similarly if the red cell ABO groups are not identical, rejection of the graft is likely. Recognition of the tissue antigens is carried out by typing the lymphocytes. This is known as tissue typing, and is a technique requiring special sera. Now answer the question.

Question Which blood cells share antigens with the kidney?

Answer 1. Platelets. Go on to **21.4**.
2. Red blood cells. Go on to **21.6**.
3. Lymphocytes. Go on to **21.7**.

21.6 Your answer – red blood cells share the antigens with the kidney. The ABO groups are important but they are not the whole story. Read **21.5** again, carefully this time.

21.7 Your answer – lymphocytes share the antigens with the kidney. You are correct. Now in siblings many antigens are shared because of common parentage. Nevertheless, tissue typing has to be carried out to make sure no major transplantation types are not equally shared. In cadaver donor grafts not only must tissue typing be done but also the time elapsing between death and insertion of the graft must be limited. This period can be divided into 2 parts – warm-ischaemia-time and cold-ischaemia-time. Warm-ischaemia-time is the time elapsing between death and the cooling of the kidney to 4°C after its removal. If this period is longer than 2 hours, there is a very little chance of the kidney functioning subsequently because of acute tubular necrosis which may be irreversible. Cold ischaemia is the time elapsing when the kidney is kept at a temperature of 4°C, and a period of up to 16 hours may be quite acceptable. Now answer the question.

Question What is meant by warm ischaemia time?

Answer 1. The time the kidney is kept at 4°C. Go on to **21.9**.
2. The time the kidney is kept from death to cooling down to 4°C. Go on to **21.11**.

21.8 Your answer – Statement 2 is true, 1 and 3 are false. No. 3 is also true. Read the chapter again from **21.11**.

21.9 Your answer – warm ischaemia time is the time the kidney is kept at 4°C. You are wrong. You should have made an intelligent guess, not a careless one. This shows, anyhow, that you have not read **21.7** properly. Read it again and answer the question correctly.

21.10 Your answer – The platelet count rises. You are wrong. The platelet count falls due to platelet sequestration; you have not read **21.11**. Go back and read it carefully, then answer the question.

21.11 Your answer – warm ischaemia is the time elapsing from death until the kidney is cooled to 4°C. You are correct.

When a cadaver kidney is grafted there is often a period of anuria due to acute tubular necrosis. This is sometimes difficult to tell from initial rejection without a biopsy of the transplant. The transplanted kidney causes a host-graft interaction resulting in rejection of the kidney sooner or later unless steps are taken to prevent this. The immunosuppressive measures include the use of predonisone, azathioprine, and anti-human-lymphocyte globulin (ALG). Nevertheless, in spite of these drugs, rejection may occur, most often in the first 3 months as an acute process, and later as a more chronic and slower phenomenon. Rejection can be recognized by swelling and tenderness of the grafted kidney, with fever and an increase in proteinuria. There is a fall in the 24 hour urine volume, creatinine clearance and urea clearance, sodium excretion, and an increase in lymphocyte excretion. The appearance of rejection is heralded by a fall in platelet count due to platelet sequestration in the kidney. In the rejection process there are platelet thrombi blocking the glomeruli as well as an inflammatory round cell exudate in the interstitium of the kidney. Later there is thickening of the basement membrane and a chronic nephritic appearance of the kidney with obliteration of the glomeruli. The arterioles are affected by a narrowing of the lumen of the arterioles, thought to be on the basis of organisation of thrombus. Now answer the question.

Question Does the platelet count rise or fall in rejection of the kidney?

Answer 1. Rises. Go on to **21.10**.
2. Falls. Go on to **21.12**.

21.12 Your answer – the platelet count falls. You are correct.
The problem of death from rejection and consequent renal failure or infection resulting from increased dosage of immunosuppressive drugs is ever present in human renal transplantation. There are several serious complications of the use of immunosuppressive drugs which contribute to the majority of the deaths following transplantation: (1) infections are the most frequent. In suppressing the rejection response the drugs also limit the normal resistance to bacterial infections and also to viral infections. Septicaemia due to bacterial infections is an ever present threat. Cytomegalic inclusion virus is present in the urine of the majority of patients on immunosuppressive drugs after transplantation. Herpes virus infections are responsible for naso-oral ulceration which may prove fatal.

Chicken pox may be accompanied by a fatal pneumonia. Tumours of the lymph glands have been reported after immunosuppressive therapy, and sarcomas of the brain and skin after ALG therapy. Now answer the question.

Question Do immunosuppressive drugs increase or reduce susceptibility to virus or bacterial infections?

Answer 1. Increase susceptibility to infections. Go on to **21.14**.
2. Decrease susceptibility. Go on to **21.16**.
3. No effect on susceptibility. Go on to **21.18**.

21.13 Your answer – urinary fistula or ureteric structure develops. You are correct. Because of the high dose of prednisone required for immunosuppressive therapy (150 mg to 30 mg per day) there is a high incidence of Cushings Syndrome with hypertension and diabetes, in patients who have received transplants. The corticosteroids are responsible for the development of peptic ulceration in transplanted patients. The ulcer may perforate or bleed, and lead to a fatal outcome. Consequently a useful procedure in screening patients for the feasibility of receiving renal transplant is to exclude the presence of peptic ulceration beforehand with a barium meal. If an ulcer is found either the patient is unsuitable for transplantation or a prior gastrectomy should be undertaken. Similarly, because of the likelihood that resistance to infections will be decreased, pulmonary tuberculosis should be excluded by X-ray of the chest. If calcified foci are found they should be carefully watched for the development of tuberculosis when the patient is given steroids and immunosuppressives. Urinary tract infection with positive urine culture before transplantation is an indication for bilateral nephrectomy. Now answer the question.

Question Would you transplant a kidney into a patient who has a peptic ulcer?

Answer 1. No. Go on to **21.17**.
2. Yes. Go on to **21.19**.

21.14 Your answer – susceptibility is increased. You are correct. The site of transplantation is the iliac fossa, with connection of the donor renal artery to the hypogastric artery of the host, and the renal vein to the internal iliac vein. The ureter is implanted into the bladder. Complications of the operation are relatively few in skilled hands. Rarely thrombosis of the renal artery or vein occurs, but leakage of urine at the ureteric anastamosis is more common. This is frequently due to an inadequate blood supply to the area of ureter implanted. Consequently a portion of the ureteric wall necroses and a urinary fistula develops. Occasionally a ureteric stricture develops at the site of implantation. Sometimes the wound breaks down. In patients in whom a second operation is necessary there is an increased incidence of death due to infection.

If a kidney is rejected it should be removed and the patient haemodialysed on a regular dialysis programme until there is a second donor graft available of suitable compatible tissue type.

In some centers the recipients own kidneys are removed before at or after transplantation, particularly if they are infected, e.g., polycystic kidneys. If left in situ they may act as a source of infection body wide when immunosuppressive drugs are given. Now answer the question.

Question What complication occurs with the ureter at transplantation?

Answer 1. Urinary fistula or ureteric structure. Go on to **21.13**.
2. Ruptured urethra. Go on to **21.15**.

21.15 Your answer – ruptured urethra develops. No. You are guessing. There is no point in reading on if you cannot concentrate. If you can concentrate please read **21.14** again.

21.16 Your answer – immunosuppressive drugs decrease susceptibility to infections. You are not correct. Your reading of **21.12** has been faulty. Try it again and concentrate on it.

21.17 Your answer – I would not transplant a kidney with a patient who has peptic ulcer. You are correct. In patients who have had renal failure following acute glomerulonephritis, renal transplantation tends often to be followed by rapid rejection of the graft due to the circulating anti-glomerular-basement-membrane antibodies which destroyed the patients' original kidneys attacking the transplanted kidney. Similarly, poor results are found in Henoch-Schönlein nephritis when these patients are grafted.

Another method of reducing the incidence of rejection of transplanted kidneys is to drain the thoracic duct and so deplete the patient of lymphocytes which are capable of mediating the rejection response of the host versus the graft. It is convenient to separate the lymphocytes from the lymph and return the lymph to the patient so that protein depletion does not occur. Thoracic duct fistulae are not easy to maintain patent, but in successful cases there is prolongation of the life of the graft, when grafts compared to implanted in a host who has not had thoracic duct drainage. The lymphocytes obtained from thoracic duct drainage can be used for the manufacture of antihuman lymphocyte globulin. Now answer the following question.

Question Does drainage of the thoracic duct prolong or shorten graft survival?

Answer 1. Shortens survival. Go on to **21.20**.
2. Prolongs survival. Go on to **21.22**.

21.18 Your answer – it has no effect on susceptibility to infections. You are guessing. Go back to **21.12** and read it more carefully. Concentrate on it.

21.19 Your answer — I would transplant a patient with a peptic ulcer. You should only do this after a gastrectomy, or at least warning the patient of the danger of the procedure. Go back and read **21.13** with care.

21.20 Your answer — thoracic duct drainage shortens graft survival. You are guessing badly and obviously have not read **21.17** carefully enough. Please go back to **21.17** and read it carefully.

21.21 Your answer — ALG is an anti-human albumin. You are wrong — it is a globulin. Read **21.22** again and don't guess.

21.22 Your answer — thoracic duct drainage prolongs graft survival. You are correct. Anti lymphocyte globulin (ALG) is a globulin antibody produced in response to injections of human lymphocytes produced in horse, goat or rabbit. It appears to cause paralysis of the mechanism the body possesses for recognizing that a protein is foreign. Injection of ALG intra-muscularly is painful, often associated with fever, and the intravenous route is preferred by many, notwithstanding the possible danger of anaphylatic shock due to the injection of a foreign protein particularly if it is obtained from a horse. At present it seems wise to reserve this powerful agent for the patient who is experiencing an acute rejection episode. When azathioprine is given to patients who have received a graft it should be given in a dose of 1.5 mg/kg body weight per day during any period of anuria, and in twice this dosage in periods in which there 200 ml or more of urine per day. Side effects include leucopenia, thrombocytopenia and anaemia, as well as reduction of resistance to infections. Hepatitis, vomiting and diarrhoea are also recognised complications.

Question Is ALG an anti human albumin raised in animals against lymphocytes?

Answer 1. Yes. Go on to **21.21**.
2. No. Go on to **21.23**.

21.23 Your answer — ALG is not an anti-human albumin. You are correct. The function of the grafted kidney may be normal from the beginning in live donor grafts but in cadaver grafts it is often poor, with a period of anuria due to acute tubular necrosis being common. After recovery there is often a marked nocturia, with a sodium diuresis at night and an oliguria during the day. Better has demonstrated that an acquired and temporary renal tubular acidosis develops after transplantation. The cause may well be tubular damage following ischaemia at the time of donor death and transplantation.

Question Is nocturia common after transplantation?

Answer 1. Yes. Go on to **21.25**.
2. No. Go on to **21.27**.

21.24 Your answer – a related live donor graft is more successful than a cadaver graft. You are correct.

After transplantation hypercalcaemia often develops due to hypertrophy of the parathyroid glands during the long period of antecedent chronic renal failure. In some patients this so called 'tertiary hyperparathyroidism' is due to autonomous parathyroid adenomas, and requires parathyroidectomy. In some patients the hyperplastic glands are not autonomous but are responsive to plasma divalent ion concentrations i.e., calcium or magnesium ions. The hypercalcaemia disappears in a few months in the majority of the patients.

Question Is hypocalcaemia or hypercalcaemia common after successful renal transplantation?

Answer 1. Hypercalcaemia. Go on to **21.28**.
2. Hypocalcaemia. Go on to **21.29**.

21.25 Your answer – nocturia is common after renal transplantation. You are correct. In all transplanted kidneys the physician has many anxieties – the first being whether the kidneys will be rejected; the second whether the complications of immunosuppressive therapy will harm the patient or even lead to his death; and the third is whether the disease process which attacked the recipients' kidneys will likewise damage or destroy the donor kidney. The chance of ultimate rejection is fairly high; and one is in an ethical dilemma about the propriety of accepting kidneys from related life donors. Kidneys from unrelated live-donors fair very little better than those from cadavers, so there is little justification for using unrelated live donors. Related live donors are often subjected to great family and social pressures to donate a kidney, and this is regrettable. In later years the donors may acquire a kidney disease or be subjected to trauma, and may have their lives shortened as a result of having donated one kidney. A prospective donor must be perfectly healthy, have no hypertension or diabetes, and have normal kidney function. For obvious reasons there should be a near perfect tissue type cross match.

Question Is a related live donor graft more likely to be successful than a cadaver graft?

Answer 1. Related live donor graft is more successful. Go on to **21.24**.
2. Related live donor graft is less successful. Go on to **21.26**.

21.26 Your answer – A related live donor graft is less successful than a cadaver graft. You are wrong. If both are of the appropriate tissue type the kidney is less likely to be rejected in a live donor because the warm ischaemia time is less. Read **21.25** again.

21.27 Your answer – nocturia is not common after transplantation. You are wrong. Nocturia is very frequent after transplantation and associated with a nocturnal sodium diuresis. Read **21.23** again carefully, then choose the correct answer.

21.28 Your answer – hypercalcaemia is common after transplantation. You are correct. Now study the following statements.

   Statement 1 Cadaver grafts are never rejected.

   Statement 2 It is important not to transplant incompatible tissue types or non-identical ABO groups.

   Statement 3 Death from infection is common in the use of large doses of immunosuppressive drugs after transplantation.

   Now choose which of the following answer you believe to be correct.

Answers 1. All the statements are true. Go on to **21.30**.
   2. All the statements are false. Go on to **21.31**.
   3. Statement 1 is true, 2 and 3 are false. Go on to **21.32**.
   4. Statements 2 and 1 are true, 3 is false. Go on to **21.33**.
   5. Statements 2 and 3 are true, 1 is false. Go on to **21.34**.
   6. Statement 3 is true, 1 and 2 are false. Go on to **21.35**.
   7. Statements 1 and 3 are true, 2 is false. Go on to **21.36**.
   8. Statement 2 is true, 1 and 3 are false. Go on to **21.8**.

21.29 Your answer – hypocalcaemia is common after transplantation. You are not correct. Hypercalcaemia is common, and the problem is whether the parathyroids are autonomous or not. Read **21.24** with more attention. Don't waste your time looking at the page. Devote yourself solely to reading the paragraph. Then answer the question.

21.30 Your answer – all the statements are true. No. This is a short chapter. Read it again from **21.1**.

21.31 Your answer – all the statements are false. You are wrong. You should read the chapter again from the beginning.

21.32 Your answer – only statement 1 is true. You are wrong. Start again at the beginning of this short chapter and concentrate this time.

21.33 Your answer – only statement 3 is false. You are wrong. Statement 2 and 3 are true; 1 is false. Start at **21.5** again and read through the chapter.

21.34 Your answer – only statement 1 is false. You are correct. References for further reading are:

Transplantation: 1964 onwards.
Van Rood J., Lancet 1969, **1**, 1142.
Calne R. Y. et al. Brit. Med. J. 1968, **2**, 404.
Starzl T. E. et al. Transplantation Proc. 1969, **1**, 448.
Gonick H. C. et al. Amer. J. Med. 1969, **47**, 410.
Murray J. E. et al, Transplantation 1971. **11**,
Hulme B. and Reeves D. S. Brit. Med. J. 1971, **3**, 610.
Starzl T. E. et al, Annals of Surgery 1970, **172**, 1.
Bell P. et al, Brit. Med. J. 1972, **4**, 408.
Lowrie et al, New Eng. J. Med. 1973, 288, 863. *This article is most important.*

21.35 Your answer − Statement 3 only is true. You are wrong. Statement 2 is true. Start at **21.1** again and read through the chapter.

21.36 Your answer − Statement 2 is false, the rest are true. You are incorrect. Start at **21.1** and read through this short chapter again.

Appendix

1. NOMOGRAM
Nomogram of body weight, body height and body surface area.

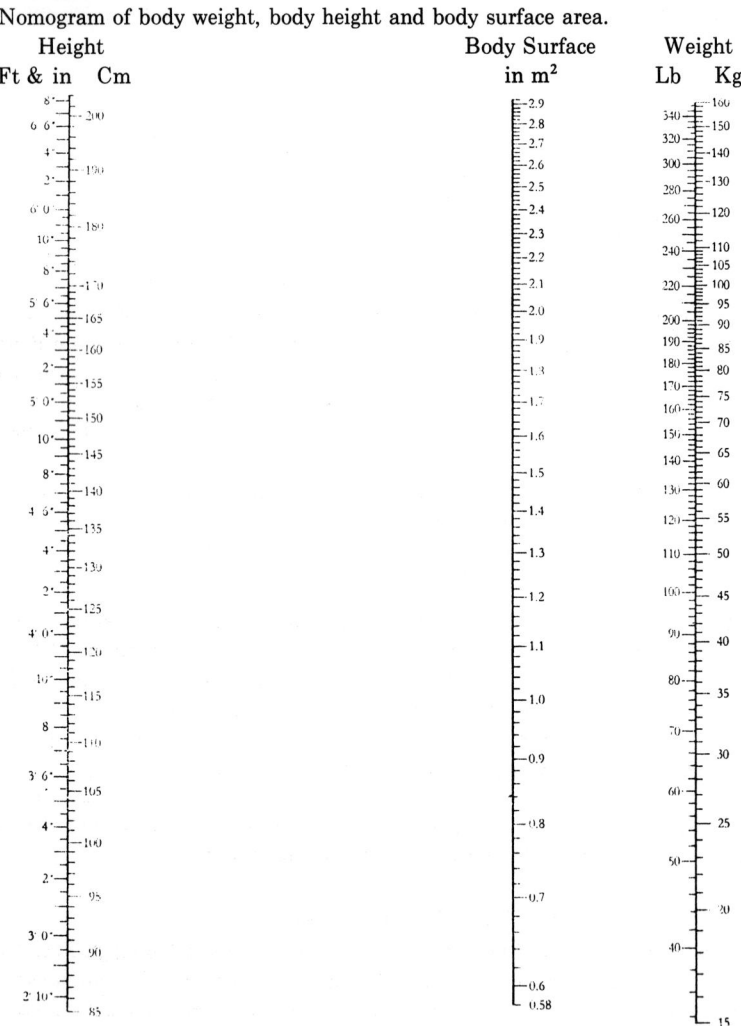

2. WRONG AND DAVIES ACIDIFICATION TEST (MODIFIED)

After a normal breakfast 2 one hourly urine specimens are collected. Ammonium chloride in a dose of 0.1 g/kg body weight is given orally in gelatin 0.5 g capsules, preferably with toast and jam, and the urine collected over the next six hours. Blood specimens are taken before, and 3 hours after, the administration of ammonium chloride. Urinary pH should fall below pH 5.3. Further details are found in the original paper of Wrong and Davies, Quart. J. Med., 1959. **28**, 259.

3. URINE TESTING

(a) Protein

1. *Heat.* Acidify the urine with 33 per cent acetic acid in a test tube three quarters full of urine. Direct the flame of a bunsen burner onto the upper quarter of the fluid column. Protein is precipitated on heating. Bence Jones protein is precipitated at first but then redissolves.

2. *Salicylsulphonic Acid* (Sulfosalicylic acid). Add 0.5 ml of 25 per cent salicylsulphonic acid to 5 ml of urine. A cloudy white precipitate forms in the presence of protein. False positives occur with uroselectan and uric acid.

3. *Albustix.* These sticks are made of cardboard, the tip of which is impregnated with tetrabromophenol blue in a buffer at pH 3. In the presence of protein the colour of the stick changes from yellow to different shades of green. The test for protein is carried out by dipping the stick into the urine and immediately withdrawing it, touching the side of the tube to remove excess urine. This test is most sensitive for albumen, and less sensitive for γ globulins, Bence Jones protein and mucoprotein. False positives are caused by highly alkaline urine and quaternary ammonium compounds. The test is sensitive to a minimum of 30 mg of protein per 100 ml and will often detect protein in the urine of normal man.

4. Bence Jones Protein – Heating Test

Adjust the urine pH until it is faintly acid to litmus, having filtered it initially. Put 5 ml of urine into three tubes, the second and third add 1 and 2 drops of 33 per cent acetic acid respectively, and put into a water bath, the temperature of which is gradually raised. Bence Jones protein first comes down between 40°C. As the heating continues the Bence Jones protein redissolves below 100 and 60°C whereas albumin and globulin only precipitate above 60°C. If albumin is also present the precipitate does not apparently redissolve, and in this case it is necessary to filter the urine through a hot filter funnel, the Bence Jones protein precipitating when the filtrate cools. The albumin remains in the filter paper.

(b) Glucose and Reducing Substances in Urine

(1) *Benedict's test.* This detects reducing substances including glucose. Add 8 drops of urine to 5 ml of Benedict's solution in a test tube. Boil for 2 minutes and then allow to cool. A blue colour indicates the absence of reducing substances, a

green precipitate indicates one plus of reducing substances, yellow brown 2 plus, reddish brown 3 plus.

(2) *Clinitest*. 5 drops of urine and 10 drops of water are placed in a test tube and one tablet added with *dry* fingers. After the boiling has subsided the colour should be compared to the chart provided.

The above tests, Benedict's and Clinitest, will detect glucose, fructose, lactose, pentose, galactose, glucuronates, salicyluric acid, homogentisic acid and concentrated solutions of uric acid and creatinine. To confirm the presence of glucose rather than one of the other causes, the use of 'Clinistix' is advised. This consists of a cardboard stick impregnated at one end with glucose oxidase and o-tolidine. When the stick is dipped rapidly into the urine, immediately withdrawn and excess urine drained off down the side of the tube, glucose is converted by atmospheric oxygen in the presence of glucose oxidase to gluconic acid and hydrogen peroxide. The latter, in the presence of peroxidase, converts the o-tolidine to a blue dye. The test requires a wait of 10 seconds after dipping. It will detect glucose down to 10 mg/100 ml.
Ascorbic acid reduces the sensitivity of the test.

False negatives may occur with ascorbic acid.

False positives may be caused by hypochlorites, bleaches, detergents containing sodium perborate, and impurities in coal gas. No sugars or glucuronates give false positives.

(c) **Blood**

The only adequate test for blood is microscopy. Free haemoglobin can be detected with the reversion spectrometer. A convenient chemical test for haemoglobin (free or in red cells) is the 'Haemastix' test in which o-tolidine and an organic peroxide are present. The stick is read 60 seconds after a rapid dip into the urine.

A positive test is indicated by a blue colour. False positives are caused by hypochlorites left in urine containers. Positive tests do not replace microscopy.

4. Dialyzing Fluid Composition for Kolff Twin Coil Artificial Kidney.

Component	Gm. per 100 L.	Milliequivalents per Litre					
		$Na+$	$K+$	$Ca++$	$Mg++$	$Cl-$	HCO_3-
NaCl	570 =	97	—	—	—	97	—
$NaHCO_3$	300 =	36	—	—	—	—	36
KCl	30 =	—	4	—	—	4	—
$CaCl_2$	28 =	—	—	5	—	5	—
$MgCl_2$	7.5 =	—	—	—	1.5	1.5	—
	Total	133	4	5	1.5	107.5	36

Dextrose 1.5 per cent.
Lactic acid to adjust pH to approx. 7.4.
To maintain the pH during dialysis, 90 per cent O_2 with 10 per cent CO_2 is bubbled through fluid.

5. DRUG EXCRETION IN RENAL FAILURE
Modified from Richet G., J. d'Urol. et Nephrol. **72**, No. 4. 1966, and Kunin C. M., Ann. Int. Med. **67**, 151, 1967.

(a) **Antibiotics and chemotherapeutic agents whose excretion is delayed in renal failure**

Streptomycin	Nitrofurantoin
Dihydrostreptomycin	Naladixic acid
Tetracycline	Isoniazid
Demethylchlortetracycline	PAS
Oxytetracycline	Cycloserine
Colimycin	Ethionamide
Polymyxin	Bismuth, Arsenic, Mercury
Kanamycin	Antimony
Short acting sulphonamides	Diamidine

(b) **Other Drugs whose excretion is delayed in renal failure**

Digoxin	Aldomet
Quinidine	Guanethidine
Most Analgesics	Pempidine
Phenobarbitone	Mercurial Diuretics
Curarising drugs	Thiazides possibly
Opiates	Cortisone
Atropine	Phenylbutazone

(c) **Dosage of Antibiotics**

(1) *Unmodified Dosage* in *renal failure* where GFR is less than 10 ml/minute:

>Chloramphenicol
>Erythromycin
>Cloxacillin
>Novobiocin

(2) *Modified Dosage:* normal initial dose and half dose as shown below

>Penicillin 8–10 hourly
>*Cephaloridin 24 hourly cephalexin
>Ampicillin 12 hourly
>Lincomycin 12 hourly

Appendix

*Tetracycline every 3–4 days
*Oxytetracycline every 3–4 days
*Demethylchlortetracycline every 3–4 days
*Methacycline   every 3–4 days
*Kanamycin   every 3–4 days
*Streptomycin   every 3–4 days
*Vancomycin   every 9 or 10 days
*Colistin   every 3–4 days
*Polymyxin B   every 3–4 days

Try to avoid using those asterisked, unless there is no alternative.

Not that Cephalexin is preferable to Cephaloridine because the former is less nephrotoxic. Under no circumstances should more than 4 G of Cephaloridine/day be given to a patient with renal failure.

(3) Avoid chlortetracycline.

(4) Gentamycin. Look up an article by R. A. Chan et al in Annals Int. Med. (1972) **76**, 773 for a nomogram detailing the dose of gentamycin at varying levels of renal function.

Index

This index should not be used until you have read the book
1st bold figure(s) indicate chapter, the non-bold figure(s) refer to the paragraph.

Abnormalities, uretero-pelvic **18**.20
Abscesses, pyelonephritis and **7**.11
Acidosis
   hyperchloraemic **18**.16
   metabolic **9**.5
   renal tubular
   systemic
      3.56, **15**.44, **15**.45, **15**.47, **15**.52, **15**,53, **15**.58
      Lignac-Fanconi syndrome and **15**.17
Actinomycosis **6**.30
Addis count **4**.11
Addison's disease **5**.57
   dilution tests **3**.60
   salt-losing nephritis and **15**.87
   sodium conservation and **3**.57
Adenocarcinoma see Hypernephroma **14**.8
Adrenal cortex, angiotensin effects **14**.15, **14**.16
AGN see Glomerulonephritis, acute
Albumin
   loss in nephrotic syndrome **6**.1
   loss in peritoneal dialysis **8**.25
   plasma clearance **6**.5
   serum, in nephrotic syndrome **6**.1, **6**.5
Albuminuria **3**.1
   amyloidosis and **6**.30
   congestive heart failure and **6**.41
   familial Mediterranean fever and **6**.30
   malignant essential hypertension and **14**.43
   nephrotic syndrome and **5**.63
Albustix Appendix **3**.3
Aldactone **14**.16
Aldosterone
   nephrotic syndrome and **6**.10
   secretion **14**.16

Aldosterone (cont.)
   angiotensin and **14**.16
   pre-eclamptic toxaemia and **13**.13
   pregnancy and **13**.7
Aldosteronism, secondary **14**.15
   essential malignant hypertension and **14**.48
ALG **21**.11
Alkalosis
   malignant essential hypertension and **14**.48
Alport's syndrome **16**.43
Aluminium hydroxide **19**.24
   in hyperparathyroidism **19**.24
Alveolitis, necrotising **17**.10
Amenorrhoea **9**.13
Amino acids
   tubular abnormalities *et seq.* **15**.1
   tubular reabsorption **21**.13
Amino-aciduria **3**.44, **3**.45
   Lignac-Fanconi syndrome and **15**.6
Amino nucleoside **20**.4
Ammonia, renal formation **2**.64
Ammonium ions **2**.64
   non-ionic diffusion and **2**.57
   renal tubular acidosis and **15**.43
   urinary excretion **2**.57, **2**.64
A M P cyclic **12**.26
Amphotericin B **20**.14
Ampicillin **20**.21
Amyloidosis **6**.30, **6**.36
   primary **6**.30
   secondary **6**.36
Anaemia
   chronic glomerulonephritis and **5**.69
   chronic renal failure and **9**.3
   iron deficiency **17**.11

Index

Aneurysms, berry **16**.11
Angina of effort **6**.6
Angiography, renal **14**.6, **14**.4
Angiotensin **14**.8
    aldosterone secretion and **14**.18, **14**.16
Antibiotics
    contraindications **8**.18, **20**.14, **20**.12, **20**.19
    in acute pyelonephritis **7**.20, **7**.25
    in haemodialysis **9**.38
Antibodies response to infection **7**.15
Antibodies to bacterial antigens **7**.11
Antibodies
    AGN and **5**.5
    Coon's technique **5**.5, **5**.8
Antibodies to DNA **10**.12
Antidiuretic hormone **2**.29, **2**.31, **2**.40
    diabetes insipidus and **3**.40, **3**.46
Antigens, HL-A **21**.5
Antigens, lymphocyte **21**.5
Antigen, soluble streptoccoccal **5**.5
Antihuman lymphocyte globulin **21**.11
Anti N A D ase **5**.44
Antistreptolysin titre in AGN **5**.23, **5**.43
Anuria
    acute, water intake **8**.17
    AGN and **5**.36
    management **8**.17
    polyarteritis nodosa and **10**.28
    renal biopsy in **4**.46
    retrograde pyelography and **4**.33
    Stamey test **3**.61
    systemic sclerosis and **10**.39
    urinary tract obstruction and **8**.2, **8**.9
Aorta
    coarctation, toxaemia and **13**.25
    surgery, oliguria and **8**.9
Arginine, tubular reabsorption **2**.13
Arteria recta vera **1**.22
Arteriography, renal **4**.38, **4**.40
Arterioles
    fibrinoid necrosis **14**.39
    hyaline thickening **14**.36
    systemic sclerosis and **10**.37
Arthritis, rheumatoid **10**.64
Artificial kidney
    kiil **9**.37

Artificial kidney (cont.)
    Kolff **9**.20
    Skeggs-Leonard **9**.37
ASO titre *see* Antistreptolysin titre
Aspirin, urinary deposits and **4**.19
Atheroma **4**.38
ATP ase **2**.43
Azathioprine **21**.22
Azathioprine, rejection reaction suppression **21**.11
Azotaemia, water deprivation and **3**.46

Bacilluria, pyelitis and **13**.4
BAL see British Anti-Lewisite
Bacteriuria, pyelonephritis and **7**.21
Bactrim **7**.25
Basement membranes **1**.16
    SLE and **10**.11, **10**.12
Bellini's papillary ducts **1**.29
Bence Jones protein **3**.6
    Appendix **3**.4
Benedict's reagent **3**.44
    Appendix **36**.1
Benemid, tubular secretion and **2**.32
Bertin's columns **1**.1
Bicarbonate
    reabsorption **2**.54, **2**.56
    urinary excretion **2**.56, **2**.57
Biopsy, renal **4**.44, **4**.46, **4**.49
    acute renal failure and **8**.46
    chronic pyelonephritis and **7**.28
    pain in **4**.57
Biuret test **3**.16
Blood flow, acute renal failure and **8**.1
Body weight nomogram Appendix 1
Bone
    chronic glomerulonephritis and **5**.63
    kidney diseases and **19**.1 *et seq.*
Bowman's capsule **11**.11
    fluid composition **2**.1
    in glomerulonephritis **5**.15
British Anti-Lewisite **8**.13, **20**.39
Bronchiectasis **6**.30

Cadaver graft **21**.1 *et seq.*

Cadmium **20**.31
   poisoning, tubular damage   **3**.45
Calciferol
   dangers of   **15**.39
   in Fanconi syndrome   **15**.20
Calcification, conjunctival   **9**.3
Calcium
   oxalate stones   **15**.26
   serum *see also* Hypercalcaemia
      chronic glomerulonephritis and   **5**.63
      idiopathic hypercalciuria and   **15**.82
   urinary   **15**.77
     see also Hypercalciuria
Calcium phosphorus product   **19**.15
Calculi
   renal
      hypercalciuria and   **15**.82
      hyperparathyroidism and   **19**.2
      medullary sponge kidney and   **16**.30
      pyelonephritis and   **7**.2
   ureteral, RTA and   **15**.53
   uric acid   **15**.95
Caloreen   **8**.16, **5**.49
Calyces, renal   **4**.25
Capillaries, peritubular   **1**.22, **1**.25
Capsule, renal   **1**.1
Carbohydrate polymer   **5**.49
Carbon tetrachloride   **20**.11
Carbonic acid, pH and   **2**.56
Carbonic anhydrase   **2**.56
Carcinoma, renal cell *see* Hypernephroma
Cardiac tamponade   **9**.16
Caronamide, tubular secretion and   **2**.32
Casts
   cellular   **4**.6, **4**.19, **4**.13
   counting   **4**.11
   granular   **4**.6
   hyaline   **4**.6
   'renal failure'   **4**.6
   tubular cell   **4**.13
   urinary, in AGN   **5**.36
Catheterisation, urinary
   hazards   **7**.28
     in diabetes   **11**.12
Cells *see also under names*
   intercalated (dark)   **1**.29
Cellulose phosphate in hypercalciuria **15**.86

Cephaloridine   **20**.21
Cerebro-oculo-renal dystrophy   **15**.29, **3**.45
Chicken pox   **21**.12
Chicken pox virus   **21**.12
Chloramphenicol   **20**.20
Cholecalciferol
   hydroxy   **19**.17
Chloride, plasma
   RTA and   **15**.45
Chlorothiazide in nephrotic syndrome   **6**.53
Chlorpropamide   **12**.26
Chlorpromazine, vomiting control   **8**.16
Chlortetracycline   **20**.19
cH_2O *see* Free water
Cholera, acute renal failure and   **8**.3
Cholesterol, serum *see also*
        Hypercholesterolaemia
   lupus nephrotic syndrome and   **6**.31, **10**.16
   SLE and   **10**.16
Cimino-Brescia, A-V fistula   **9**.20
Citrates
   excretion, RTA and   **15**.53, **15**.69
   in osteomalacia   **19**.31
Clinistix   **3**.44
Clinitest Appendix   **3**.62
Cloxacillin   **20**.21
C3NeF   **6**.12
Coagulopathy   **10**.68
Cold ischaemia   **21**.7
Collagen diseases   **10**.7
Complement
   fraction in AGN   **5**.5 *et seq.*
   serum
     in basement membranes
       10.12   S.L.E.   **6**.25
Congo red test   **6**.36
Conjunctival calcification   **9**.3, **19**.24
Conjunctival injection   **19**.24
Conn's syndrome, aldosteronism and   **14**.15
Coon's fluorescent antibody technique   **5**.5
Copper   **20**.45
Cortex, renal   **1**.1 *et seq.*
   collecting ducts   **1**.29
   necrosis *see* Necrosis

Index

Cortex, renal (cont.)
    thinning   **4**.25
    tramline calcification   **8**.9
Corticosteroids in nephrotic syndrome
    6.67
Counter current multiplier system   **2**.35
Creatinine
    GFR and   **3**.27 *et seq.*
    endogenous   **2**.5
    plasma, measurement   **3**.27
Crohn's disease   **6**.30
Cushing's syndrome   **18**.7
Cystine
    deposits in Lignac-Fanconi syndrome
        15.14
    reductase   **15**.6
    stones   **4**.28
        radio-opacity   **15**.9
        solubility   **15**.1
Cystine-penicillamine diamer   **15**.4
Cystinosis *see* Lignac-Fanconi syndrome
Cystinuria   **15**.1 *et seq.*
    inheritance   **15**.4
Cystoscopy, hazards   **7**.22
Cytomegalus virus   **21**.12

Deafness, nerve   **16**.43
Decadurabolin   **8**.16
Diabetes insipidus
    nephogenic   **12**.8, **7**.31
    congenital   **12**.8
    pituitary, hydronephrosis and   **4**.36
    plasma ADH and   **3**.40
    vasopressin and   **12**.8
    water deprivation and   **3**.40 *et seq.*
Diabetes mellitus   **11**.1 *et seq.*
    see also Glomerulosclerosis
    glycosuria and   **3**.44
    urinary tract infection and   **11**.12
Dialysis   **4**.46 *see also* Haemodialysis
    acute tubular necrosis and   **8**.25
    indications for   **8**.25
    peritoneal   **8**.31, **8**.23
        fluid osmolality   **8**.23
        indications for   **9**.27

Dialysis (cont.)
    protein loss   **8**.31, **8**.25
    vomiting and   **8**.25
Diamer   **15**.4
Diet, low protein   **3**.49
    in uraemia   **9**.21
Digoxin   **20**.24, **20**.51
Dilution tests   **3**.60
Diodrast, tubular secretion   **2**.32
Dimercaprol   **8**.13, **20**.39
Disequilibrium syndrome   **9**.22
Diuresis, osmotic   **2**.29
    chronic renal failure and   **9**.1
Diuretics
    in malignant hypertension   **14**.48
    in nephrogenic diabetes insipidus   **12**.26
    mercurial, nephrotic syndrome and   **6**.41
DNA   **10**.12
Duct thoracic   **9**.41
Duct, thoracic, drainage of   **21**.17
Dwarfism   **15**.31
Dysproteinaemia   **15**.19
Dysuria, acute pyelonephritis and   **7**.15

Eclampsia   **13**.10
Encephalopathy, hypertensive   **5**.49
Endocarditis, subacute bacterial
    (SABE)   **17**.17 *et seq.*
Endothelial cells   **5**.12, **1**.19
    pre-eclamptic toxaemia and   **13**.10
Enuresis, nocturnal   **9**.6
    urine culture   **7**.15
Epithelial cells   **1**.12
    in Bowman's space   **5**.15
    squamous   **4**.13
    tubular   **4**.13
        AGN and   **5**.15
Epithelial crescent   **5**.15
ERPF *see* Renal plasma flow
Erythema multiforme   **6**.25
Erythrocytes *see* Red cells
Esbach's test   **3**.20
Escherichia coli, pyelonephritis and
    7.1
Ethacrynic acid   **8**.3

Fanconi syndrome **3**.45
  see also Lignac-Fanconi
    syndrome
  amino-aciduria and **3**.45
  clinical features **15**.25
  genetic aspects **15**.19
  osteomalacia and **15**.25
  proteinuria and **3**.5
Fibrin **10**.68
Fibrin split products **5**.8, **10**.68
Fibrin and fibrinogen
  thrombotic thrombocytopenic purpura
    and **10**.43
Fibrosis, periureteric **8**.2
Fick principle **2**.24
Filtration fraction **2**.24, **2**.32
Fingers, pseudo-clubbing **19**.21
Fistula, subcutaneous A-V **9**.20
Fluorescent granular deposits **10**.12
Fluorescent, granular deposition **5**.5
Foam cells, urinary **16**.43
Foetal survival, glomerulonephritis and
  13.29
Foot processes **1**.12
Free water clearance **2**.29 *et seq.*
Frusemide (furosamide) **5**.49, **8**.13, **8**.3
Frusemide in acute renal failure **8**.3
Fructose **2**.12
Furosemide *see* Frusemide

Galactosaemia **3**.45
Galactose **2**.12
Giordano-Giovannetti diet **9**.21
Glitter cells **4**.13
Globulin
  AGN and **5**.7
  Goodpasture's syndrome and **17**.10
  loss in peritoneal dialysis **8**.31
  SLE proteinuria and **10**.8
Glomeruli
  blood supply **1**.22
  electron microscopy **1**.12 *et seq.*
  filtration rate **2**.1 *et seq.*
    AGN and **5**.36
    blood urea and **3**.16
    body surface area and **2**.5

Glomeruli (cont.)
  creatinine clearance and **3**.27
  free water reabsorption and **12**.7
  pre-eclamptic toxaemia and **13**.13
  pregnancy and **13**.1
  Henoch-Schönlein purpura and **17**.3
  hyalinised **5**.19
  permeability in nephrotic syndrome **6**.5
Glomerulitis
  focal **10**.11
  lupus **10**.11
  post-streptococcal **5**.12
Glomerulonephritis
  acute **5**.1 *et seq.*
    anuric **5**.15
    clinical features **5**.24
    differential diagnosis **5**.41
    polyarteritis and **10**.23
    treatment **5**.45
  chronic **5**.19, **5**.55
    acute exacerbation **5**.23
    differential diagnosis **5**.67
    prognosis **5**.57
    treatment **5**.57
  diffuse, SABE and **17**.17
  foetal survival and **13**.26
  haemorrhagic **16**.43
  Henoch-Schönlein purpura **10**.49
  lupus **10**.1 *et seq.*
    prognosis **10**.16
    treatment **10**.24
  membranous **6**.14 *et seq.*
    prognosis **6**.12
    'no light microscopical change' **6**.14,
      6.12
    prognosis **6**.12, **6**.65
    pregnancy and **13**.26
    proliferative **6**.12
    prognosis **6**.65
    proteinuria and **3**.5
  Focal sclerosing **6**.14
  lobular **6**.14
  membrano proliferative **5**.19, **6**.12,
    6.14, **6**.65
  mesangio-capillary *see* membrano-
    proliferative
  renogram in **3**.68

Index

subacute **5**.15
    prognosis **5**.46
Glomerulosclerosis
    diabetic **11**.1 *et seq.*
        nodular **11**.3
        prognosis **11**.6
        treatment **11**.12
Glucose
    hyperkalaemia and **8**.14
    oxadase sticks **3**.44
    tolerance test **3**.44
    tubular reabsorption **2**.8, **2**.10
    phlorizin and **2**.12
    urinary tests **3**.44
Glutaminase **2**.64
Glycine
    tubular reabsorption **2**.13
    urinary **3**.45
Glycinuria, hereditary **15**.26
Glycol
    ethylene **20**.11
    propylene **20**.11
Glycosuria **2**.12
    heavy metal poisoning and **3**.44
    Lignac-Fanconi syndrome and **15**.25
    nephrotic syndrome and **6**.17
    pregnancy and **13**.1
Gold **20**.41
Goodpastures's syndrome **17**.10 *et seq.*
Gout, uric acid stones **15**.95
Grafts — cadaver **21**.1
    live donor **21**.1
    rejection **21**.5
    survival chances **21**.1
GTT *see* Glucose, tolerance test
Guanethidine **20**.24
Guanidino succinic acid **8**.23
Gynaecomastia **9**.13

Haemastix Appendix **3**.0
Haematoma, femoral **4**.40
Haematoxylin bodies, SLE and **10**.11
Haematuria
    aspirin ingestion and **4**.11
    focal nephritis and **17**.3

Haematuria (cont.)
    malignant essential hypertension and **14**.43
    microscopic
        focal embolic nephritis and **17**.21
        Henoch-Schönlein purpura and **17**.3
    polycystic kidneys and **16**.9
    streptococcal infection and **5**.3
    transitory, IVP and **18**.7
Haemodialysis **9**.28 *et seq.*
    acute renal failure and **8**.14
    chronic **9**.28
        indications for **9**.27
        Kiil machine **9**.37
Haemolytic-uraemic syndrome **10**.68
Haemopericardium **9**.16
Haemoptysis, Goodpasture's syndrome and **17**.10
Haemorrhage
    gastrointestinal **3**.16
    subarachnoid **16**.11
    uraemia and **9**.19
Haemosiderosis
    pulmonary **17**.10
    transfusion **17**.10
Heart disease, benign hypertension and **14**.33
Heart failure
    AGN and **5**.31
    congestive **5**.24
        creatinine and inulin clearance **3**.27
        proteinuria and **6**.41
        uraemia and **9**.16
Henle's loop **1**.25
    as counter current multiplier system **2**.35
    water deprivation and **2**.40
Henoch Schönlein purpura **17**.3
Heparinisation, whole body **9**.16
Hepatosplenomegaly **6**.25
Herpes virus **21**.12
Histidine **13**.1
Histidine
    tubular reabsorption **2**.13
    urinary **3**.45
Hodgkin's disease **6**.30
Hump **5**.5

Hyaline casts **3**.1
Hycal **8**.16
Hydrocalycosis **13**.4
Hydrogen ions
  excretion **2**.56 *et seq.*
Hydronephrosis **18**.20, **3**.57, **15**.45
  diabetes insipidus and **12**.1 *et seq.*
  pregnancy and **13**.4
  puerperal **13**.4
  urine concentration and **3**.40
Hydropelvis **12**.21
  ureterosigmoidoscopy and **18**.16
Hydroureter **12**.20
  pregnancy and **13**.4
  ureterosigmoidostomy and **18**.16
Hydroxyapatite **9**.3
Hypercalcaemia
  diabetes insipidus and **12**.21
  hyperparathyroidism and **19**.9
  post-transplantation **21**.24
  vitamin D and **15**.37
Hypercalciuria, idiopathic **15**.82
Hypercholesterolaemia **6**.1
  lupus erythematosus and **10**.16
Hyperglycaemia, uraemic **6**.22 *et seq.*
Hyperkalaemia
  acute renal failure and **8**.14
  dialysis and **8**.14
  treatment **8**.14
Hyperlipaemia, nephrotic syndrome and **6**.1
Hypernephroma **6**.42
  diagnosis **18**.1
  metastases **18**.7
  pyelography in **4**.18, **4**.40
  treatment **18**.10
Hyperoxaluria, primary **15**.99
Hyperparathyroidism **19**.1 *et seq.*
  diagnosis **19**.2 *et seq.*
  hypercalcaemia and **19**.2
  osteomalacia and **19**.11
  renal tubular acidosis and **15**.52
  secondary **19**.14
    chronic renal failure and **9**.3
  tertiary **21**.24
Hyperphosphaturia **2**.16
Hypertension

Hypertension (cont.)
  AGN and **5**.24 *et seq.*
  chronic pyelonephritis and **7**.26
  duplex kidney and **16**.40
  essential
    benign **14**.26
    malignant **14**.26
      haematuria and 181
  glomerulonephritis and **5**.41
  polycystic diseases and **16**.22
  pregnancy toxaemia and **13**.10 *et seq.*
  renal **14**.1 *et seq.*
  renin and **14**.1
  secondary malignant **14**.22
Hyperuricaemia, pre-eclamptic toxaemia and **13**.14
Hypervitaminosis D **15**.34 *et seq.*
Hypervolaemia, AGN and **5**.28
Hypoalbuminaemia **6**.1
  nephrotic syndrome and **6**.1
  peritoneal dialysis and **9**.19
  relationship with hyperlipaemia **6**.5
Hypokalaemia
  diabetes insipidus and **12**.17
  malignant essential hypertension and **14**.48
  polyuria and **14**.15
  ureterosigmoidostomy and **18**.16
Hypophosphataemia **2**.16
  RTA and **15**.52
  vitamin D resistant rickets and **15**.32
Hypopituitarism **3**.60
Hypoproteinaemia **6**.1
Hyposthenuria **3**.60
Hypotensive agents, pyelonephritis and **7**.38
Hypovolaemia **8**.3

IgA focal nephritis **17**.1
Imuran (azothiaprine) **10**.24
Incontinence *see also* Enuresis duplex ureter and **16**.38
Infarction, renal **8**.9 *et seq.*
  panarteritis and **10**.22
  pyelonephritis and **14**.29
  SABE and **17**.17

Insulin, hyperkalaemia and **8**.14
   'Intact nephron hypothesis' **9**.1
Inulin **2**.12
   renal clearance **2**.2, **2**.12
   stop flow experiments **2**.44
Iodine, protein-bound **6**.10
Ion exchange, RTA and **15**.47
   see also Ammonium ions;
      Hydrogen ions
Iron sequestration, Goodpasture's syndrome
   and **17**.11
Ischaemia cold **21**.7
Ischaemia, renal **14**.3 *et seq.*
   IVP and **4**.38
   pyelonephritis and **14**.27
Ischaemia warm **21**.7
Isoleucine, tubular reabsorption **2**.13
Isoniazide **20**.24
Isosthenuria **3**.60

Juxta-glomerular apparatus **1**.22, **1**.26
   renin production **14**.1 *et seq.*

Kanamycin **20**.20
Karyorrhexis **10**.11
Katonium, sodium removal **6**.60
Keratopathy, band **9**.3
Kidney *see also under* Renal
   anatomy **1**.1 *et seq.*
   artificial *see* Artificial kidney
   duplex **16**.38
   embryology **16**.5
   enlargement, polycystic disease and
      16.6
   failure
      acute **8**.1 *et seq.*
         extra-renal causes **8**.3
         pre-renal **8**.3
      amyloidosis and **6**.30
      anaemia and **9**.3
      chronic **9**.1 *et seq.*
      hyperparathyroidism and
         19.1 *et seq.*
      malignant essential hypertension and
         14.26

Kidney (cont.)
   plycystic disease and **16**.16
   post partum **13**.34
   pyelonephritis and **7**.25
   SABE and **17**.17
   salt-losing nephritis and **16**.36
   long axis length **4**.21
   oxygen consumption **2**.43
   physiology **2**.1 *et seq.*
   polycystic **16**.6
      IVP and **4**.18
   positioning **4**.45
   space occupying lesions **4**.18
      see also Hypernephroma; Tumours
   tissue osmolality **2**.40
   transplantation **21**.1 *et al.*
      rejection reaction **21**.11
         drug suppression **21**.11
   weight 1 **1**.1
Kiil artificial kidney **9**.37
Kimmelstiel-Wilson syndrome **11**.3 *et seq.*
Kjeldahl nitrogen estimation **3**.20
Kolff artificial kidney **9**.20
   fluid composition
      appendix 4

Lasix in acute renal failure **8**.3
Lead **20**.32
Leucine, tubular reabsorption **2**.13
Leucocytes see Polymorphs; White cells
Leucocytosis, polyarteritis nodosa and
   10.22
Lignac-Fanconi syndrome
   see also Fanconi syndrome
Limbal arc, calcification **19**.24
Linear fluorescence **5**.8
Lipids, metabolic disorders **6**.5
Lipoproteins **6**.5
Liver
   amyloidosis **6**.42
   cirrhosis **6**.79
   secondary neoplasms **6**.42
Lobectomy **18**.5
Lobular glomerulonephritis **6**.14
Looser's nodes **19**.14
Lowe's syndrome **15**.29

Lung
  abscess **6**.30
  'bat's wing' **9**.16
Lupus erythematosus **10**.1 *et seq.*
  clinical picture **6**.25
  complement fraction in **6**.25
  nephrotic syndrome and **10**.8 *et seq.*
  renal involvement **10**.1
  sex incidence **10**.1, **6**.25
  systemic
    focal nephritis and **17**.1
    pregnancy and **13**.31
    renal biopsy in **4**.48
    urinary deposit **4**.1
Lupus nephritis *see* Nephritis
Lymph gland tumours **21**.12
Lysine
  stones **15**.1
  tubular reabsorption **2**.13
Lysozyme **15**.82

Macroglobulin **6**.5
  glomerular disease and **3**.6
Macula densa **1**.22
Malaria
  nephrotic syndrome **6**.50
Mannitol **8**.13
Mediterranean fever, familial amyloidosis and **6**.30
Medulla, renal **1**.1
  cystic disease **16**.32
  RTA and **15**.62
Medullary sponge kidney **16**.25 *et seq.*
Megacystis **18**.20
Megaureter **18**.20
Membrano-proliferative **5**.19, **6**.14, **6**.12, **6**.65
Mental retardation, diabetes insipidus and **12**.14
Mercuric chloride poisoning **8**.9
Mercury **20**.39
  nephrotic syndrome and **6**.41
Mesangial (axial) cells **1**.19
Mesonephric bud **16**.5
Metals, heavy, toxicity **3**.45
Metanephros **16**.5

Methicillin **20**.21
Methionine **7**.25, **2**.13
α methyldopa **20**.24
Methylsergide **18**.20
Microglobulin $\beta + \gamma$ **3**.5
Mineralocorticoid
  unknown
    180H DOC precursor **2**.45
Moniliasis, diabetes and **11**.19
Muscle paralysis, RTA and **15**.47
Myeloma **3**.6, **3**.45
  multiple **4**.20, **6**.30
Myocardial infarction **6**.6
Myocarditis, toxic serous **5**.28
Myxoedema **6**.79

Na-K A T Pase **2**.43
Nandralone decanoate **8**.16
Necrosis
  acute tubular **4**.46, **8**.9
    dialysis in **8**.16 *et seq.*
  cortical **4**.46
    prognosis **8**.9
Neomycin **20**.14
Nephrectomy
  chronic pyelonephritis and **7**.38
  duplex kidney and **16**.40
  hypernephroma and **18**.10
  renal artery stenosis and **14**.27
Nephritis
  acute type 1 *see* Glomerulonephritis, acute
  drug induced **17**.29
  Ellis classification **5**.1, **6**.14
  familial **16**.43
  focal **17**.1 *et seq.*
    embolic **17**.21
  hereditary haematuric **16**.43
  interstitial **17**.29
  lupus **10**.1
  salt-losing **5**.57
    chronic pyelonephritis and **5**.57
    chronic renal failure and **9**.5
Nephrocalcinosis **4**.28
  hyperparathyroidism and **19**.25
  RTA and **15**.53
Nephronophthisis **16**.53

Nephrons **1**.1 *et seq.*
  cystic **16**.1
Nephrosclerosis, benign **14**.36
Nephrosis, lower nephron *see* Necrosis,
  acute tubular
Nephrotic syndrome **6**.1 *et seq.*
  chronic glomerulonephritis and **5**.55
  congenital **16**.53
  diabetes and **11**.6
  differential diagnosis **6**.83
  lupus erythematosus and **10**.8
  'no light microscopical change' type **6**.6
  polyarteritis nodosa and **10**.28
  pregnancy and **13**.28
  prognosis **6**.65
  proteinuria and **4**.48, **3**.6
  renal biopsy in **4**.48
  treatment **6**.65, **6**.67
Nerve, 8th **20**.14
Neuropathy
  diabetic **6**.17
  uraemia and **9**.13
Nitrofurantoin **20**.24
Nocturia **9**.6
  renal disease and **12**.2
Non-ionic diffusion **2**.64
Norethandrolone **8**.16

Oedema
  cerebral **9**.22
  facial, AGN and **5**.24
  peripheral **6**.1
Oliguria **6**.10
  aortic surgery and **8**.13
  cystoscopy in **8**.2
  hypertension and **5**.24
  oedema and **5**.24
Opiates **20**.24
Osmolality **2**.36 *see also under* Plasma;
  Urine
Osmolarity **2**.36
Osteitisfibrosa cystica **19**.1 *et seq.*
Osteoarthritis, rickets and **15**.34
Osteomalacia **19**.11
  chronic renal failure and **9**.3
  Fanconi syndrome and **15**.25

Osteomalacia (cont.)
  RTA and **15**.58
Osteomyelitis **6**.30
Osteoclasts, bone erosion **19**.21
Osteodystrophy, renal **19**.11 *et seq.*
Oxalosis **15**.99

PAH *see* Para-amino hippurate
PAS **20**.24
Panarteritis, infarction and **10**.22
Papillitis, necrotising **7**.2
  blood urea in **7**.15
  diabetes and **11**.12
Papilloedema, malignant hypertension
  and **14**.45
Para-amino hippurate
  renal blood flow and **3**.61
  stop flow studies and **2**.44
  tubular secretion **2**.21 *et seq.*
Paracetamol **20**.5
Parathyroid
  see also Hyperparathyroidism
  hormone levels **19**.2
  hormone, phosphate
    reabsorption and **2**.16
  neoplasms **2**.16
Parathyroidectomy **19**.24
Parenchyma, renal
  in acute pyelonephritis **7**.11
  in chronic pyelonephritis **7**.28
Pempidine **20**.24
Penicillamine **15**.4, **20**.45
Penicillin **20**.21
  tubular secretion **2**.32
Peptic ulcer, hyperparathyroidism and
  19.9
Pericardial effusion, uraemia and **9**.16
Pericarditis **6**.25
  uraemia and **9**.16
Perirenal fascia **1**.1
Phenacetin **20**.1
Phenacetin addiction
  nephritis and **20**.1
  medullary concentration **20**.1
Phenindione toxicity **17**.32
Phenobarbitone **20**.24

Phenol red, tubular secretion   **2**.32
Phenolsulphonphthalein test   **3**.38
Phenylalanine, tubular reabsorption   **2**.13
Phenylbutazone   **20**.24
Phlorizin, glycosuria and   **2**.12
Phosphatase, serum alkaline hyperparathyroidism and   **19**.2, **19**.5
  osteomalacia and   **19**.15
Phosphate
  as urinary buffer   **2**.16
  tubular reabsorption   **2**.16
    in RTA   **15**.43, **15**.45
    rickets and   **3**.36
  urinary   **4**.1
Picrate, plasma creatinine and   **3**.14
Pink disease   **20**.39
Pitressin *see* Vasopressin
Plasma
  cells, parenchymatous infiltration   **7**.28
  coagulation factors, uraemia and   **9**.13
  glomerular ultrafiltration   **2**.1
  osmolality   **2**.36
  volume in AGN   **5**.31
Platelet count   **21**.11
Pleurisy   **6**.25
Pneumaturia   **11**.15
Pneumonia, focal nephritis and   **17**.10
Polyarteritis nodosa   **10**.34
  'microscopic form'   **10**.23
Polyarthritis   **6**.25
Polycythaemia   **16**.22
Polydipsia
  hypervitaminosis D and   **12**.18
  hysterical   **12**.29
Polymorphs
  acute pyelonephritis and   **7**.11
  AGN and   **5**.15
  chronic pyelonephritis and   **7**.28
Polymyxin B   **20**.20
Polyuria   **12**.1 *et seq.*
  hypervitaminosis D and   **12**.18
  hypokalaemia and   **12**.28
Portillovirus   **10**.68
Post γ globulin   **3**.6
Post partum renal failure irreversible   **13**.34
Potassium

Potassium (cont.)
  perchlorate   **20**.4
  solution osmolality and   **2**.39
  tubular conservation   **3**.61
  tubular reabsorption   **2**.52
Potomania, pitressin response   **12**.29
'Prediabetes'   **11**.1
Prednisone
  in Goodpasture's syndrome   **17**.12
  in Henoch-Schönlein purpura   **17**.9
  in lupus glomerulonephritis   **10**.24
  in nephrotic syndrome   **6**.65 *et seq.*
  in polyarteritis nodosa   **10**.34
  in pyelonephritis   **4**.19
  rejection reaction
    suppression   **21**.11
Pregnancy
  glomerulonephritis and   **13**.26, **13**.28
  hydronephrosis and hydroureter   **4**.36
  kidney in   **13**.1
  lupus erythematosus and   **13**.31
  nephrotic syndrome and   **13**.28
  pyelonephritis and   **7**.26
  prevention   **7**.22
Product, CaXP   **19**.15
Protein
  Bence Jones   **3**.6
    Appendix 4
  dietary *see* Diet
  differential clearance   **6**.5
  'error of indicators'   **3**.7
  in acute renal failure   **8**.14
  loss in peritoneal dialysis   **8**.31
  Tamm-Horsfall   **3**.1
  urinary tests   Appendix 4
    see also Proteinuria
  urine concentration and   **2**.70
Proteinuria   **3**.1 *et seq.*
  AGN and   **5**.36
  asymptomatic   **4**.48
  chronic glomerulonephritis and   **5**.55
  chronic pyelonephritis and   **7**.32
  congestive heart failure and   **6**.41
  diabetic glomerulosclerosis and   **11**.6
  functional
    kidney transplantations and   **9**.44
  nephrotic syndrome and   **6**.1 *et seq.*

Index

plasma albumin and **6.**61
polyarteritis nodosa and **10.**28
postural (orthostatic) **3.**5
qualitative tests **3.**7
selective **6.**5
non-selective **6.**5
SLE and **10.**8
thrombotic thrombocytopenic purpura and **10.**44
Pseudo-nephrotic syndrome **10.**16
Purpura *see* Henoch-Schönlein purpura; Thrombotic thrombocytopenic purpura
Pyelography
  intravenous **4.**20 *et seq.*
    hypernephroma and **18.**6
    medullary sponge kidney and **16.**30
  retrograde **4.**33
Pyelonephritis **7.**1 *et seq.*
  acidosis and **3.**57
  acute
    aetiology **7.**1
    clinical features **7.**15
    pathology **7.**11
    recurrent **7.**20
    sex incidence **7.**2
    treatment **7.**20
  chronic **5.**67
    clinical features **7.**28
    diagnosis **7.**28
    IVP and **4.**40
    ischaemia and **14.**27
    tests for **4.**21
  diabetes insipidus and **12.**21
  diagnosis from AGN **5.**41
  duplex kidney and **16.**38
  hypertension and **14.**29
  interstitial nephritis and **17.**29
  pregnancy and **13.**4
  ureterosigmoidostomy and **18.**16
  vesico-ureteric reflux and **4.**30
Pyelovenous backflow **4.**33
Pyramids, renal **1.**1 *et seq.*
  distortion **4.**25
'Pyrexal' test **4.**19, **7.**32
Pyuria

Pyuria (cont.)
  chronic pyelonephritis and **7.**32
  sterile, renal tuberculosis and **18.**15

Quinine **20.**24

Red cells
  casts **4.**19
    in AGN **5.**13
  urinary **4.**1
    in AGN **5.**36
Red eyes **19.**24
Rejection **21.**5, **21.**11
Renal angles, in pyelonephritis **7.**11
Renal artery **1.**7
  fibromuscular hyperplasia **4.**38
  occlusion and hypertension **14.**4
  radiography **4.**40
  stenosis **4.**38
    hypertension and **14.**4
    indications for surgery **14.**22
    treatment **14.**22
Renal colic **15.**53
'Renal failure casts' *see* Casts
Renal function
  pre-eclamptic toxaemia and **13.**13
  pregnancy and **13.**7
  tests, divided **3.**61
Renal impairment
  malignant hypertension and **14.**26
Renal pelvis **1.**1
  tumours **18.**1 *et seq.*
Renal plasma flow (RPF) **2.**21, **2.**24
Renal vein **1.**1
Renal vein renin **14.**22
Renin **14.**1 *et seq.*
  secretion **14.**22, **14.**8
  aetiology of acute renal failure **8.**9
  plasma, in rapidly progressive G N **14.**29
  renal vein **14.**22
Renography
  in urinary tract obstruction **8.**9
  radioactive **3.**68

Resins
Resins, resonium A **8**.14
  calcium cycle **8**.14
Resonium A
  sodium plasma exchange **8**.14
Retinopathy, diabetic **6**.17
Rheumatoid arthritis **6**.30
Ribonuclease **15**.82
Rickets *see also* Osteomalacia
  Lignac-Fanconi syndrome and **15**.11
  vitamin D resistant **15**.32 *et seq.*
Ring shadows **11**.14
Rovsing's operation **16**.19
RPF *see* Renal plasma flow
RTA *see* Acidosis, renal tubular
  distal **15**.44, **15**.47, **15**.53, **15**.59, **15**.61, **15**.64
  proximal **15**.44, **15**.45, **15**.71

SABE *see* Endocarditis
Salicylsulphonic acid test **3**.7
Shunt, Scribner **9**.28
Shohl's solution
  in chronic pyelonephritis **7**.38
  in medullary sponge kidney **16**.36
Scintillography **4**.57
Sclerosis, systemic **10**.37
  acute renal failure and **10**.39
Scribner shunt 'bridge' **9**.28
Siderophilin **6**.5
Skeggs-Leonard artificial kidney **9**.37
Skin lesions, streptococcal **5**.44
SLE *see* Lupus erythematosus
Slit pores **1**.12
Sodium
  exchangeable, pregnancy and **13**.7
  intake, nephritic oedema and **5**.31
  loss **9**.5, **15**.87, **15**.91
    chronic pyelonephritis and **7**.31, **7**.38
    infantile RTA and **15**.61
    medullary sponge kidney and **16**.25
    osmotic diuresis and **9**.1
  phytate, in hypercalciuria **15**.86
  removal by katonium **6**.60
  retention, pre-eclamptic

Sodium (cont.)
  toxaemia and **13**.13
  tubular conservation **3**.57
  tubular reabsorption **2**.45, **2**.43
Sodium iothiomalate **2**.32, **2**.5
Sodium potassium ATP ase **2**.43
Sodium pump **2**.43
Soluble streptococcal antigen **5**.5
Stamey test **3**.61 *et seq.*
  disadvantages **3**.64
  renal artery stenosis and **14**.22
Steroids, in nephrotic syndrome **6**.12
Stomatitis, uraemia and **9**.13
'Stop flow' experiments **2**.44
Streaming, renal vein thrombosis and **6**.44
Streptococcal infection **5**.5, **5**.23, **6**.12
Stretococci, haemolytic
  glomerulonephritis and **5**.5, **5**.23
Streptomycin **18**.15, **20**.14
  contraindications in uraemia **20**.14
Stricture, ureteric **21**.14
Sulfosalicylic acid *see* Salicylsulphonic acid
Sulphacetamide **20**.12
Sulphadimidine **20**.12
Sulphonamides, in pyelonephritis **7**.25
Syndrome, Alport's **16**.43
Syndrome, haemolytic-uraemic **10**.68
Syphilis **6**.30

Tamm-Horsfall protein **3**.1, **4**.6
Taurine, urinary **3**.45
Tetrabromphenol blue **3**.7
Tetracyclines **20**.19
  contraindications in renal failure **8**.18, **20**.19
Thiazide, hypokalaemia and **14**.48
Thiosulphate, renal clearance **2**.5
Third factor **2**.45
Thoracic Duct drainage **21**.17
Thrombocytopaenia **6**.25
  uraemia and **9**.13
Thrombosis, renal vein **6**.35, **6**.67
Thrombotic thrombocytopenic purpura **10**.44 *et seq.*
Thyroid hormone **6**.10
Time, cold ischaemia **21**.7

Time, warm ischaemia **21**.7
'Titratable acidity' **2**.57, **15**.43
Tm **2**.8
TmG **2**.8, **2**.10
Toxaemia of pregnancy **13**.1 *et seq.*
  nephrotic syndrome and **13**.28
TPR *see* Phosphate, tubular reabsorption
Transplantation **21**.1 *et seq.*
Transplantation site **21**.14
  antibodies, anti G B M **21**.17
  antilymphocytic globulin & A L G **21**.22 **21**.22
  azathioprine (imuram) **21**.22
  donor, live **21**.23
  hypercalcaemis, post transplantation **21**.24
  hyperparathyroidism tertiary **21**.24
  nephrectomy, bilateral **21**.13
  nocturia, post transplantation **21**.23
  peptic ulceration **21**.13
  thoracic duct **21**.17
  ureteric fistula **21**.14
Tridione **6**.50
Trimethoprim **7**.25
Tritiated insulin **3**.33
Tryptophane, tubular reabsorption **2**.13
Tuberculosis **4**.18, **6**.30, **18**.15
Tubular cells *see* Epithelial cells
Tubules **1**.10 *et seq.*, **2**.8
  acidosis *see* Acidosis
  acute necrosis *see* Necrosis
  brush border **1**.25
  clearance **2**.8
  disorders **15**.1 *et seq.*
    hydronephrosis and **18**.20
  distal, function tests **3**.40 *et seq.*
  embryology **16**.5
  Lowe's syndrome and **15**.29
  malformation **16**.2
  maximum transport rate (Tm) **2**.8
  potassium conservation **3**.61
  proximal, function tests **3**.36
  reabsorption **2**.8 *et seq.*
  secretion **2**.24 *et seq.*
  sodium conservation **3**.57
  'swan-neck' deformity **15**.6
Tumours, renal **18**.1 *et seq.*

Ulceration peptic **21**.13
Ultra-filtration theory (Ludwig) **2**.1
Uraemia
  amyloidosis and **6**.30
  'bat's wing' lung and **9**.16
  benign hypertension and **14**.33, **14**.39
  cardiovascular changes **9**.16
  clinical features **9**.13, **9**.16
  glucose tolerance test **6**.22
  low protein diet and **9**.21
Urates, urinary **4**.1
Urea
  blood
    glomerular filtration rate and **3**.16, **3**.12
    IVP and **4**.20
    renal osteodystrophy and **19**.11 *et seq.*
    tetracyclines and **20**.19, **8**.18
  clearance **3**.16, **3**.12
  urinary **8**.1
  urine concentration and **2**.70
  vasopressin and **2**.70
Ureter **1**.1
  duplex **16**.38
    obstruction **3**.68
      calculous **4**.33
  oedema **3**.64
  tumours **18**.20
Ureteric anastamotic leakage **21**.14
Ureterosigmoidoscopy **18**.16
Uric acid stones **15**.94, **15**.96
Urinary tract
  changes in pregnancy **13**.4
  obstruction, acute renal failure and **8**.2 *et seq.*
Urine
  acidification **2**.54, **2**.57
    chronic pyelonephritis and **7**.31
  biochemical investigation **3**.1 *et seq.*
  buffers **15**.43
  composition, water deprivation and **2**.40
  concentration **2**.35
    chronic pyelonephritis and **7**.31
    renal disease and **12**.2
    RTA and **15**.71

Urine (cont.)
    tests **3**.46, **3**.62
    daily volume **12**.1 *et seq.*
        osmotic load and **12**.1, **12**.2
    in isosthenuria **3**.46, **3**.60
    microscopy **4**.1 *et seq.*
        tumours and **18**.1 *et seq.*
    osmolality **2**.35, **2**.40
        diabetes insipidus and **12**.8
        phenindione and **17**.32
        urea and protein effects **2**.70
        water deprivation and **2**.40 pH **2**.66, **3**.56
        Lignac-Fanconi syndrome and **15**.16
        RTA and **15**.43
    sediment in AGN **5**.36
    stasis, pregnancy and **13**.4
    telescoped deposit **4**.19, **10**.8
    testing Appendix 3
    titratable acidity **2**.57, **15**.43
    two-hourly collection **4**.11

Van Slyke standard urea clearance **3**.12
Vancomycin **20**.14
Vasa recta **1**.1, **1**.3
Vasopressin
    diabetes insipidus and **12**.7, **12**.8
    duct permeability and **2**.35, **2**.70
    urine concentration test **3**.46 *et seq.*
Vena cava, hypernephroma metastasis **18**.1
Venography, renal vein thrombosis and **6**.42
Vesico-ureteric reflux **4**.30
    pyelonephritis and **7**.20
Virus, Chicken pox **21**.12
Virus Coxsackie **10**.68
Virus cytomegalus **21**.12
Virus herpes simplex **21**.12

Vitamin B_{12}, GFR measurement and **3**.33
Vitamin D
    intoxication **15**.39
        diabetes insipidus and **12**.18
    osteomalacia and **19**.17
    rickets and **3**.36, **15**.39
Vitamin D_3
    metabolites
        $1:25(OH)_2D_3$ **2**.16, **19**.7
Vitamin D 25 hydroxycholecalcuferik **19**.17
Vomiting, anuria and **8**.16

Warm ischaemia **21**.7
Wasserman test, lupus nephrotic syndrome and **6**.25
Water *see also* Free water
    absorption **2**.29, **2**.35, **2**.36
    deprivation **2**.36, **2**.35, **2**.40
        diabetes insipidus and **12**.8
    intake
        in AGN **5**.45
        in anuria **8**.18, **5**.49
    maximal tubular reabsorption **12**.7
Wegener's syndrome **10**.29 *et seq.*
White cells
    casts **4**.19
        in AGN **5**.13, **5**.36
    cystine infiltration **15**.6
    urinary **4**.13
        AGN and **5**.36
        'pyrexal' test and **4**.19
Wilson's disease **3**.36, **20**.45
Wrong and Davies test **3**.56
    Appendix 2

Xylose **2**.12